To Carol

DESIGNING USABILITY INTO MEDICAL PRODUCTS

DESIGNING USABILITY INTO MEDICAL PRODUCTS

Michael E. Wiklund, P.E.
Stephen B. Wilcox, Ph.D.

FOREWORD BY
Matthew B. Weinger

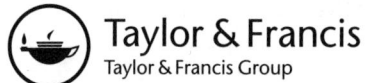

Taylor & Francis
Taylor & Francis Group

Boca Raton   London   New York   Singapore

A CRC title, part of the Taylor & Francis imprint, a member of the
Taylor & Francis Group, the academic division of T&F Informa plc.

Library of Congress Cataloging-in-Publication Data

Designing usability into medical products / edited by Michael E. Wiklund, Stephen B. Wilcox.
   p. cm.
  Includes bibliographical references and index.
  ISBN 0-8493-2843-8 (alk. paper)
   1. Medical instruments and apparatus--Design and construction. 2. Design. 3. New products--Evaluation. 4. Medical instruments and apparatus--Quality control. I. Wiklund, Michael E. II. Wilcox, Stephen B.

R856.D473 2004
610'.28--dc22

2004048932

This book contains information obtained from authentic and highly regarded sources. Reprinted material is quoted with permission, and sources are indicated. A wide variety of references are listed. Reasonable efforts have been made to publish reliable data and information, but the author and the publisher cannot assume responsibility for the validity of all materials or for the consequences of their use.

Neither this book nor any part may be reproduced or transmitted in any form or by any means, electronic or mechanical, including photocopying, microfilming, and recording, or by any information storage or retrieval system, without prior permission in writing from the publisher.

The consent of CRC Press does not extend to copying for general distribution, for promotion, for creating new works, or for resale. Specific permission must be obtained in writing from CRC Press for such copying.

Direct all inquiries to CRC Press, 2000 N.W. Corporate Blvd., Boca Raton, Florida 33431.

Trademark Notice: Product or corporate names may be trademarks or registered trademarks, and are used only for identification and explanation, without intent to infringe.

Visit the CRC Press Web site at www.crcpress.com

© 2005 by CRC Press

No claim to original U.S. Government works
International Standard Book Number 0-8493-2843-8
Library of Congress Card Number 2004048932
Printed in the United States of America 1 2 3 4 5 6 7 8 9 0

Dedication

To Amy and my children, Ben, Ali, and Tom

M.W.

To Stephanie

S.W.

Contents

About This Book xi
About the Authors xv
Acknowledgments xix
Foreword xxi

General Principles and Processes

1. The Rising Bar — Medical Product Design Excellence 3
   Michael E. Wiklund

2. The Role of Industrial Design and Human Engineering in the Design of Software-Driven Medical Products 11
   Stephen B. Wilcox

3. Is Your Human Factors Program Ready for FDA Scrutiny? 21
   Michael E. Wiklund

4. Human Factors Roundtable 31

5. User-Centered Medical Product Development and the Problem of Egocentrism 55
   Stephen B. Wilcox

6. Ethnographic Methods for New Product Development 61
   Stephen B. Wilcox

7. Time-Lapse Video Offers More Information in Less Time 73
   Stephen B. Wilcox

8. Finding and Using Data Regarding the Shape and Size of the User's Body 77
   Stephen B. Wilcox

9. Can You Trust What People Say? 85
   Stephen B. Wilcox

10. Eight Ways to Kill Innovation 93
    Stephen B. Wilcox

11. Developing Testable Product Simulations:
    Speed Is of the Essence 103
    Stephen B. Wilcox

12. Patient Simulators Breathe Life into Product Testing 113
    Michael E. Wiklund

13. Return of the Renaissance Person: A Valuable Contributor
    to Medical Product Development 125
    Stephen B. Wilcox

14. Patenting Software User Interfaces 131
    Michael E. Wiklund

Design Methods and Guidance

15. The Vision Statement for Product Design —
    In Your Mind's Eye 145
    Michael E. Wiklund

16. Making Medical Device Interfaces More User-Friendly 151
    Michael E. Wiklund

17. Controlling Complexity 161
    Michael E. Wiklund

18. Eleven Keys to Design Error-Resistant
    Medical Devices 169
    Michael E. Wiklund

19. Designing a Global User Interface 181
    Michael E. Wiklund

20. Why Choose Color Displays? 193
    Michael E. Wiklund

21. Intuitive Design: Removing Obstacles
    Also Increases Appeal 203
    Michael E. Wiklund

22. Medical Devices That Talk 215
    Michael E. Wiklund

23. Home Healthcare: Applying Inclusive Design Principles
    to Medical Devices 227
    Stephen B. Wilcox

24. Designing Usable Auditory Signals 235
    Stephen B. Wilcox

25. Medical Device User Manuals:
    Shifting toward Computerization 245
    Michael E. Wiklund

Corporate Human Factors Programs

26. User-Centered Design at Abbott Laboratories 257
    Edmond W. Israelski and William H. Muto

27. User-Centered Design at Ethicon Endo-Surgery 269
    Larry Spreckelmeier

Product Design Case Studies

28. Case Study: Personal Hemodialysis System 283

29. Case Study: Patient Monitor 291

30. Case Study: Development of a Contrast Medium Injector
    System for CT Scanning 299

31. Case Study: Remotely Controlled Defibrillator 307

Resources 317

Index 323

About This Book

This book is co-authored by good friends who are also arch competitors. Both Michael and Steve lead human factors research and design practices — one in Concord, MA, the other in Philadelphia, PA — focused on medical technology development. On several occasions, their firms have bid on the same projects. Fortunately, each firm has won its share of bids, so there have been no hard feelings. In fact, the competition, as well as the authors' participation in special professional activities, has generated mutual admiration.

Michael and Steve have served together as judges for the Medical Design Excellence Awards. They have authored separate portions of a human factors design standard published by the Association for the Advancement of Medical Instrumentation. And they have both led professional interest sections of the Industrial Designers Society of America. Over the course of several committee meetings and dinners, Michael and Steve have enjoyed comparing notes about managing consulting practices and the challenges of working in the medical technology industry.

The idea of writing a book together did not surface until one summer day in New York City. The authors were in the city to attend a Medical Design Excellence Awards ceremony, but not before an early lunch at the Carnegie Deli (see Figure). Steve ordered a monster-sized hot pastrami with a side of bacon. Michael ordered an omelet (no cheese) and a bottomless cup of coffee (decaffeinated). When the waitress delivered the food, she commented, "You guys look like the types to co-author a book about medical technology design." Imagine that!

OK. The waitress was not our muse. Actually, the authors were discussing — between mouthfuls — how much they enjoyed writing articles about medical product development and how much fun it would be to collaborate. And that is when one of the authors (identity intentionally withheld) said, "We could get filthy rich writing a nonfictional account about the design of user-friendly infusion pumps, defibrillators, and patient monitors!"

So, this is the book conceived in a New York deli. Many of the chapters first appeared as articles in *Medical Device & Diagnostic Industry, Appliance Manufacturer, and Innovation*. As a result, each chapter stands well on its own, and readers should feel free to jump to the chapters that interest them. Being hardworking and responsible individuals, the authors updated each chapter to reflect their current thinking and the latest facts. They also added several new illustrations to clarify the written material and present examples of good design. For people who like shortcuts, the authors have even added a list of key points to the end of each chapter.

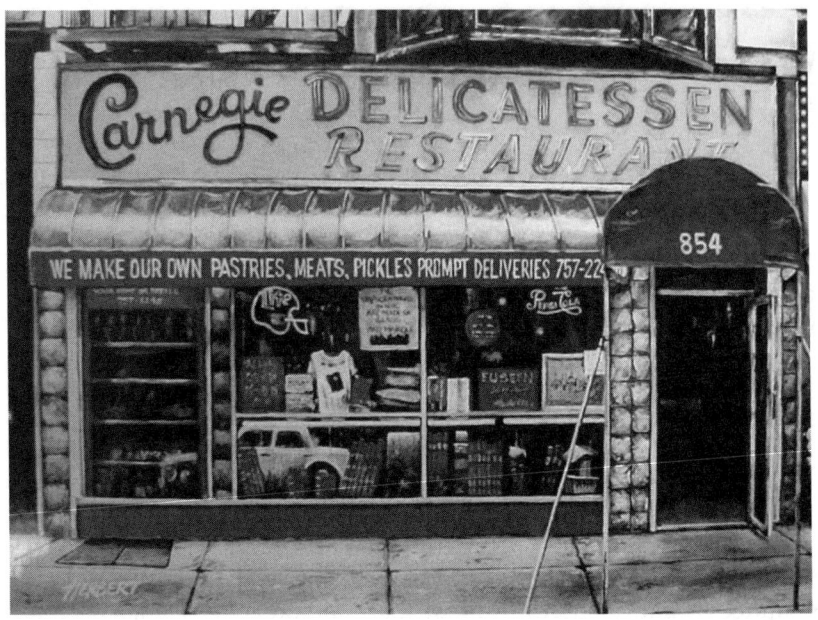

Carnegie Delicatessen Restaurant in New York City. Source: www.asahi-net.or.jp/~rn8t-nkmr/family/NY/carnegie-deli.jpg

The early chapters discuss broad concepts pertaining to making medical devices safe and effective by involving users in the design process. The middle chapters discuss more specific design and evaluation methods and tools. The later chapters present case studies of user-friendly medical technologies and corporate human factors programs, as well as related resources for medical design professionals.

The authors hope that readers will draw useful guidance from the book on an as-needed basis. They see limited value in reading the book chapters in a particular order. Rather, they encourage people to take what they need from the book when they need it. One reader may seek advice about conducting ethnographic research. Another may seek guidance on designing medical device alarms. Yet another may seek guidance on designing an intuitive user interface. Meanwhile, reading the whole book will give the reader a comprehensive understanding of designing medical devices in a manner that places users' needs front and center — not a bad outcome.

Michael and Steve do not suggest taking their advice as the gospel, particularly because they do not agree on every technical issue. Michael is a human factors engineer and Steve is a psychologist, by training. They do practically the same thing professionally, but have very different perspectives. Enough said? The studious reader will note areas of minor disagreement in the authors' preferred approaches to user research. This divergence may be the book's greatest strength or weakness. But either way, the authors' sometimes divergent views reflect the fact that user-centered design is part science and part art. The authors present some information as fact. For example, government requirements to conduct human factors studies in the course of medical device design are fact. The rest of the authors' guidance draws upon their professional opinions, making the guidance subject to debate.

Michael and Steve will continue to debate the fine points and encourage readers to draw their own conclusions.

About the Authors

Michael E. Wiklund, P.E.

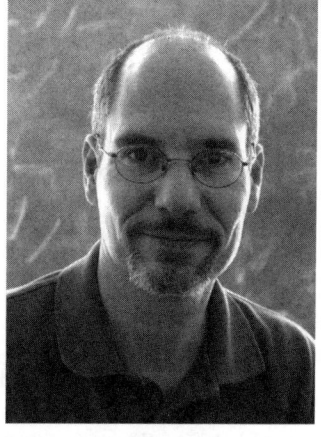

Michael has been a practicing human factors engineer for 22 years and counting. He loves his profession because it enables him to work closely with people as well as up-and-coming, exciting technology. He was originally drawn to the medical industry because it affords the opportunity to create designs that make a difference in people's lives — making people safer, healthier, and more comfortable.

Michael received his master's degree in engineering design (human factors) from Tufts University, where he is now an adjunct associate professor. His graduate course, Applied Software User Interface Design, has evolved over more than a decade to keep pace with changing technology and a growing job market for engineers and designers, with a sympathetic attitude toward the needs and preferences of real people.

Michael has spent the majority of his career as a consultant specializing in user-interface research, design, and usability testing. In addition to contributing individually to medical product development projects, he has built a large consulting practice and helped other organizations build their own internal consulting groups. Following a long tenure with American Institutes for Research, he recently launched his own consulting practice.

His recent projects have involved the development of advanced technologies, such as patient monitors, dialysis machines, infusion pumps, and medical information management systems. However, his professional interests extend beyond medical product development to include consumer and household products, aviation and automotive applications, and business and personal software applications (including Web sites). Accordingly, he has recently worked on wireless communication devices, commerce and health-related Web sites, and even garden tractors. His medical clients have ranged from large, multinational companies with broad product lines to startup companies developing novel technologies, each interested in improving the quality of interaction between their products and customers.

This is Michael's third major publication. Previous publications include *Medical Device and Ergonomic Design: Usability Engineering and Ergonomics* and *Usability in Practice*. He has also written more than 50 technical articles for assorted design and technology publications. Someday, he would like to try his hand at a children's story or a novel that does *not* include the words "human factors" or "usability." We'll see about that. It may not be possible.

Michael holds multiple user-interface design patents and was named one of *Medical Device and Diagnostic Industry* magazine's 100 Notable People in the medical device industry (2004).

Outside work, Michael enjoys spending time with his wife (Amy) and children (Ben, Ali, and Tom), as well as dabbling in digital photography and painting — his favorite motifs being designed objects such as fire hydrants and industrial gear.

Michael hopes this book inspires readers to create medical products that work well for every person who interacts with them.

Stephen B. Wilcox, Ph.D.

Steve began his professional life as an academic psychologist, teaching and doing research on visual perception, the psychology of language, and cognitive psychology. In 1984, he joined Herbst LaZar Bell, a product development consulting firm headquartered in Chicago, to create a design research and human factors capability for them. In 1991, he founded Design Science, based in Philadelphia. Design Science is a 20-person consultancy that specializes in user research, human factors, and interaction design, with a particular focus on medical products. Steve has worked on a wide variety of projects with clients including Ethicon Endo-Surgery, Baxter, Becton-Dickinson, Alaris, Guidant Corporation, Hill-Rom, Roche, Steris, Medrad, Inc., Laerdal, and Datascope.

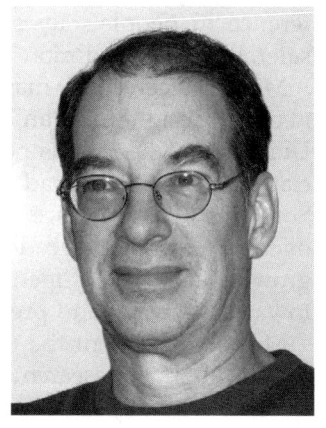

Steve was recently a vice president of the Industrial Designers Society of America (IDSA) and chairs IDSA's Human Factors Professional Interest Section. He was recently included among the 100 Notable People selected by *Medical Device and Diagnostic Industry* magazine for his "contributions to the medical device and healthcare industries." In 2003, he was a delegate representing the U.S. in Berlin at the biannual meeting of the International Council of Societies of Industrial Design. In 2001, he was elected to IDSA's Academy of Fellows. He has received awards from and served as a judge for the annual design competitions of both IDSA and *International Design* magazine. He is also one of the judges (from 2003 to 2005) for the Medical Design Excellence Awards. In 2000 he chaired the IDSA national conference in New Orleans. He has also been a guest editor of *Innovation*, a publication of IDSA. Steve is a member of AAMI's (Association for the Advancement of Medical Instrumentation) Human Factors Engineering Committee, which has created the Standard, HE74 (*Human Factors Design Process for Medical Devices*).

Steve has taught human factors courses in the design departments of the University of the Arts and Carnegie Mellon University, and he has authored more then 50 articles in various professional publications.

Steve holds a B.S. in psychology and anthropology from Tulane University, a Ph.D. in experimental psychology from Penn State, and a Certificate in Business Administration from the Wharton School of the University of Pennsylvania.

Steve's other passions include New Orleans music, opera, Japanese prints, real ale, and anything French. He occasionally even has time to pursue these passions.

Acknowledgments

We have many people and organizations to thank for making this book a reality.

Our spouses were wonderfully supportive. Amy Allen, Michael's wife and quite conveniently a professional editor, was a constant source of encouragement and made lots of editorial suggestions that made the book far more readable. Stephanie Knopp, Steve's wife and quite conveniently an accomplished graphic designer, was also a constant source of encouragement and designed the book cover as well as the chapter title pages.

A considerable portion of this book's content originally appeared in *Medical Device & Diagnostic Industry*, published by Canon Communications (Los Angeles, CA). The publisher was extraordinarily generous to grant us permission to use the material. We owe a special thanks to Canon's John Bethune (editorial director), who has supported our writing for several years and has poured considerable editorial resources into making our words read better. Thanks also go to Canon's Steve Halasey (editor-in-chief), who invited both of us to serve as jurors for Canon's Medical Design Excellence Awards program, which helped us develop some of the insights shared in this book.

We thank Kristina Goodrich, executive director and CEO of the Industrial Designers Society of America (IDSA) and Karen Berube, managing editor and designer of IDSA's bi-monthly magazine entitled *Innovation*. They also granted us access to material previously published in *Innovation* and have been a continuing source of professional support and encouragement.

Similarly, we thank *Appliance Manufacturer* and Joe Jancsurak (editor) for their permission to use material previously published in their magazine.

We appreciate the support we have received from professional colleagues at American Institutes for Research and Design Science, members of the Association for the Advancement of Medical Instrumentation's Human Factors Engineering Committee, and members of the U.S. Food & Drug Administration's human factors staff.

Thank you to Matthew Weinger (Vanderbilt University), Ed Israelski and Bill Muto (Abbott Laboratories), and Larry Spreckelmeier (Ethicon Endo-Surgery, Inc.) for the book's insightful foreword and corporate case studies. We are also grateful to the companies that invited us to write case studies about their product development efforts, including Aksys, Ltd., Datex–Ohmeda–Division of Instrumentarium Corporation, Guidant Corporation, and Medrad, Inc.

Finally, thank you to the myriad organizations that granted us permission to use images of their products or working environments, and to Kristin Leclerc, Joy Arsenault, and Karen King — colleagues who helped us secure permissions and provided logistical support.

Foreword

A Clinician's Perspective on Designing Better Medical Devices

Matthew B. Weinger, MD

Dr. Weinger was a professor of anesthesiology at the University of California, San Diego and the director of the San Diego Center for Patient Safety based at the VA San Diego. He practices anesthesia, teaches, and conducts patient safety research with a focus on medical device design and evaluation. Dr. Weinger is also the user chair of the Association for the Advancement of Medical Instrumentation (AAMI) Human Factors Committee that is developing national standards for the design of medical device user interfaces. He is currently Professor of Anesthesiology, Biomedical Informatics, and Medical Education at Vanderbilt University, Nashville, TN.

As a practicing clinician who also conducts human factors research, I want to provide the reader with a rationale for the guidance in this book. In my medical practice, I routinely encounter usability problems while operating equipment. Throughout this foreword, I will discuss these problems and what I consider to be some of their major causes and effects. While many of these examples focus on operating room equipment, my observations apply to nearly all medical devices and users, and the full spectrum of likely environments in which devices will be used. After all, medical device usability is just as important to the elderly patient with poor eyesight and short-term memory loss who is measuring her blood sugar level with a portable glucometer while sitting in a dimly lit room as it is to the highly trained medical professional who is delivering anesthesia to a heart patient experiencing operative complications.

From my perspective — as a frontline clinician who wears scrubs and must make life-affecting decisions every day — medical devices are only valuable if they make the job of taking care of patients better, easier, and more satisfying. Therefore, if a new device increases my workload, creates new opportunities for error, or reduces my efficiency without offsetting benefits, I will not tolerate it; it has no place in my OR. Even when a device offers important clinical advantages, any deficiencies in the device's design or implementation may offset those benefits, leading to underuse, misuse, or detrimental changes to concurrent care processes.

As an example, bar-code medication management systems are increasingly being implemented to reduce the incidence of medication errors. With these systems, before nurses give a medication, they must bar-code scan the patient's identification bracelet, as well as the medication. The system assures that the medication the doctor ordered is being administered via the correct route (e.g., oral versus intravenous) to the correct patient, in the correct dose, and at the correct time. But, the potential patient safety benefits of bar-code systems have been partially offset by system design attributes that reduce nurses' task efficiency. As a result, nurses have been observed intentionally using work-around strategies and circumventing some of the safety features in order to "get the job done." For example, a nurse taking care of eight patients may administer all of their medications and then batch scan at a central station after the fact, using copies of ID bracelets and medication labels. Thus, well-intentioned efforts to enhance safety through the implementation of technology can be undermined by system designs that do not fully account for user needs and preferences.

Modern medical practice has become extremely complex over the past couple of decades. For economic reasons, the healthcare system is relying increasingly on lower-skilled personnel with limited healthcare education and training. For example, medical assistants, often with little more than a high school education, are now handling clinical tasks previously performed by registered nurses. At the same time, the requisite amount of medical knowledge clinicians must absorb and apply is already enormous and growing exponentially. With modern advances in sophisticated technology (e.g., gene chip arrays to screen for inherited diseases), most clinicians do not understand the science underlying many of the electronic medical devices in daily use. Given these disconcerting trends, it is troubling that many medical device user interfaces are poorly designed, fail to adequately support the clinical tasks for which they are intended, and frequently contribute to medical error. And, until recently, most design and manufacturing companies gave only limited attention to the human factors engineering of medical devices.

Human Factors Engineering and Medical Devices

This book uses the term *medical device* to describe an object, tool, or piece of equipment that clinicians or patients use to accomplish medical diagnostic or therapeutic tasks or activities. This definition is consistent with those used by the U.S. Food and Drug Administration (FDA), the federal agency responsible for the oversight of medical devices, as well as national and international consensus standards-making bodies. However, the principles pertaining to medical devices apply as well to the design and evaluation of clinical processes and integrated care environments (e.g., medical systems like hospital emergency rooms or inpatient pharmacies).

Human factors engineering (HFE) may be defined as the application of knowledge about human characteristics and abilities (physical, emotional, and intellectual) to the design of tools, devices, systems, environments, and organizations. The development of usable medical devices requires the adherence to HFE principles and processes throughout the entire design cycle, beginning with the earliest concepts and continuing after the device is released for commercial use. The FDA has mandated that medical device manufacturers use HFE design principles and adhere to standard "Good Manufacturing Practices." Additionally, national and international committees have recently published consensus standards (e.g., AAMI/ANSI HE-74: 2001 and i.e., IEC 60601-1-6) for a rigorous HFE design process for all medical devices.

User Error or Use Error?

Traditionally, many errors associated with medical devices were blamed on "user error." Clinicians were faulted for inadvertently pushing the wrong buttons, loading infusion pump cartridges incorrectly, or misinterpreting onscreen information. Inanimate devices were considered innocent. Users were expected to be responsible for flawlessly mastering every device's operation, regardless of design shortcomings, because they were the highly trained professionals. More recently, the approach of holding the user fully responsible for mishaps has proved to be both wrong and nonproductive.

One device that appears to be prone to use errors is the infusion pump. Inadvertent overdoses of pain relievers delivered via patient-controlled analgesia (PCA) infusion pumps have caused hundreds of deaths of hospitalized patients. PCA pumps provide better pain relief than other delivery methods because they allow patients to control their own pain medication (typically opiate drugs like morphine) administration. In the case of the most commonly documented type of error, clinicians inadvertently entered an inappropriately low drug concentration during initial pump programming. In the device's drug concentration "setup" screen, the clinicians accepted the "default" choice provided by the pump interface of the minimum drug concentration (e.g., 0.1 mg/ml of morphine) although the actual drug loaded into the device was actually 10 times more concentrated (e.g., 1.0 mg/ml). Consequently, a 10-fold *higher* dose than expected was administered because the device divides the desired unit dose (e.g., 2 mg per activation) by the concentration (e.g., 0.1 mg/ml programmed) to calculate the drug volume administered with each pump activation (e.g., 20 ml). As a result, the patient received 20 mg of drug instead of the intended 2 mg.

Another common scenario involving infusion pump use error has been the acceptance of settings appropriate for one drug (e.g., morphine) when a different, more potent opiate (e.g., hydromorphone) is actually being administered. In many cases, otherwise healthy patients stopped breathing (opiates cause respiratory depression) and either died or suffered irreversible brain damage. Neither the display of the programmed settings nor the operator manual's instruction to verify settings prior to use were sufficient to prevent fatal overdoses.

The typical response to these kinds of events has been censure (and often firing) of the nurse who programmed the pump, additional training of other nurses, admonitions by hospital administrators for clinicians to be more careful and to try harder, and legal action by the affected patients and their families. The manufacturer of a device involved in such mishaps has usually responded by adding warnings to the device and the associated user manual and by altering in-service training to alert clinicians of the risks. However, history has shown that, in the absence of redesign of the device and the associated care processes in which it is used, these actions are not likely to prevent such errors.

A new paradigm has evolved, based on HFE principles and empirical evidence that defines these events as use errors — without placing blame directly on the users — and provides methods to understand how to reduce their incidence. According to this new paradigm, users are invariably fallible and are constantly subjected to many types of "performance shaping factors," often beyond their direct control, that will affect their ability to perform tasks correctly. Additionally, devices are never used in isolation and must be considered as an integral part of a broader system (Figure 1).

When the design of the user interface of a medical device is flawed, the design is more likely to promote use error, reduce the chance of recovery if an error occurs, or impede an effective clinical response during an emergency or unusual situation. When a use error occurs, it is necessary for the clinician to detect the error and "recover" before the patient experiences adverse consequences.

Device use errors can trigger a cascade of events that ultimately leads to patient injury. Recovery from error cannot only be impeded by device design features but also by myriad factors related to the clinician, the immediate clinical environment, and wider system issues (e.g., availability of training, work schedules, etc.). The best way for device designers to minimize the incidence of use errors and, more importantly, the associated hazards to patients and clinicians, is to employ a formal HFE process that focuses on meeting users' needs and requirements during actual device operation in the anticipated use environments. Such an approach will also improve device use efficiency and user satisfaction.

Designing for the Intended Use Environment

I strongly advocate taking a systems approach to the design of safe and effective medical devices. A medical device *cannot* be properly created and evaluated without carefully considering where it will be used as well as who will use it and how they will use it. The medical use environment includes not just the attributes of the immediate physical surroundings (e.g., lighting, noise levels, furniture) that can vary appreciably from one care environment to another (picture an intensive care unit vs. a nursing home), but also the other devices that will be used concurrently, the other individuals in the environment (e.g., the patient), and the broader healthcare milieu.

The typical care environment contains many types of medical (and non-medical) devices that often interact (Figure 2). There are multiple competing

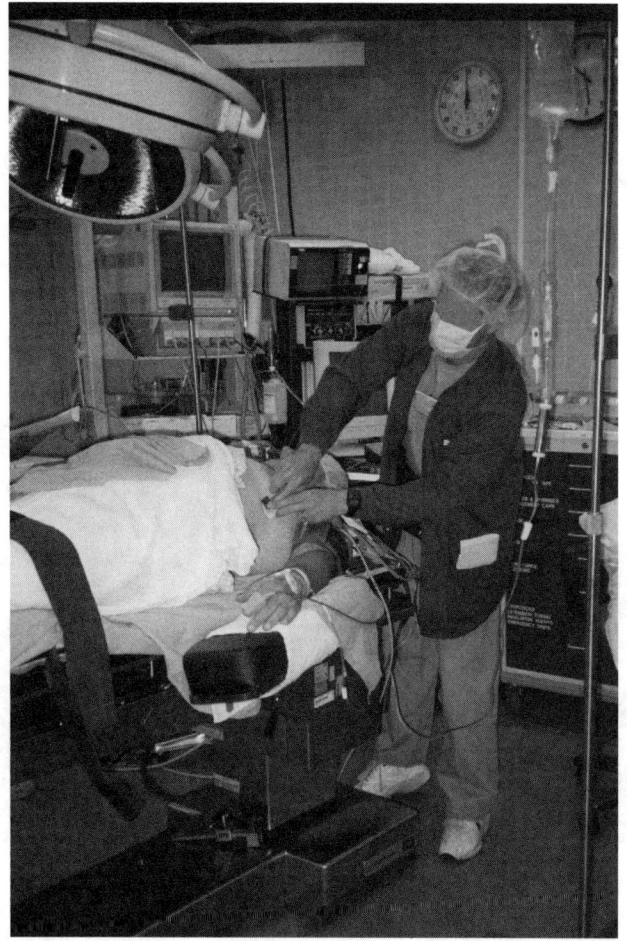

FIGURE 1
The operating room is an example of a complex care environment where multiple devices interact, sometimes in unpredictable ways. These devices range from simple disposable leads to sophisticated electronic monitoring and anesthetic delivery systems. Testing devices in their actual use environment will help to identify potentially important design flaws.

demands for users' time and attention as well as frequent distractions and interruptions. The designer must be cognizant of institutional structures, such as policies, procedures, available staffing, and training, as well as higher-level "system factors," such as the social and political attitudes within the care environment; professional and organizational culture (e.g., regulations, conventions, and values), and legal and governmental constraints.

Medical devices often end up being used in environments that were not envisioned by their initial designers. For example, sophisticated devices like medication infusion pumps, mechanical ventilators, and dialysis machines that were originally designed for use by experienced nurses and physicians in intensive care settings, are now being used in patients' homes. This *technology*

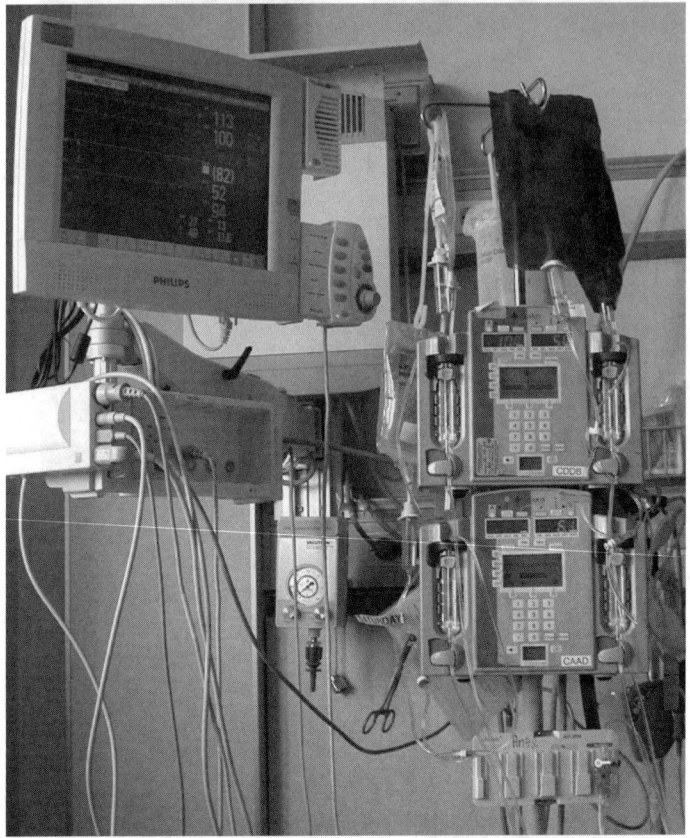

FIGURE 2
In the intensive care unit, multiple diagnostic and therapeutic devices are often used together. Their design attributes can interact in both desirable and undesirable ways: Data from the physiological data display devices help to guide adjustments in the therapeutic medication infusions systems, but multiple conflicting alarms and warnings can be distracting and confusing.

creep can lead to serious use errors because the devices were neither designed nor tested to ensure their suitability to these unanticipated users, uses, and use environments.

Understanding the User

A cardinal tenet of human factors engineering is that a failure to understand the needs and requirements of the ultimate device users will preclude effective design and increase the likelihood of use error, device misuse, and adverse events. This has led to the promotion of "user-centered design" (there are other names and flavors of this concept), whereby the user is the focus of the design process. With this approach, user input and formal user

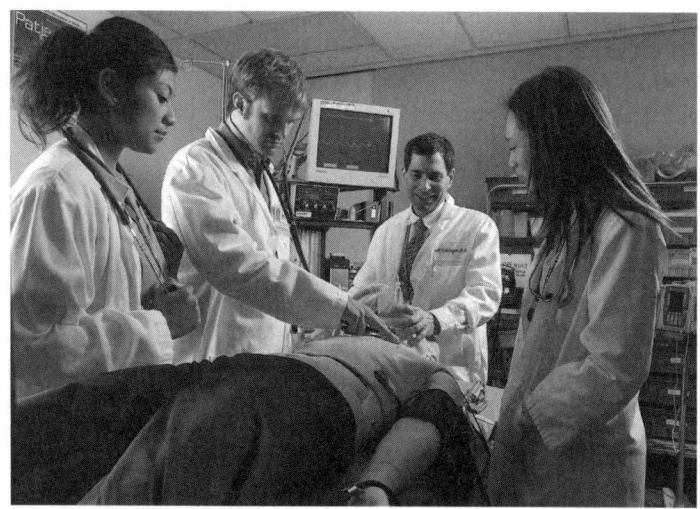

FIGURE 3
Medical devices are typically used by teams of physicians, nurses, respiratory therapists, and even patients. Teams can be trained to work together, for example, in this realistic patient-simulation training facility.

testing starts at the earliest conceptual stages and then continues throughout the design process, thereby facilitating iterative design improvement.

A single medical device can be used by a wide variety of users, from highly educated physicians to patients and caregivers. When trying to design the best device possible, it is advantageous to define device users broadly as all individuals who may interact with the device. Clinicians often work together in teams (Figure 3), and increasingly patients (and their families) are being asked to actively participate in care decisions and management. Thus, users would include not just primary device operators (usually clinicians but sometimes patients), but also those who unpack, transport, maintain, clean, and test the device, as well as the patients or other individuals who are directly affected by the device's use. Note that this definition is more inclusive than the definitions used in international standards documents for either *user* (the authority responsible for the use and maintenance of equipment) or *operator* (the person handling the equipment).

There are many ways to obtain reliable user information. Some traditional methods of soliciting user input, such as customer calls by sales personnel, market surveys, and focus groups are notoriously unreliable and, if used in isolation, can lead to serious design flaws (not to mention market failures). The focus must be on actual user needs: "What do clinicians really *need* to provide better, safer, and more efficient patient care?" To answer this question, one must understand what clinicians do, and how and why they do it. This can best be accomplished through a structured approach to user testing that employs rigorous HFE methods.

Companies are often disappointed when devices do not yield expected sales, or device features are not utilized, despite designers' careful compliance with the results of an exhaustive marketing survey that suggested that clinicians wanted the particular device or feature. While the problem can be ineffective implementation of a viable concept, it is just as likely that the development process depended too heavily on unreliable clinician input. What users say they want can be appreciably different than what they actually need. In other words, both users and designers tend to confuse clinicians' ultimate goals with the means of accomplishing those goals. The status quo is a powerful anchor that makes it difficult to envision and implement innovative solutions. A related problem is that companies may conduct exhaustive product testing with users, but fail to effectively determine whether their product will actually work effectively in the real world. For example, testing will be much less useful if subjects are asked if they *like* a feature or interface attribute ("preference testing") rather than measuring if users can successfully accomplish specific realistic tasks (or series of tasks) in an acceptable amount of time without use errors (functional testing).

Some Principles of a User-Centered Device Design Process

Human factors engineering espouses certain principles of good design. Unfortunately, in my experience, many of these principles are routinely ignored or violated by modern medical devices. For example, many microprocessor-controlled medical devices have hidden modes of operation, ambiguous alarm messages, and complex and inconsistent control actions.

I recall a respiratory gas analyzer that had a hidden calibration mode that rendered it unusable if the disposable sampling tubing was not attached when the unit was initially powered up. At least two different tourniquet controllers had no indicator showing that the cuff was inflated, although this impression was mistakenly given by a display of "cuff pressure" and a running timer on the front panel. In addition, I have encountered several physiological monitors that could be placed, through a nonobvious sequence of control activations, into a "demonstration mode" whereby, in the absence of a patient, normal and unchanging vital signs were displayed. While this feature was intended for sales personnel, on several occasions, clinicians inadvertently placed these monitors into demo mode while they were connected to patients, making the devices insidiously nonoperative.

Fundamentally, an effective device will communicate and collaborate with its human user as if it were a well-trained member of the clinical team; one that shares common goals and requirements. A well-designed interface between human and machine conveys to the user the device's purpose, operational modes, and controlling actions. With most devices, a number of user actions are possible at any given time. The allowable commands often depend on the current operational mode. The user should be able to tell

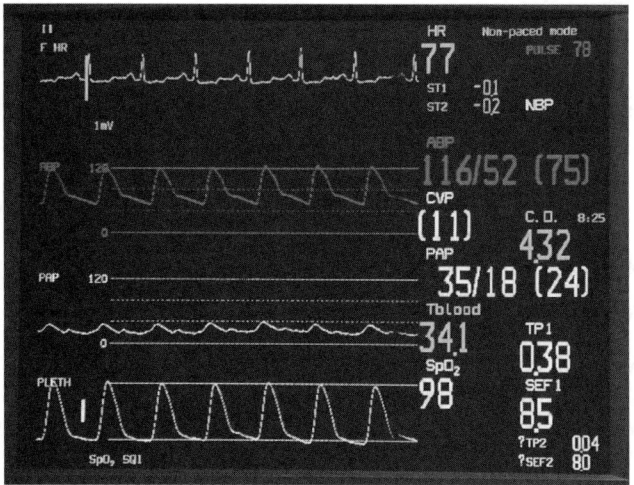

FIGURE 4
Modern physiological displays such as the one depicted here are rich in complex analog and numeric data but do not adequately support clinicians' need for knowledge about patient status, particularly during acute crisis situations. For example, if the patient's blood pressure suddenly decreases, the clinician must determine the possible cause by locating, memorizing, and integrating the many other data elements displayed.

what actions are possible at any given instant and understand the consequences of those actions.

Therefore, user feedback is critical. After each device interaction, I need to know if the device understood what I wanted it to do and to tell me if it performed the action. And, if it didn't complete the expected action, I need it to tell me why and what it intends to do next. Busy clinicians cannot be expected to remember the minute details of a device's operation. We must be able to readily accomplish key device functions, especially during emergency or crisis situations when short-term memory and attention will invariably be impaired. This principle is even more important when considering the design of medical devices to be used by patients at home. For example, it is unrealistic to expect that an 85-year-old patient with bronchitis will remember how to perform a multistep process to calibrate an electronic inhaled bronchodilator delivery system. And, if occasional calibration is necessary to assure safe dosing, then use errors will be inevitable, despite the provision of training videos and user instructions.

Physiological monitors that display patient data often violate these principles. People are not very good at monitoring tasks. They get bored, don't pay attention, are easily distracted, forget things, and can have trouble identifying and following trends in complex data streams. Modern physiological monitors (Figure 4) present too much data in a complex and poorly integrated manner that is not consistent with clinicians' mental models of human physiology. These information- and content-intensive devices demand excessive user attention, frequently distracting them from other clinical tasks. In addition, key functions and data are often hidden in nested menus requiring unique and nonobvious control activation or navigation. Therefore, when multiple parameters are abnormal and the patient is doing poorly, the device may not adequately support the users' clinical requirements and may actually promote use error.

Consistency of design, both within a device and across devices, is quite important for reducing use error. Mosenkis suggested that healthcare providers use medical devices in the same way they use their automobiles — they *expect* that a new device will work more or less the same as equivalent older devices.[1] To accomplish this, the designer must understand how users think and work. Established conventions and expectations must be discerned and accommodated. Conformation to national or international consensus design standards can help assure consistency as well as assist in the shaping of user expectations about how device controls and displays will function.

Limiting the Consequences of Use Error

A designer is responsibile for anticipating use errors and minimizing the risk that any error will produce ill effects. Actions with potentially undesirable consequences should be reversible. If an action is clearly undesirable, then the system should prevent the user from performing that action.

Some medical device companies take a design approach that fails to identify critical use errors until very late in the development process, perhaps during final validation testing of production models. By that point, it is very expensive — both politically and economically — to make major design changes. Design-related sources of error need to be detected early in the design process when there is time to pursue a better design and validate its effectiveness.

All of this requires effort, particularly with regard to engaging the end-users in the design process. Toward that end, I want to describe an effective partnership between clinicians and medical device manufacturers. Beginning in the middle of the past century, anesthesiologists recognized the problem of inadvertently delivering a hypoxic gas mixture (insufficient oxygen) to anesthetized patients. This problem occurred because, while anesthesia machines were designed to make it easy to change the flow of inhaled gases (oxygen, nitrous oxide, air, and others) to the patient, there were no safeguards to prevent the user from accidentally turning the oxygen flow down or off. What followed was a fruitful collaboration between clinician users and anesthesia machine manufacturers to make these devices safer.

At first, redesign efforts led to the introduction of tactile cues (e.g., shape, position, and location of the oxygen flow control knob), visual cues (oxygen is always labeled with a green color), physical constraints (e.g., bars in front of the oxygen knob to prevent inadvertent bumping) and, most importantly, standardization among manufacturers (oxygen always on the right, always turn clockwise to increase flow, etc.). Next, manufacturers introduced both new and improved monitoring devices with associated alarms to measure delivered and inspired oxygen concentration and to assure continued ventilation. Finally, manufacturers developed technological constraints that made the delivery of a hypoxic gas mixture virtually impossible. For example, a physical linkage of oxygen and nitrous oxide flow control mechanisms prevents the delivery of nitrous oxide without concurrently delivering a minimal concentration of oxygen. Also, modern anesthesia machines are designed to always deliver at least the minimal amount of oxygen sufficient to keep a patient alive. These design enhancements — a direct response to a clearly defined user need — have virtually eliminated the occurrence of hypoxic brain injury due to inadequate oxygen in the delivered gas mixture.

The Design of Complex Microprocessor-Based Devices

An increasing number of medical devices are microprocessor-controlled. Modern technology allows the designer to cost-effectively incorporate far more clinically useful features. In fact, this has led to a situation (also seen in consumer electronics) where the device can contain virtually all of the features that any anticipated user might theoretically want. The resulting medical device can become quite complex, incorporating a large number of controls and functions (Figure 5).

But, in reality, the majority of users need only a small subset of all of the device's features and, when users operate such a device, most of the time they only use a few of the available features. In the worst cases, users are stuck with an overly complex device that imposes excessive training requirements, slows and complicates tasks, and places undue cognitive demands on the clinician. Some designers recognize this problem and respond by making the device appear less complex, perhaps through the use of a small number of primary controls and displays. However, this can be problematic because it leads to hidden modes of operation and faulty user mental models of how the device functions. The real solution is to get rid of features that have marginal, if any, value to the preponderance of users.

Documentation and Training

I will conclude by discussing a topic that receives insufficient attention from medical device designers. In reality, clinicians almost never read device manuals (I suspect this is also true for many patients) and typically receive minimal if any training on how to use devices, despite what a manufacturer may recommend. Medical personnel often rotate through clinical sites at a pace that leaves little time for training, even if there is time and funds available for training, which is not always the case. Additionally, medical device manuals are usually collecting dust on a shelf in the clinical engineer's basement office, not exactly a location accessible to busy clinicians. Moreover,

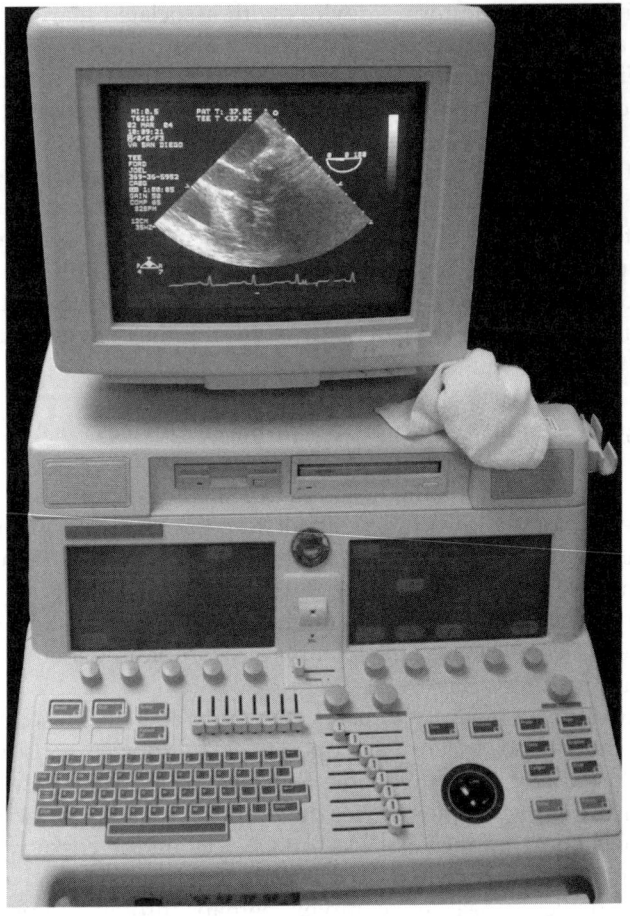

FIGURE 5
New microprocessor-controlled devices have become increasingly complex with a dizzying array of controls and displays. This ultrasound device is used in the operating room by anesthesiologists as they are trying to accomplish many other clinical tasks. My laboratory has data to suggest that use of this type of complex medical device may increase workload or impair vigilance.[2]

even if clinicians had ready access to the manuals, they are not likely to be useful. Medical device user manuals are rarely written to meet the real needs of end-users.

A helpful user manual could answer questions, such as:

- Even though I have used many previous models of this kind of device, how do I use *this* particular brand I've never seen before on this patient *right now*?
- How do I view the ST segment trends *right now* to see if my patient is having a heart attack?

- Why can't I synchronize the defibrillator so I can shock this patient out of atrial fibrillation to get her blood pressure up so she doesn't have a stroke?

However, most manufacturers write user manuals to satisfy regulatory requirements. To my disappointment, the most salient aspects of many manuals are warnings to "be careful" and descriptions of formalized "workaround procedures" to help users avoid previously identified use errors that could not be mitigated by design changes. Yet, plaintiff lawyers will tell you that no statement intended to protect the manufacturer, whether placed on the device or in the accompanying documentation, is likely to preclude product liability in the event of an adverse event, particularly if the device has clearly demonstrated usability problems. Therefore, while there is ample opportunity for improving user manuals, a far better solution is to design devices that the intended users can operate effectively *without any training at all!*

Conclusions

Designing for the medical domain is challenging. Poorly designed medical devices, whether disposable syringes or complex imaging systems, can cause clinicians to make errors that lead to adverse patient outcomes. Devices intended for use by patients can similarly foster adverse outcomes if not designed properly.

Designers must be cognizant of the fact that even experienced clinicians will commit use errors. Therefore, the design focus should be on minimizing the chance of use errors, giving users the opportunity to recover from errors when they occur, and mitigating the adverse consequences of use errors when they cannot be prevented.

While clinicians are highly trained personnel who can handle any technological challenge, that is not how they want to spend their time. Clinicians want to focus on patient care instead of fiddling with devices that are difficult to use. The medical device's design should allow it to become a natural extension of the users' cognitive and physical capabilities — one that augments rather than diminishes the user's ability to function as demanded by their needs and environment.

A goal of excellent medical device design should be to allow clinicians to use a device correctly and safely *the very first time* they interact with it, preferably without training or reading the manual. The most reliable method to accomplish this laudable goal is to implement a structured human factors engineering program that stretches from the beginning to the end of the development process. Such a program must take a user-centered approach that focuses on users' needs and requirements, considers the complexities of the device's likely use environments, and involves continual user input and evaluation of the evolving design. Clinicians and patients are invaluable partners in this quest for design excellence.

References

1. Mosenkis, R., Human factors in design, *Medical Devices*, van Gruting, C.W.D., Ed., Elsevier, Amsterdam, The Netherlands, 41–51, 1994.
2. Weinger, M.B., Herndon, O.W., and Gaba, D.M., The effect of electronic record keeping and transesophageal echocardiography on task distribution, workload, and vigilance during cardiac anesthesia, *Anesthesiology*, 87, 144–155, 1997.

General Principles
and Processes

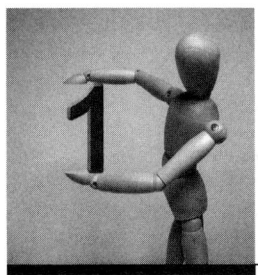

The Rising Bar — Medical Product Design Excellence

Michael E. Wiklund

It does not get much better than working on life-saving medical devices — a defibrillator that corrects dangerous heart arrhythmias, a respiratory therapy device that helps newborn babies to breathe, and a hemodialysis machine that people can operate at home, thereby improving both their health and their lifestyle. It is fulfilling work because you know you are helping people. Indeed, helping people (and perhaps making a living) seems to be the primary factor that draws design professionals into medical product development and keeps them there.

There is no question that an intensive-care ventilator is going to save many lives during its service life of a decade or more (see Figure 1.1). Consequently, designers have a solemn responsibility to get the design right. There is little room for design mediocrity or negligence, considering the heavy marketplace competition and the potentially dire consequences of misuse.

Getting the design right means exhaustively investigating the product's functional requirements and the users' needs and preferences. Today, products such as programmable infusion pumps may have a host of users, including physicians, nurses, technicians, and patients. Defining and meeting users' needs is a tall but necessary order. If designers fail to consider the needs of all user groups, some may ultimately struggle to use the given product. Worse, they may commit errors leading to an adverse outcome — the medical industry's jargon for hurting or killing someone.

The potential consequences of inadequate design lead progressive designers of medical devices to invest substantially in human factors analyses. This is the only reliable means to ensure that users will be able to perform key tasks during extremely stressful, not to mention tedious, times using advanced technology (see Figure 1.2a,b,c). Progressive designers have to

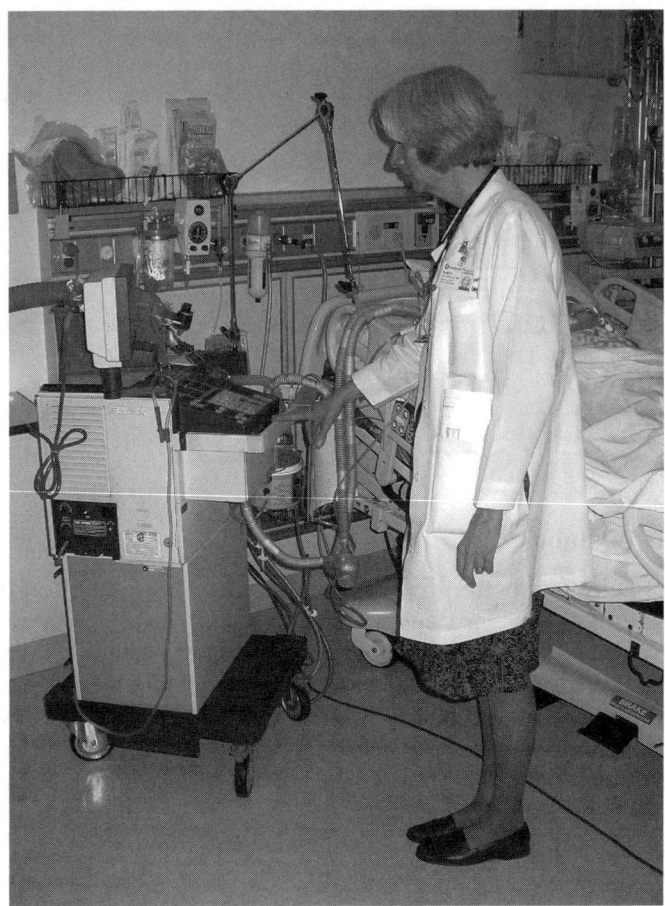

FIGURE 1.1
Intensive care unit nurse attends to a patient on a ventilator. Photo courtesy of Emerson Hospital (Concord, MA).

know the users and the possible uses — unintended as well as intended. They also have to understand the environment and how it will influence interactions between users and the product. Then, they must integrate all of the accumulated insights to generate viable design solutions that fit the users' mind and body and that work effectively under all potential circumstances, including unusual or unlikely circumstances.

Despite the average designer's propensity for spontaneous, creative expression, designing medical products calls for a disciplined design approach. The Food and Drug Administration's (FDA) regulations prescribe specific development steps and call for extensive documentation. Medical product designers must come to terms with taking things step by step and allowing empirical data to drive the design, while still seizing opportunities to be creative and innovative.

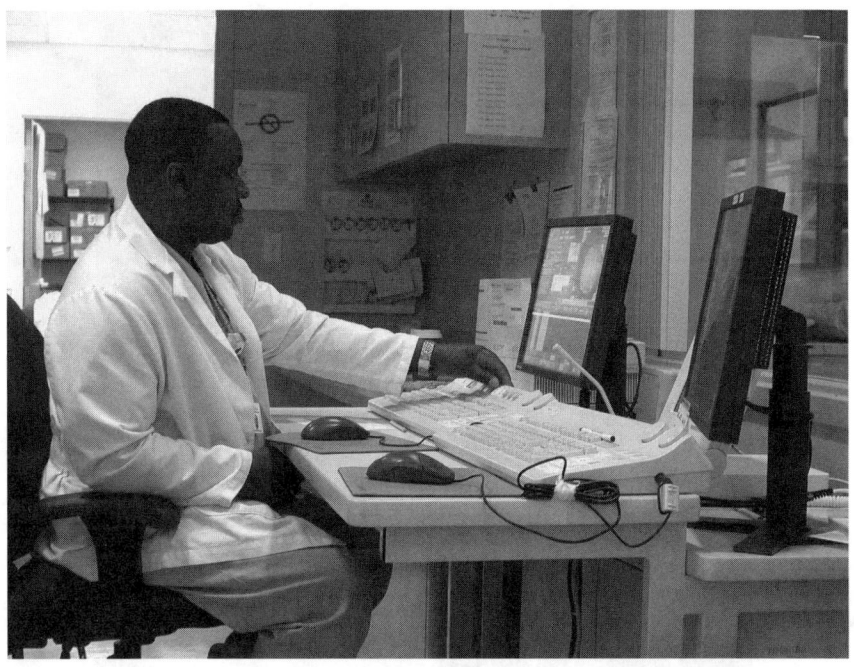

FIGURE 1.2a
Hospital personnel interacting with a diagnostic scanner. Photo courtesy of Emerson Hospital (Concord, MA).

The good news is that many manufacturers are producing excellent medical products (see Figure 1.2a,b,c), and their designs are collecting awards. Healthcare workers will eagerly point out the products they love to use. Usually the best-loved products are the ones that make the caregivers' jobs easier, enabling them to spend more time with their patients and less time making the devices work properly. It is these products that give healthcare professionals confidence in their ability to render safe and effective patient care, particularly during stressful moments, which for some caregivers is all the time.

Of course, design excellence extends well beyond user interaction quality. An increasing number of medical devices have shapes and materials that add a touch of class and enhance user task performance. This is particularly true of products intended for use by people at home. For example, today's blood-testing devices look more like sleek cellular phones (see Figure 1.4). Patient monitors are styled like computers and televisions. Breathing masks use soft, compliant materials usually associated with high-quality scuba gear.

So look for the market to demand increasingly sophisticated medical devices that safely and effectively perform the requisite functions but do so in a way that satisfies users on many levels. The days of crude metal boxes decorated with a confusing array of controls and displays are numbered. Industrial and human factors design professionals are finally making their mark in an industry that is starting to set some trends of its own.

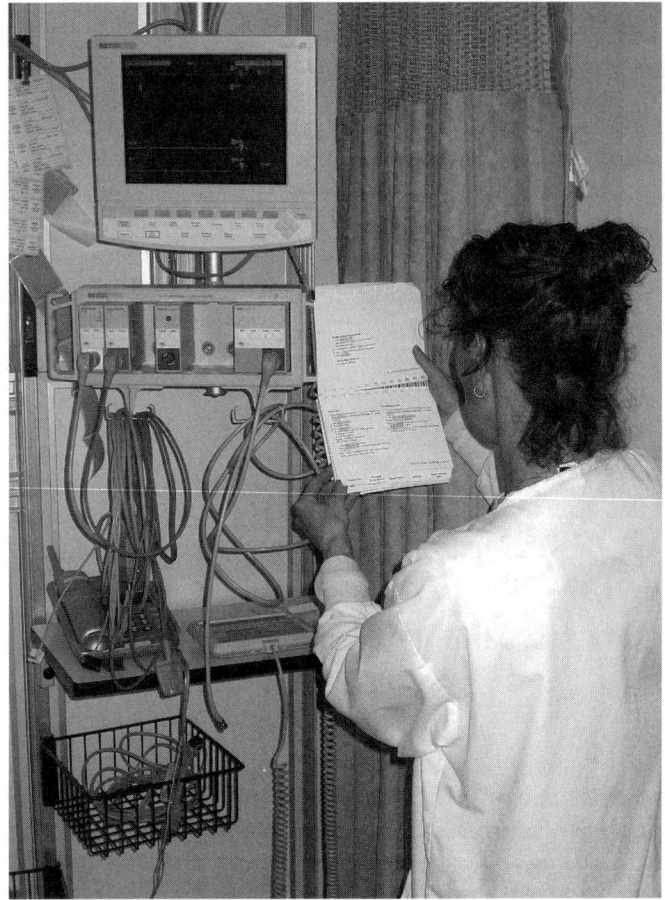

FIGURE 1.2b
Hospital personnel interacting with a patient monitor. Photo courtesy of Emerson Hospital (Concord, MA).

More about FDA Requirements

The high rate of medical device use errors causing patient injury or death led the FDA in 1997 to establish stiffer regulations pertaining to the user interface development process. Today, the FDA expects manufacturers to explicitly define user requirements and then demonstrate the link between the requirements and the design solution. The agency also expects manufacturers to conduct tests to determine if users are able to perform tasks effectively. To learn more about the FDA's requirements, see www.fda.gov/cdrh/humanfactors.

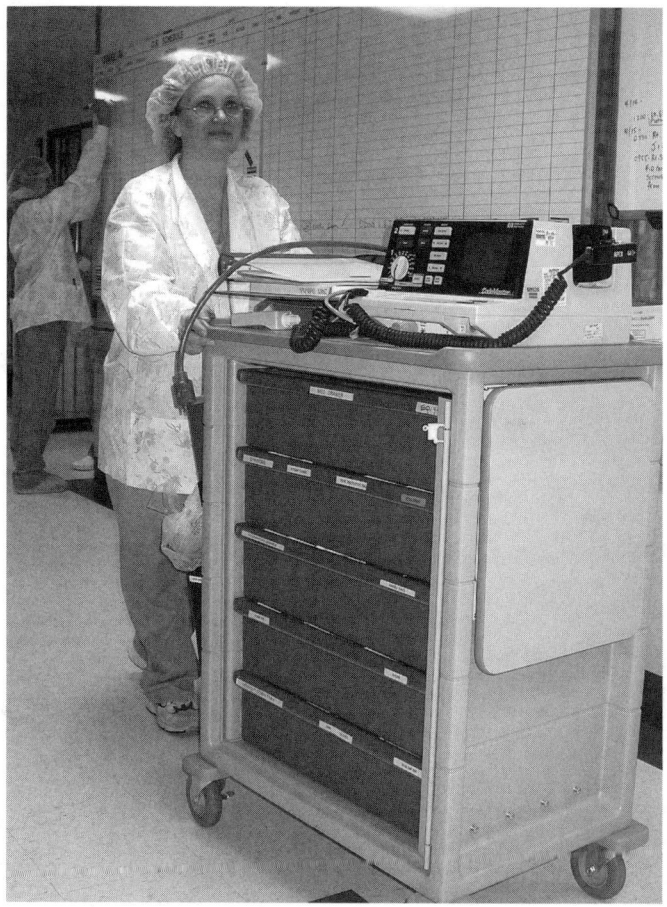

FIGURE 1.2c
Hospital personnel pushing a "crash cart" that includes a defibrillator. Photo courtesy of Emerson Hospital (Concord, MA).

The FDA has endorsed the Association for the Advancement of Medical Instrumentation's publication, *Human Factors Design Process for Medical Devices* (ANSI/AAMI HE74: 2001). This is a good reference for those planning a medical device design effort.

Key Points
- Medical device designers have a solemn responsibility to get the design right in order to protect patients from harm. Getting the design right means exhaustively investigating the product's functional requirements and the users' needs and preferences.

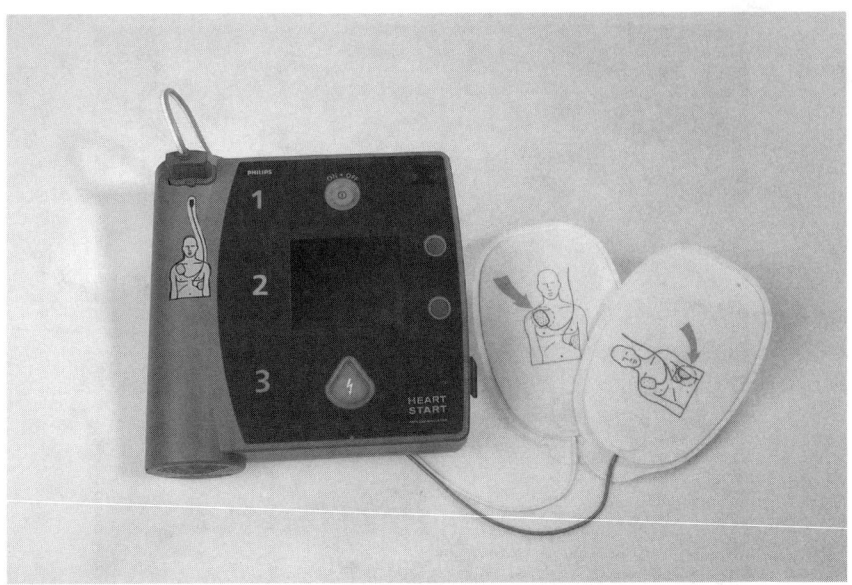

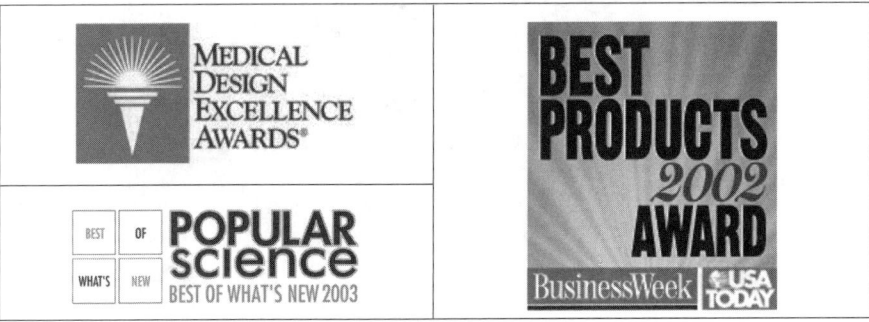

FIGURE 1.3
HeartStart Home Defibrillator has received several awards for design, engineering, and overall technological innovation. Photo courtesy of Philips Medical Systems. All rights reserved. The Medical Design Excellence Awards logo and logotype are registered trademarks of Canon Communications LLC. The Best of What's New 2003 logo courtesy of Popular Science (Time Warner Inc.). The Best Products of 2002 Award logo courtesy of BusinessWeek (The McGraw-Hill Companies Inc.).

- Helping people and making a living seem to be the primary factors that draw design professionals into medical product development and keep them there.
- Despite the average designer's propensity for spontaneous, creative expression, designing medical products calls for a disciplined design approach.
- The FDA expects manufacturers to explicitly define user requirements and then (1) demonstrate the link between the requirements and (2) conduct tests to determine if users are able to perform tasks effectively.

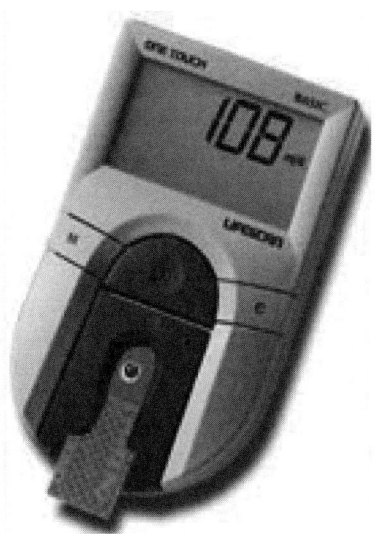

FIGURE 1.4
LifeScan's OneTouch® Basic® Blood Glucose Monitoring System's size and shape is comparable to a cellular phone.

- The marketplace demands increasingly sophisticated medical devices that safely and effectively perform the requisite functions but do so in a way that satisfies users on many levels.
- Usually the best-loved products are the ones that make the caregivers' jobs easier, enabling them to spend more time with their patients and less time making the devices work properly.

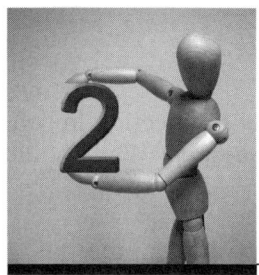

The Role of Industrial Design and Human Engineering in the Design of Software-Driven Medical Products

Stephen B. Wilcox

Software is aggressively cannibalizing hardware everywhere, including in medical product development. The reasons for this, we think, have to do with flexibility, the ability to handle variation, including:

- **Variation in skill levels.** Particularly in diagnostic equipment, there is constant pressure to reduce the skill level required to use products. Thus, products which used to be used by physicians or Ph.D.s are now required to be used by technicians as well. Software allows a product to have "multiple faces," so the physicians will not be insulted, but the uneducated technician can still use it relatively free of error.
- **Variation in languages.** Software interfaces can be produced in any language you want. It is a lot easier to send out a software update than to alter the labeling on traditional displays and controls.
- **Variation in functions.** Through software, a device can be altered to perform multiple functions, a capability much more difficult to achieve with "physical" products.
- **Variation in componentry.** Upgradeability is much easier with software.
- **Variation in conditions of use.** Software can learn from past mistakes or contain automatic adjustment to different conditions.

Why Not Software Engineering Alone?

In discussing the role of industrial design and human engineering in software product design, it is only fair to answer the question: Why should software engineers not do it alone? Our answers are as follows:

- **Bridging of software and hardware design.** A typical approach is for different teams to handle software and hardware. The problem is that hardware decisions affect software and vice versa. For example, the ideal control solution may be "soft keys," which can be altered, based upon the tasks to be performed. However, for soft keys to work, both the software and the hardware have to be appropriate. Industrial designers and human engineers can bridge this gap by treating the product as an integrated software/hardware combination.
- **Creating an elegant product.** For software as well as hardware, engineers do not need industrial designers to make a manufacturable product that works. However, without the designer's input, visual elegance becomes a rare commodity, and it is visual elegance that often provides the competitive edge, particularly in product areas where performance and price have converged.
- **Addressing usability.** A central theme of this volume is that usability of a product can be designed in just as any other characteristic can. However, doing so requires the specific technical skills of the human engineer to truly optimize usability and to avoid unnecessary trial and error in the process.

How Do Industrial Design and Human Engineering Integrate into Product Development with Software-Driven Products?

Figure 2.1 is a (simplified) summary of the design process for a typical product. What follows is a description of several steps of the process.

Field Research

Starting with a marketing/engineering design brief, which lays out the central goals and constraints for a new product, the first step is to go into the actual environment of use (see Chapter 6 for a detailed discussion of ethnographic field research). Such field research is the best antidote in the world for what we have come to call "corporate lore," an incorrect vision of how

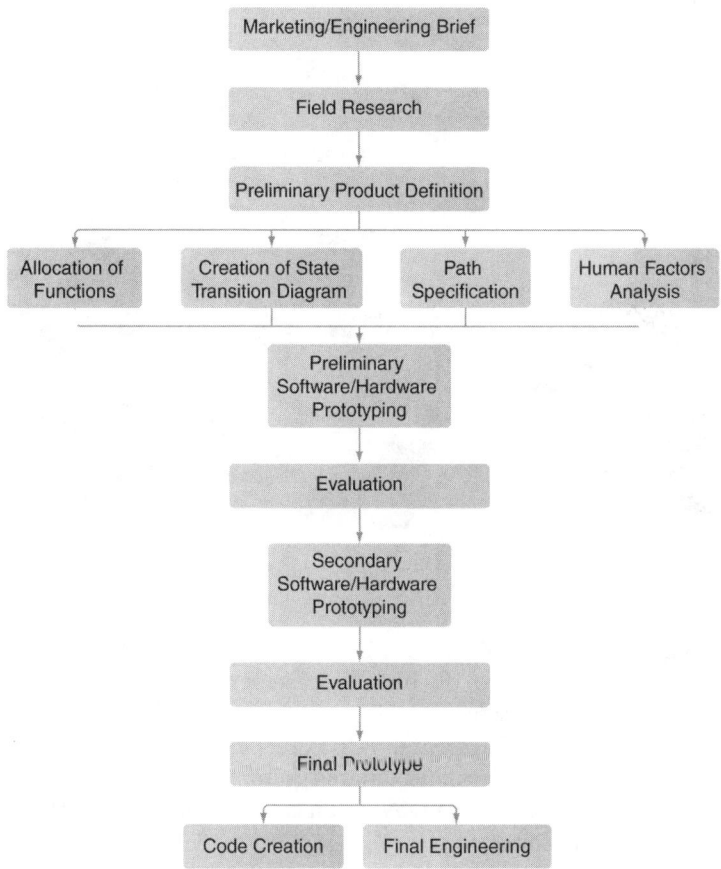

FIGURE 2.1
A simplified summary of a user-centered product design process.

products are used caused by intense focus on the product without adequate information. It is crucial to find out how products are used and misused, what users like and do not like, what odd biases and misconceptions users have, what constraints are imposed by the environment of use, and so on. Such research involves on-site interviews with users as well as careful observation.

As one example, Figure 2.2 shows a laparoscopic surgical suite. It is easy to describe some of the basic differences between laparoscopic and open surgery, but only through spending significant amounts of time there can

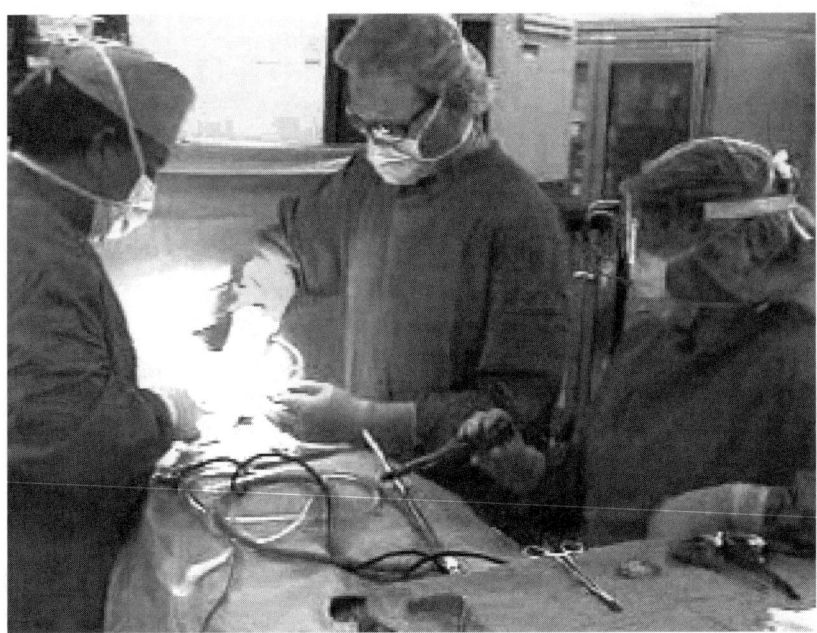

FIGURE 2.2
A laparoscopic surgical suite.

one begin to understand the implications of the relatively dark environment, with the physician focused on the video screen while placing his or her hands and arms into very awkward postures.

The hard part about field research is looking carefully enough and probing deep enough to really understand what is going on, while, at the same time, collecting information in such a way that it can be rigorously communicated, as discussed in Chapter 6.

Preliminary Product Definition

The preliminary product definition combines the initial specifications contained in the brief with the customer/user information obtained from field research. It lists the functions that the product will perform and any constraints imposed by marketing, engineering, or customer/user needs. It forms the basis for product design.

Allocation of Functions

As indicated in Figure 2.1, this step and the next three steps are logically performed in parallel.

Dealing with hardware and software as an integrated whole provides the opportunity to allocate functions in a "scientific" way — which functions are to be performed by hardware and which are to be performed by software. This often seems to take the form of allocating everything to software that can be safely allocated to it, given the advantages of software over hardware. Nothing is worse than committing to a hardware solution just before a competitor comes out with a product with the flexibility and cost reduction associated with software.

Creation of a User-Centered State Transition Diagram

Figure 2.3 shows an example of a user-centered state transition diagram for a simple product. It differs from the diagrams typically used by software engineers in that it maps out states from the user's point of view, not from the point of view of the underlying tasks and functions of the device. The diagram summarizes each state the product has to achieve and the pathways between those states. The state transition diagram provides the blueprint for the development of the software interface. A useful exercise is to create a state transition diagram for an existing product. It can help in identifying awkward or error-inducing characteristics of the product.

Path Specification

In creating prototypes, which will be described subsequently, it is normally impractical to model the whole system. Thus, there has to be a decision about what will be contained in the prototype. Path specification involves choosing key procedures for initial development and testing. They are typically based upon which functions are the most important vis à vis the user and which functions are similar enough, from the user's perspective, that the prototype of one should shed light on the others. Path specification is extremely important in that specifying too many paths slows the product development program, but specifying too few can allow problems to slip through. Let us emphasize, though, that the key to path specification is to think of it as a crucial part of usability testing.

Human Factors Analysis

Once the preliminary product definition has been produced, the process of making human factors decisions can begin. This is where we rely upon databases of human sizes and shapes (*anthropometry* — see Chapter 8), technical documents about strength and range of joint motions, and all sorts of technical information about cognitive characteristics, such as learnability. With regard to software, information is available about what works best for many of the decisions that have to be made — screen layout, timing, choice of pointing devices, and so on. Such information is far from the whole story, but it can eliminate a good deal of trial and error by providing research-based guidelines.

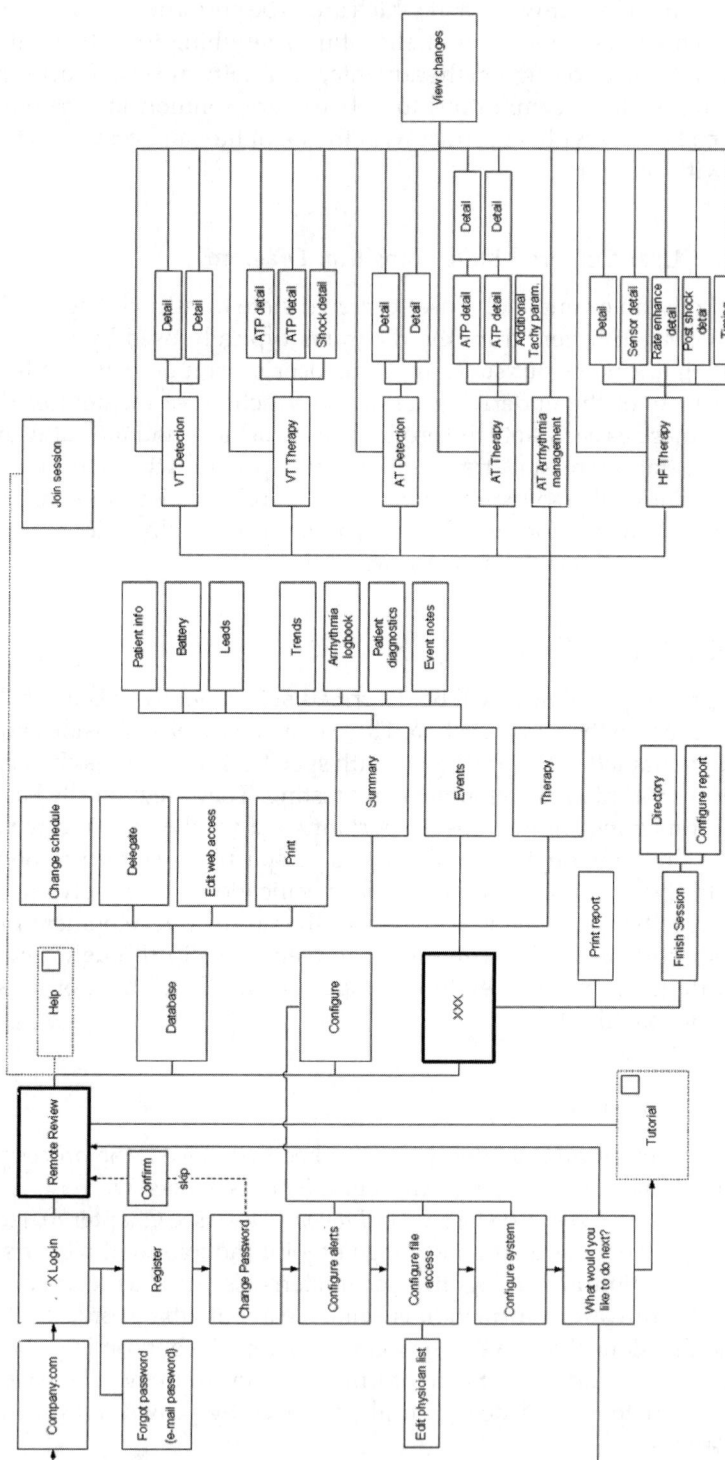

FIGURE 2.3
A user-interface state transition diagram.

Preliminary Software and Hardware Prototyping

For many designers, this is the fun part. This step involves "conceptual design," but we have called it *prototyping* to emphasize the importance of creating prototypes that can be subjected to user testing as soon as possible. In the case of software, there is no way to know what you have until the dynamic dimension is added, something that cannot be done without a working prototype. In the case of hardware, prototyping involves everything from quick foamcore sketch models to cast parts. Also, the advantages of creating software simulations of hardware should not be overlooked as a way of creating really early testable prototypes prior to any physical models. Using simulation/animation software, you can create screen simulations of moving parts and incorporate sound. Chapter 12 discusses prototyping in detail.

The key is to use software prototyping tools that are as fast as possible so there is less psychological investment in them. A prototype that only takes a few hours to create is psychologically easier to redo a few times than a prototype that takes a long time to create and that will be used as the actual product.

Usability Testing

The general idea is to take advantage of the various rapid prototyping tools (for both hardware and software) now available to produce working prototypes much earlier in the process than they used to be produced. As soon as they are created, they can be tested with users. Usability testing involves having potential users of a product "use" the prototype. Some key issues for usability testing include the following (see Nielsen's *Usability Engineering*,[1] for a good overview of usability testing):

- **What to test.** Usability testing requires a working prototype. Rely on drawings or verbal descriptions only as a last resort. In a pinch, a shortcut is a *Wizard-of-Oz* simulation, in which you manipulate the system yourself (hiding inside the box if it is big enough) to make it simulate the way it would operate in response to user input.
- **How to test.** The obvious thing to do is to simply put people in front of the prototype and see what happens. However, there are a number of other techniques that can be useful under certain circumstances, including:

    Constructive interaction, in which people use the prototype in groups of two or more. The great advantage is that you can record what they say to provide additional insight.

    Coaching, in which you allow people to ask you questions when they have problems. Coaching yields additional information, and it is useful when you find that the prototype has problems that keep people from getting to square one with the system.

Speaking aloud, in which people explain what they are doing as they do it. The advantage to this is that you can find out what the perceived problems are instead of having to infer them. The disadvantage is that use of the system may be altered.

Retrospective testing, in which you record the test, then review the tape with the person. This takes more time, but it is a good way to hear what the person has to say in a way that does not alter the initial testing.

- **What to measure.** *Time* and *errors* are the classic measures. Other possibilities include such things as physiological or biomechanical measures (e.g., heart rate or range of joint motion), the amount of time reading instructions, or subsequent recollection of procedural steps.
- **Who should do the testing.** It is crucial for members of the design team not to administer the test. There are too many ways that bias can be introduced.

Another important aspect of usability testing is to record the sessions for future reference and to communicate the results to others. Figure 2.4 shows, in diagrammatic form, a usability testing system. It involves recording multiple video and audio channels simultaneously, which are amplified, then fed into a mixer. The idea is to get a good view of the person's face, his or her hands, what is happening on the screen, etc., while recording what he or she says and the tester's comments. The recording of a single tape with a split-screen image avoids the problem of synchronization, which would be caused by trying to record a session without a mixer.

As illustrated in the diagram of product development, there is usually more than one cycle of usability testing. The goal of each session is to identify problems with the prototype. The problems are then addressed by redoing the prototype, and, if necessary, the cycle is repeated. The number of cycles depends upon the complexity of the system, among other things. However, despite the time it takes (days or weeks), identifying problems with usability testing is much faster and cheaper than using the medical marketplace as a usability testing system.

Conclusion

Industrial design and human engineering have contributions to make to the design of software-driven medical products that cannot be replaced by other professionals. Although it is certainly possible to create a software-driven product without industrial designers and human engineers, the resulting design is inevitably compromised in the very aspect of a medical product that is often crucial to its success.

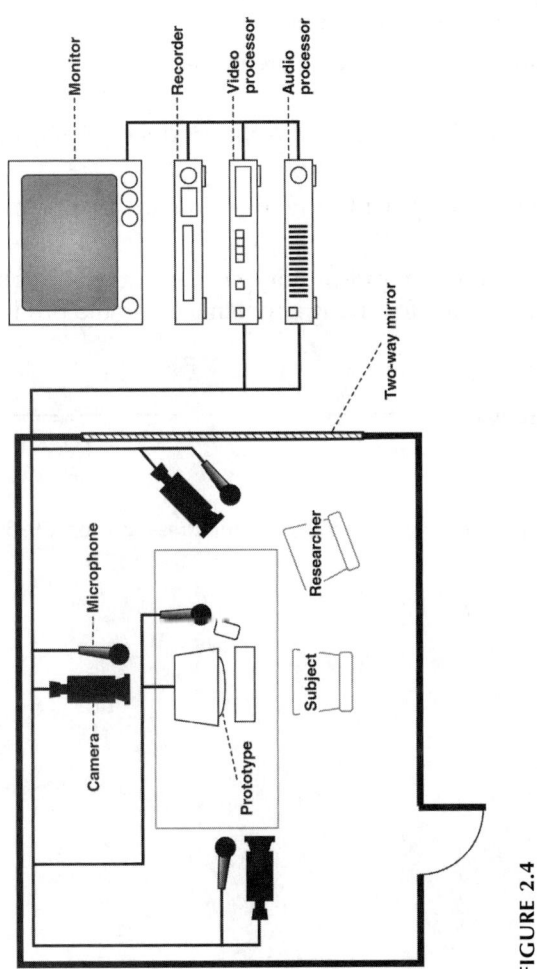

FIGURE 2.4
A usability testing recording system.

Key Points

- Software-driven products provide great flexibility, but require particular attention to usability.
- Incorporating industrial design and human engineering is particularly important for software-driven products in order to create products that users want and can use.
- Field research is an important preliminary to good product development.
- Systematic attention to the user as the product is designed is equally important.
- As product development unfolds, human factors data can be applied.
- The combination of rapid-prototyping and good usability testing provides the means for fixing problems *before* the product is introduced.

References

1. Nielsen, J., *Usability Engineering*, Academic Press, Boston, 1993.

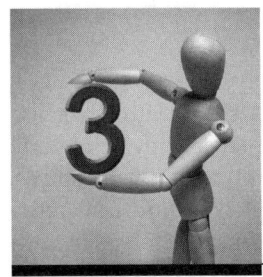

Is Your Human Factors Program Ready for FDA Scrutiny?

Michael E. Wiklund

For the agency, human factors is more than a buzzword. Manufacturers lacking a comprehensive approach to user-centered design are likely to find this out firsthand.

Manufacturers planning to bring a medical device to the U.S. market should ask themselves the following questions: Are we ready for the FDA to inspect our human factors program? Will our user-interface designs and related test data easily navigate the premarket review process? How a company answers these queries will reveal a great deal about its likely success in dealing with the FDA and appealing to the marketplace.

If the answers are an honest yes, this is probably a company that has made a deliberate and thoughtful investment in a human factors program. It is likely to encounter few problems with the FDA, at least with respect to human factors design, and can expect to enjoy a competitive advantage in the marketplace.

If the answers are no, or even maybe, the company may be in for trouble. This may be a company that has paid too little attention to the regulation requiring companies to utilize a systematic design process in the course of product development. As a result, it may have left itself open both to trouble with the FDA and to liability claims related to use error.

Background

Since June 1997, the FDA quality system regulation's design controls section has required manufacturers of Class II and Class III medical devices (along with certain Class I devices) to demonstrate adherence to good design practices. According to FDA human factors scientists Peter B. Carstensen and Dick Sawyer (now retired), the critical language with respect to human factors is including the needs of the user and patient. The FDA's objective is to improve the quality of user-interface design in order to reasonably minimize the incidence of use errors that could cause patient injury or death. Examples of common use errors include placing a device on the wrong setting, misprogramming its automated behavior, or improperly connecting its components.

In the ensuing five years, many manufacturers have responded positively to the requirement by establishing robust human factors programs. Others have been less responsive. Their hesitance may be due to a lack of technical understanding or to a lack of commitment — whether philosophical, financial, or both — to setting up an effective human factors program. Some companies seem to be taking a wait-and-see approach, unsure how serious the FDA is about enforcing its human factors mandate.

Along with the Association for the Advancement of Medical Instrumentation (AAMI), the FDA has taken steps to address these barriers, through education, standards development, and enforcement measures. In 2001, AAMI sought to improve the level of understanding of the new regulations among manufacturers by publishing a new national standard entitled AAMI HE74:2001 Human Factors Design Process for Medical Devices (see Figure 3.1). This new standard replaces in part AAMI HE48:1993 Human Factors Engineering Guidelines and Preferred Practices for the Design of Medical Devices.

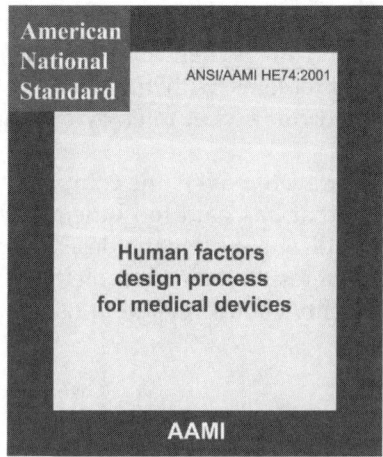

FIGURE 3.1
ANSI/AAMI HE74:2001 describes a human factors design process for medical devices. Photo courtesy of the Association for the Advancement of Medical Instrumentation.

Endorsed by the FDA, the standard delineates the appropriate steps toward producing a user-friendly and error-resistant design. It acknowledges that human factors research, design, modeling, and testing activities should be scaled to match the complexity of the device and its manner of use. As such, a hemodialysis machine would probably warrant a more substantial investment than a pulse oximeter, due to the extent of user interactions and the opportunity for detrimental use errors (see Figure 3.2).

The FDA is increasingly holding manufacturers accountable to its human factors expectations through field inspections, product reviews, and post-market surveillance. The agency's human factors specialists speak passionately and often about protecting the public against products with human factors shortcomings. At industry conferences and sponsored workshops, they cite numerous examples of patient injury and death attributable to user-interface design flaws. The agency points to the design processes described in AAMI HE74:2001 as an important part of the solution. They also rattle the saber a bit, noting that the FDA now has the regulatory responsibility to take action in cases of bad user-interface design.

Field Inspections

Every facility inspection by the FDA brings with it a chance that field investigators will ask to see evidence of the company's human factors program. Depending on the situation, field investigators may ask to review examples of human factors analyses and tests associated with products already on the market or currently under development. In such cases, manufacturers should be prepared to open up their design history files, which might include the following items:

- Human factors program plan
- User research reports and videotapes
- Task analysis report
- User requirements specification
- Conceptual, preliminary, and final design drawings and descriptions
- Computer-based prototype software files
- Usability test reports and videotapes
- User-interface style guide

Field investigators may also ask to meet the company's human factors specialists, who may be formally trained staff, professionals in related disciplines who learned human factors on the job, or consultants.

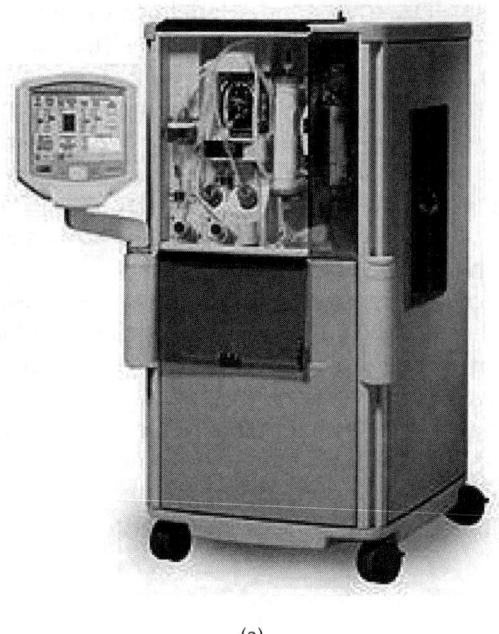

(a)

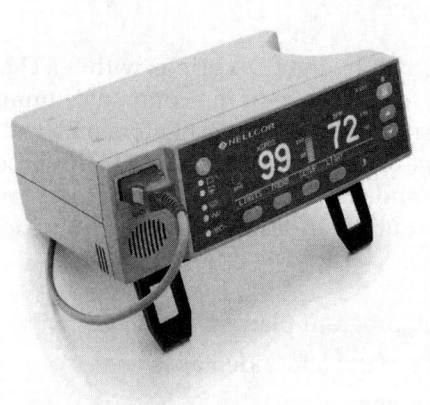

(b)

FIGURE 3.2
The hemodialysis machine (a) may require a greater investment in human factors research and design than the simpler pulse oximeter (b). Photo courtesy of Tyco Healthcare.

Notably, few if any of the FDA's field staff have hands-on experience or degrees in human factors or even related disciplines, such as psychology or industrial design. To some extent, this limits their ability to identify subtle issues related to the design process and user-interface design. However, the agency provides its field staff with basic human factors training and background materials to distinguish a good human factors program from a bad one, assuming one exists at all. If an investigator finds cause for concern, he or she may investigate the matter more deeply, drawing support from the agency's experts as needed. Thus, field inspectors will at least catch gross human factors deficiencies.

If a company is unable to demonstrate proper attention to human factors, the FDA is empowered to issue a warning letter, a uniformly dreaded outcome among medical device developers. Warning letters give manufacturers a deadline to correct documented problems before the agency imposes a severe penalty.

Carstensen spearheads the agency's human factors efforts. He says that a company can be written up for not having the necessary design controls in place, even if the device appears to have a good user interface. The company must have a design control process in place — one that includes the required human factors steps, he says. Sawyer points out that device developers must verify the match between design inputs (users' needs identified through research) and design outputs (specific user-interface design characteristics).

Premarket Reviews

The FDA has asked many companies that are seeking premarket clearance for their products to supplement their applications with additional proof that the device can be used safely by typical users working under the normal range of use conditions. Such proof often includes findings from evaluations of device operation conducted early in the design process using relevant use scenarios, effectively requiring usability tests of computer-simulated or working prototypes. And of course, discovering design deficiencies in a prototype will save the manufacturer the money and time that might be spent redesigning a production model.

The rigor of a human factors review is proportionate to the complexity of the device's user interface and the potential for deleterious use errors. According to Carstensen, reviewers may flag a particular product as having a relatively complicated user interface, perhaps because it has numerous controls or unusual interaction mechanisms. In such a case, the reviewer may contact CDRH's human factors group, and a staff member will be assigned to the review team. He or she will perform a more intensive analysis that pays particular attention to submission materials related to hazards, use errors, design requirements, design features, and user instructions. In more focused reviews, the FDA staff seeks answers to basic questions, such as the following:

- Does the device adhere to basic human factors design principles?
- Does the device preclude use errors that could lead to patient injury or death?
- Has the manufacturer tested the user interface with representative users to demonstrate its operability?

Review of a device's human factors aspects may raise concerns about specific features. For example, the reviewers may be concerned about the design of the imbedded alarm system or cable connections to peripheral devices. They may question whether users will be able to hear a high-pitched alarm tone, noting that older men suffer a predictable degradation in their ability to hear high-pitched sounds. Or they may be concerned about whether the device's cable connections provide sufficient tactile feedback to confirm that the connection is complete and secure.

Considerable attention is focused on usability test reports because many usability problems become evident only when representative users perform representative tasks. For example, the task of programming a single-channel infusion pump may seem logical according to a flow diagram. However, users may struggle to perform the task correctly, even after receiving training, due to the need to convert units of measure as part of a complicated dose calculation. This kind of problem could lead to an accidental patient overdose, but it is difficult to spot on a paper review. Therefore, the FDA looks to manufacturers to conduct rigorous, dynamic usability tests to reveal such problems.

In fact, a glance at the FDA's human factors guidance documents or its Web page (see Figure 3.3) reveals the agency's view that usability testing is the cornerstone of any human factors program. The FDA's human factors team strongly encourages manufacturers to invest in a series of usability tests during the course of product development in order to make the product review process go more smoothly.

Postmarket Investigations

Occasionally, the agency's human factors staff may be called upon by the agency's Office of Surveillance and Biometrics to evaluate the human factors suitability of a device involved in an incident leading to a patient injury or death. In the past, they have scrutinized various catheters, glucose meters, infant apnea monitors, ventilators, infusion devices, and many other devices involved in multiple incidents.

According to Carstensen, these human factors reviews typically begin with an ad hoc meeting to discuss the given incident as well as concerns about

Is Your Human Factors Program Ready for FDA Scrutiny?

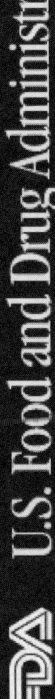
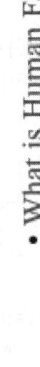
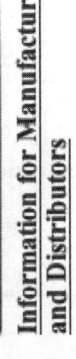

FIGURE 3.3
The FDA's Web site (www.fda.gov/cdrh/humanfactors/) offers extensive human factors guidance. Web site posted by the U.S. Food and Drug Administration (as of April 2004).

the device's design. The discussion may escalate to include follow-up design analyses by the FDA's human factors experts and a request for the manufacturer to conduct studies to address a specific concern. A particularly severe problem could trigger a device recall. However, according to Sawyer, "In the case of an obvious and serious user-interface deficiency, manufacturers often will be the first to recognize a problem and take necessary corrective and preventive actions on their own."

International Perspective

Recent changes to the good manufacturing practice regulations and AAMI HE74:2001 establish a clear mandate for U.S. medical device companies to focus on human factors. But many companies first introduce their products in Europe in order to accelerate market entry and build a base of clinical experience. What are the expectations abroad? Are the requirements significantly different?

In fact, the expectations are quite similar. For starters, the International Electrotechnical Commission is expected to incorporate an adapted version of AAMI HE-74:2001 as a collateral standard to IEC 60601: IEC 60601-1-6, Edition 1, medical electrical equipment Part 1–6: General requirements for safety Collateral standard: Usability (currently under development, second draft circulated for comment in July 2002). Therefore, organizations such as TÜV, which evaluate medical devices against applicable standards, will also be seeking evidence of good human factors design.

Conclusion

Who should care about human factors? Certainly, any quality-conscious engineer or designer should. User interfaces are a particularly visible sign of design excellence and warrant close attention from the technical staff. Marketers should also be concerned. More than ever before, customers are able to distinguish good user interfaces from bad ones and choose to purchase devices with good ones.

But it is top management and the staff in a firm's regulatory affairs department that hold the final responsibility for demonstrating a good faith response to the FDA's mandate. In the absence of such a response, not only is the FDA regulatory action a real possibility, but marketing problems and liability concerns could arise as well.

Key Points

- Manufacturers should ask: "Are we ready for the FDA to inspect our human factors program? Will our user-interface designs and related test data easily navigate the premarket review process?"
- A company that has made a deliberate and thoughtful investment in a human factors program is likely to encounter few problems with the FDA, at least with respect to human factors design, and can expect to enjoy a competitive advantage in the marketplace.
- Since June 1997, the FDA quality system regulation's design controls section has required manufacturers of Class II and Class III medical devices (along with certain Class I devices) to demonstrate good human factors engineering practices.
- In 2001, AAMI sought to improve the level of understanding among manufacturers of the FDA's human factors engineering-related regulations by publishing a new national standard entitled AAMI HE-74:2001 Human Factors Design Process for Medical Devices.
- The FDA is increasingly holding manufacturers accountable to its human factors expectations through field inspections, product reviews, and postmarket surveillance.
- Every facility inspection by the FDA brings with it a chance that field investigators will ask to see evidence of the company's human factors program.
- The FDA has asked many companies that are seeking premarket clearance for their products to supplement their applications with additional proof that the device can be used safely by typical users working under the normal range of use conditions.
- The rigor of a human factors review by the FDA is proportionate to the complexity of a device's user interface and the potential for deleterious use errors.
- Occasionally, the agency's human factors staff may be called upon by the agency's Office of Surveillance and Biometrics to evaluate the human factors suitability of a device involved in an incident leading to a patient injury or death.
- The International Electrotechnical Commission is expected to incorporate an adapted version of AAMI HE74:2001 as a collateral standard that calls for good human factors practices in the development of products intended for use in Europe.
- Top management and the staff in a firm's regulatory affairs department hold the final responsibility for demonstrating a good faith response to FDA's human factors-related regulations.

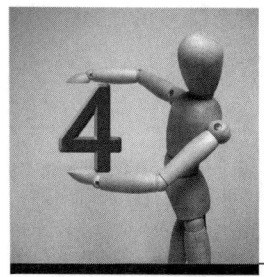

Human Factors Roundtable

Part I: The Regulatory Imperative

Human factors can be defined as knowledge regarding the characteristics and capabilities of human beings that is applicable to the design of systems and devices of all types. In the medical industry, there is increasing awareness of the importance of good human factors practices in the design of safe, effective, and commercially successful products — especially in the wake of the FDA's adoption of the quality system regulation. In the special roundtable discussion that follows, *Medical Device & Diagnostic Industry* (MD&DI) magazine has brought together a varied group of human factors specialists — regulators, consultants, device industry experts, clinicians — to explore how companies can promote better product design and excel in the new product development environment.

The roundtable (see Figure 4.1), which took place in late 2000, was organized with the assistance of MD&DI contributing editor Michael E. Wiklund. Like the other participants, Wiklund has played a prominent role as a member of the Human Engineering Committee of the Association for the Advancement of Medical Instrumentation (AAMI), which has prepared a standard for medical device design that was expected to be approved in the summer of 2001. Joining Wiklund in the roundtable were Peter B. Carstensen, a systems engineer who is the human factors team leader at the FDA's Center for Devices and Radiological Health (CDRH); Rodney A. Hasler, senior technical field response manager at ALARIS Medical Systems, Inc. (San Diego, CA); Dick Sawyer, now retired, a human factors scientist at CDRH; and Matthew B. Weinger, M.D., formerly professor of anesthesiology at the University of California, San Diego and staff physician at the San Diego VA Medical Center, who is also co-chair of the AAMI committee. Dr. Weinger is currently Professor of Anesthesiology, Biomedical Informatics, and Medical Education at Vanderbilt University, Nashville, TN.

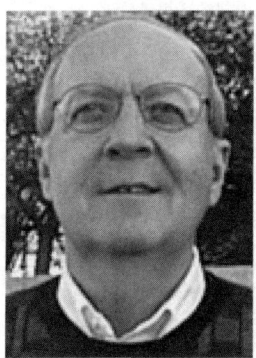
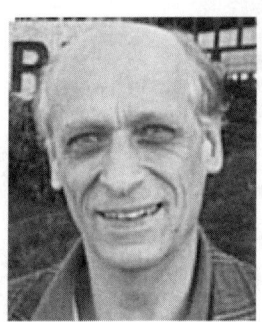
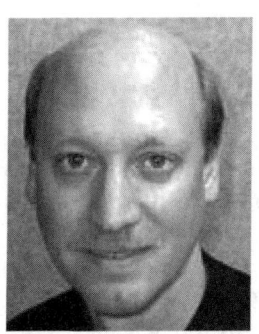
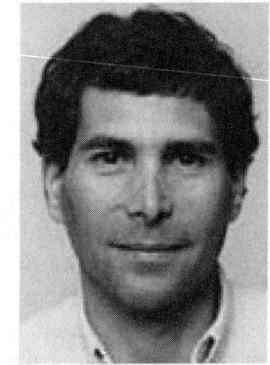
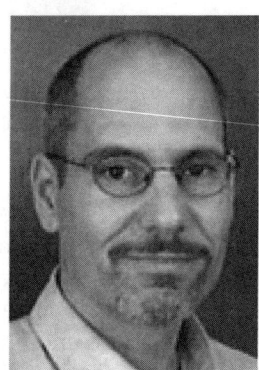

FIGURE 4.1
Roundtable participants (from left to right): Peter B. Carstensen (FDA), Dick Sawyer (formerly with the FDA), Rodney A. Hasler (ALARIS Medical Systems), Matthew B. Weinger (Vanderbilt University), and Michael Wiklund.

MD&DI: The first question is directed to our participants from the FDA. Current GMPs make good human factors practice a regulatory imperative. Can you give a short history lesson on how we got to this stage?

Carstensen: I think it really had its beginnings back in 1974–75. I joined the agency in 1974, as the agency was anticipating the Medical Device Amendments of 1976, and got involved right out of the gate with an ancillary committee that had been working on a standard for anesthesia gas machines for a number of years. At that point the standard had specified about 80% of the requirements and was beginning to deal with what were essentially human factors issues, and I introduced the committee to MIL STD 1472, which is the military version of an AAMI guideline. That gave rise to the organizing of the AAMI human factors committee. I managed to convince the future chairman of that committee — designated Z79 — to approach AAMI and get a human factors committee set up and write general standards for guidance for human factors in medical equipment.

And then around 1984 we had a major anesthesia incident, and the subsequent congressional oversight hearings revealed the significant extent to which human error contributed to such incidents. Jeff Cooper up at Harvard had done a study on critical anesthesia incidents, a 1984 study, in which he had talked about as many as 20,000 avoidable anesthesia deaths every year, with 90% or more of those caused by or related to human error. That got the FDA's attention, and we organized a human factors group — the agency's first identifiable human factors group — in 1993. The group comprised Dick Sawyer, myself, and a couple of other people, and the whole human factors program at the FDA really grew out of that.

So it was in the wake of those congressional hearings that the FDA first talked about adding design control to the good manufacturing practices regulation. A further impetus was the Lucian Leape study of human error in hospitals in New York state, which I believe came out in 1991. Leape later published an article in *JAMA*, called "Error in Medicine," in which he extrapolated the New York data across the country and talked about anywhere from 44,000 to 98,000 avoidable deaths every year in the United States. By the way, many people actually think those are very conservative numbers, as staggering as they are.

In 1995, we held an AAMI/FDA conference on human factors in which we really laid out our strategy and our new human factors program. Two years later, the National Patient Safety Foundation was created. And then this dynamite report came out from the National Academy of Sciences — the Institute of Medicine (IOM) report, "To Err Is Human" — which was really based on the earlier Leape study. So these were the crucial events driving our program.

Sawyer: In conjunction with what Pete's talking about, you may remember the recall study the FDA carried out in the late 1980s — I believe it was completed in 1990 — indicating that about 44% of manufactured recalls were due to design problems. A case-by-case examination of those recalls indicated the prevalence of design-in errors, or errors induced by bad design. So this really gave us the leverage to introduce design issues into the Safe Medical Devices Act of 1990. I think the center had to fight very hard to get the word *design* into that document — which then served as a basis for getting design into our GMP regulation as part of the design controls.

MD&DI: Did we really need new design controls in the GMP regulations, as opposed to allowing industry or the marketplace to provide the impetus for better human factors?

Wiklund: I think the gist of this question goes to political views regarding whether regulation is the way to effect change in an industry as opposed to letting change be driven by the marketplace.

Carstensen: I think you could make a case that it could be marketplace driven to some extent. There certainly are companies that do human factors for marketing reasons — perhaps in addition to liability concerns. Clearly, there are companies I know that invest a lot of resources to get a marketing advantage. But yes, I think that in our judgment a regulation was needed, if for no other reason than to get the attention of the industry and give companies the good news that it is in their self-interest to have a strong human factors program.

Sawyer: In most other critical industrial arenas — the military, air-traffic control, transportation, and so forth — there has been a need for some regulation to get things off the ground so that companies really start paying attention to human factors issues. There are clearly precedents in other sectors for regulation.

Carstensen: I would add one other thing. I think we still see plenty of evidence that companies aren't doing as good a job as they should. But we are convinced that it's more a result of ignorance than of any effort to evade their responsibilities. Getting the attention of companies through the regulation enables us to provide the education and guidance that can help them do what really is in their self-interest.

MD&DI: For readers unfamiliar with the discipline, how would someone define *human factors*? How does the application of good human factors practice make medical devices better?

Wiklund: Today, more and more people are probably familiar with the term *human factors* because of the impact that good human factors practice is having in making things like consumer software applications or electronic devices more usable. Many companies in the commercial sector are promoting good human factors as equivalent to good design or good-quality consumer experiences. As far as defining the discipline, I consider human factors to be the application of what we know about human characteristics to the design of products and systems, including, of course, medical devices. Human factors considers people's mental and physical capabilities as well as their perceived needs or preferences, and tries to accommodate these in the development of good designs that will be safe, usable, efficient, and satisfying. Obviously, when you're talking about medical devices — which serve a life-critical function — there is an inherent justification for a very strong focus on human factors to help achieve important design objectives, especially safety.

Given the proper attention to human factors, one would expect that a medical device could be improved in myriad ways. For example, it would be more ergonomic, which means that it's better suited to the physical interactions of those exposed to it. If it's something you pick up, the handle will be properly shaped so it's comfortable, so that you don't accidently drop it. When you design a display according to good human factors principles, the display is readable from the intended viewing distance and the information is organized in a fashion that is complementary to the task at hand. Controls will be laid out, shaped, and labeled in a manner that is as intuitive as possible, so that the threshold for learning how to use the device is lower and long-term usability is assured.

Hasler: I would agree with the definition we just heard. I also think it reflects the dichotomy of human factors. There are two distinctive components to human factors. The first is ergonomics, which applies human physical capabilities to the device. The second is the cognitive component, which applies the human thought process to the device design.

Weinger: The second part of the question asked how using good human factors processes makes devices better. Mike described the outcomes and how they can be improved through good design, but I think another key element is that a good process involves users — via testing and other techniques — throughout both the initial and iterative design stages. One could very well assemble a good human factors team in terms of knowledge or data and put them together with a bunch of talented engineers and they could design a device that from a theoretical standpoint should have good usability, but until you actually get users in there to use it, you don't know that your solutions are correct. I think that's a key element that needs to be part of that description.

Wiklund: That's a good point. Some of the work that the AAMI committee on human factors is doing hinges on trying to get companies to adopt a human factors process that includes early and continual involvement of the end-users, whether they be physicians, nurses, or patients using medical devices in their own homes. The objective is to get users involved in the process of coming up with good designs that meet their needs and preferences.

Weinger: You can get users involved, but if you simply do focus groups you may end up with a less-than-optimal outcome. And so another element of a successful human factors design process is applying not only the knowledge, but also the tools that will actually describe or verify usability and efficacy in all these critical elements — in other words, usability testing.

MD&DI: Do the people who use medical devices on a daily basis think that there's a usability problem? Do they recognize good human factors design from bad?

Weinger: At present, there is much greater recognition of human factors design than there was 5 or 10 years ago by clinicians across the board. However, those clinicians that have been interacting with medical devices in high-stress, rapid-tempo types of environments like the operating room or the emergency room have recognized problems for quite a few years, and in fact have played a key role in moving both the standards-making and regulatory processes forward. More generally, when clinicians use a device, they may not know about human factors, but most of us know how to cuss at a product when it doesn't make our job easier but rather makes it more difficult, or makes us more error-prone, or prevents us from doing what we want to do, or slows us down. As soon as you tell someone what human factors and usability are they say, "Oh that's the problem with this or that device!" So they may not know the word, but they certainly know what the problems are.

MD&DI: How would you gauge the magnitude of the problem? You spoke about cussing at devices, and those of us not in the clinical environment every day don't have a real good sense of whether this is an unusual or a very frequent event.

Weinger: The answer to that is rather interesting, in that toward the latter part of the 1980s things were actually somewhat better, and then in the last 10 years they've gotten worse again — and the reason for that is computers. Basically, mechanical devices like the old anesthesia machines had gone through 40 years of iterative design to make them more usable (see Figure 4.2). And it's only been in the last 10 or 15 years that we've progressively introduced microprocessor-based devices throughout healthcare, and the human-computer interface has now become a real problem and it's not just in medicine. I'm frequently aggravated with my desktop computer when it crashes suddenly and I lose my work. And from a practical standpoint, there's actually been more time to develop usability of consumer devices. In the operating room, you could imagine that if you're trying to take care of a patient and your monitor suddenly freezes up, that would be a very bad thing. In fact, I've personally seen it happen.

MD&DI: Is there a particular class of devices that are hard to use and vulnerable to user error?

Weinger: Although all types of devices pose a risk, the more complex the device, and the more microprocessor-based technology it includes, the greater the risk. The criticality of the device is also paramount. A device whose failure means that a patient could die — for example, a cardiopulmonary bypass machine — obviously carries tremendous risk. Generally, devices that incorporate both control and display pose a greater risk than ones that are simply used for displays, but it also depends on the condition of the patient. For example, intravenous infusion pumps have received a lot of negative press recently. I think that's partly because they're so widely used and because they have both control and display components and are employed in high-acuity situations. They are probably the one device that

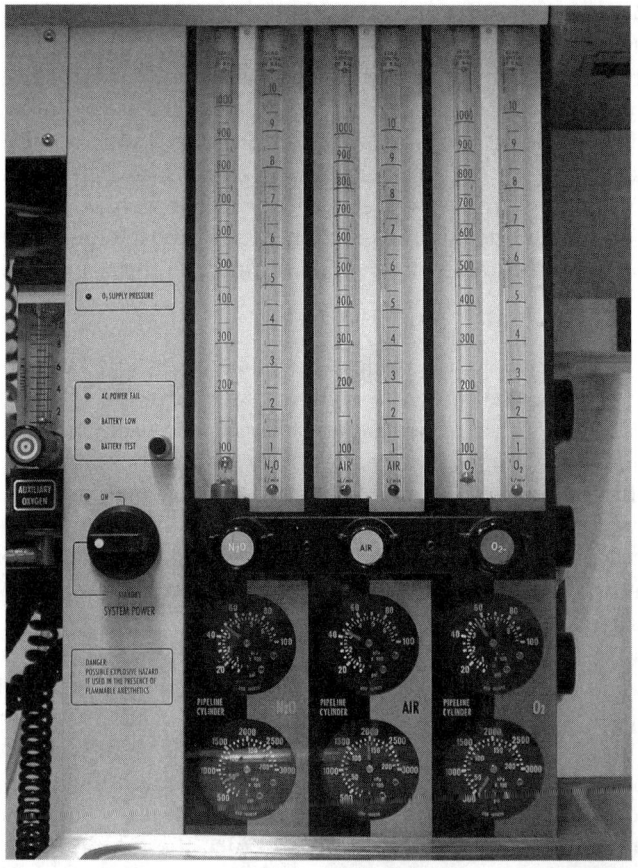

FIGURE 4.2
This anesthesia machine incorporates flow tubes and associated pressure gauges to confirm the availability and delivery of anesthesia gases (N_2O, air, and O_2). Photo courtesy of Emerson Hospital (Concord, MA).

comes most readily to mind, but I don't think that pumps are an isolated phenomenon, by any means.

MD&DI: In terms of the FDA's overarching view of all the medical device reports and so forth, which categories of devices does the agency point to as more generally problematic?

Sawyer: There's such a huge range of devices that it's hard to characterize. The problems that we commonly see are with devices such as infusion pumps, ventilators, and other intensively interactive kinds of devices. The more a user manipulates or responds to a device in addition to merely reading it, the more there is to go wrong and the more obvious any error. Conversely, if somebody misreads a monitor that is not interactive, the FDA will probably never know about it, since it's unlikely to be reported.

Weinger: It's a more widespread problem than what the FDA sees, because things that get reported to the FDA are generally safety related. But, as Mike pointed out earlier, human factors encompasses more than just safety — it has to do with efficacy and efficiency and satisfaction. When you're sitting in your office working on your computer and the thing crashes, there's no safety issue involved, but your efficiency, efficacy, and satisfaction are all reduced. And many times in the medical environment, devices make our jobs more difficult rather than easier. This isn't going to get reported to the FDA, but it probably adds to overall healthcare costs, both directly and indirectly.

Wiklund: Let me ask you a follow-up question, Matt. Let's assume that clinicians recognize that they are well served by devices in which there's a substantial investment in good human factors. Do manufacturers expect that, if they invest heavily in human factors, they'll actually see a tangible benefit in terms of the popularity of their device in the marketplace — how well it sells relative to a device that did not benefit from a comparable attention to human factors? In other words, do you think clinicians have a strong enough voice in getting their institutions to buy products that reflect good human factors design?

Weinger: A year or two ago, I would have been more hesitant to say yes. As everyone knows, the economic pressures in the healthcare marketplace are extremely powerful. A very well-designed device that has good usability but is more expensive than a competitive product might be more difficult to purchase, even if the clinicians want it. But the IOM report and the increased emphasis on safety have begun, I think, to turn the tide in favor of devices supported by the kind of clinician input that says, "This device is easier to use and, we believe, is going to be safer." Such consensus carries much more weight now than it might have even two years ago.

Hasler: I absolutely agree. As Matt mentioned, there are mitigating problems and institution-specific issues — which can include group purchasing contracts and things like that — but, given a level playing field, when you're talking about sales opportunities, a product that is well designed has a powerful advantage with human factors.

MD&DI: Matt, how would you respond to the statement that the ultimate responsibility for the proper use of medical devices — for avoiding user error — rests with the caregivers?

Weinger: The succinct response would be "yes, but," so let's talk about the "but." If a patient is injured during device use, the manufacturer is likely to be as liable as the clinician from a medical, legal, and regulatory standpoint — particularly if the clinician points out that the device contributed to the adverse event. Because there are many other impediments to safe practice besides the device, the clinician doesn't always have the opportunity or time to deal with a device that is poorly designed. The goal for both device manufacturers and clinicians is patient safety and good outcomes, and they should work together to those ends. It's not productive either to point a finger at manufacturers and say it's entirely their responsibility to produce the best possible device, or to target clinicians and insist that they bear the sole responsibility to make sure the device is used correctly. There needs to be a collaboration.

MD&DI: Does the FDA find that medical device manufacturers are aware of the new regulations? Are manufacturers responding to the FDA's satisfaction?

Carstensen: Well, they're probably not aware to the extent that we'd like. I think we've come to that conclusion, but it's difficult to measure the industry as a whole. We do see some encouraging signs showing that many companies are putting more effort into human factors. But we also see key indications that there are a lot of companies out there that still don't understand what's needed.

MD&DI: What are those encouraging signs?

Carstensen: We get to look at a limited number of the premarket applications, and I'm really basing my comment on that: what we've experienced in terms of looking at the device descriptions that come in as part of the premarket approval program.

Sawyer: People like Mike and other consultants or designers also have told us that they're seeing more and more business, getting more and more opportunities. In the year following the design control development requirements going into effect, the FDA did a sampling study by field investigators that indicated that somewhat more than half of the companies out there were doing human factors. How well we don't know, but there were early indications that companies were actively looking at human factors issues. Again, how completely and how well is going to vary tremendously, no question about that.

MD&DI: Awareness among manufacturers is important. Could you point to a few of the things the FDA has done to this point to maximize awareness? For companies that are just now discovering there's a human factors imperative, where can they turn to get up to speed quickly?

Sawyer: The FDA is doing a number of things. Of course, we put out guidance documents, which were disseminated some years ago, on design controls. Another guidance, on device use safety, just came out recently. We have teleconferences on human factors; there's one coming up in the near future. We're putting out a video for field investigators that tries to get them to understand the linkage between design and errors, to have a feel for when human factors input is necessary in the design process. We do presentations at industry trade events such as MD&M or the ASQC meetings. More and more, we're actually getting involved in giving talks to practitioners or those in industry — to doctors, nurses, biomedical engineers. And of course we monitor the results of human factors practices in regulatory efforts such as premarket review.

Carstensen: For promoting human factors, the premarket review activities contribute in a very limited way. We reach many more people through conferences and articles or through the FDA Web site. We have a pretty robust human factors section up on our site. It includes a great deal of information for manufacturers, and we find that most manufacturers are well aware of the FDA site and have taken time to explore it. And also you could say that the AAMI human factors standard itself is an educational tool that the FDA plans to promote. Once that standard is published under our standard-recognition program it will be granted official FDA recognition, which I think will make manufacturers more inclined to pay attention to it. Most of what we've done that has been effective has really been educational in nature.

MD&DI: Moving beyond education, what is the FDA's stance on enforcement and what are the consequences of noncompliance with the regulations?

Sawyer: That's a difficult one. Companies are obviously at risk if they don't comply with the design control requirements. The FDA can act with regard to premarket approval if a company hasn't followed the design practices, produces an overtly bad design, and is unwilling to respond. What we really try to accomplish is to educate not only people in industry, but those at the FDA, at the CDRH — through presentations, device evaluations, and similar means. In terms of enforcement, however, it's a slow, progressive effort. We do find that most companies, when they know there's a real safety problem with a device, will try to do something. There are always exceptions, but most companies are responsive.

Carstensen: The odds of a company getting cited for failing to comply are difficult to quantify. You have to recognize that the field is understaffed and the premarket reviewers are not all up to speed on human factors issues. So there's probably not a high risk for a noncompliant company of being discovered and getting nailed, but that's going to change over time. As we educate more and more of the reviewers and get the field more up to speed, I think companies that ignore human factors will be putting themselves at increased risk.

Weinger: What is the FDA's mechanism for responding to a situation in which a human factors or usability problem with a device manifests itself in the marketplace, through comments by users or in the literature?

Carstensen: It depends on the severity of the problem and on how much information is available.

Sawyer: We do get involved, and it's a very difficult area. First of all, most devices that get in trouble, so to speak, were designed prior to design controls. So very often it's hard in an inspection, for example, to follow up on a given postmarket problem — it's difficult to find a procedural violation of, say, design controls. Although we may get a lot of reports on a device, there's tremendous underreporting: we may hear that there's been one death, when in fact there may have been 10. We don't really know how much underreporting there is. In addition, the depth of the reports we receive is highly variable. Often, a report doesn't really isolate the problem for us, doesn't tell us precisely what the design problem is or specify the linkage of that problem to the error and the linkage of the error to the injury or death.

Nonetheless, we do pursue postmarket problems when there are injuries, or potential injuries. Often, we'll get together with manufacturers; if the manufacturer recognizes that there's a safety problem, it's likely that they will try to do something about it. I don't know if "gentle persuasion" is the right term to use, but especially with older devices for which design controls were not involved in the original design or modifications, it's kind of an iterative process trying to persuade the company to correct a problem.

Carstensen: Postmarket enforcement is probably the least effective way for the FDA to encourage the industry to address human factors. Once you get into a postmarket action, the stakes are so high for the company and the difficulty so significant for the FDA that huge amounts of resources are consumed on both sides just dealing with the situation. It's really an object lesson for everybody, I think, that one needs to prevent these kinds of incidents that are so devastating to a company and so resource-intensive to deal with for the FDA. It's just not worth it, so we need to be putting the right stuff in at the front end, getting the job done correctly the first time. Companies need to have good design controls and validation before they start marketing a device.

Part II: Standards Development and Implementation Issues

A little more than one year ago (prior to late 2000), Americans were shocked to learn that medical errors in U.S. hospitals were responsible for more deaths annually than were highway accidents, breast cancer, or AIDS. The significant number of ongoing references in the popular press to the Institute of Medicine's now one-year-old report on medical errors is a clear indication of the impact of the study on the consciousness of the general public. The fact that the study's findings attributed a considerable percentage of errors to product-design problems has also caught the attention of the device industry.

More and more, companies are realizing the importance of creating and following a coherent human factors program with the same diligence they might devote to instituting a Web strategy or preparing for ISO certification. Although it can be difficult to identify clear trends in the design world, there is definite movement toward an earlier and more intensive consideration of human factors issues in the product development process. As reflected in the discussion that follows, the imminent release of the AAMI human factors standard makes it even more urgent for firms to have a viable human factors program currently under way — if a company's not up to speed now, they're already late.

MD&DI: In the area of standards development, could someone give us a short history lesson on the AAMI human factors committee standards development efforts, and tell us when we might expect to see these standards published by AAMI?

Weinger: For more than 20 years, there has been a very close relationship between standards-making activities — both national and international — and regulatory activities by the FDA. The AAMI human factors guidelines were first approved in 1988, but there was a period of approximately five years of activity prior to that approval. The guidelines were revised over the five-year period after 1988 by a committee that included several members of the present panel. The main changes reflected in the current version (in 2000) — which is designated HE-48 1993 and is an AAMI/ANSI standard — are the inclusion of human-computer interaction guidance with regard to designing microprocessor-controlled devices, and the inclusion of a brief description of the human factors engineering process. Beginning in 1996, the committee began deliberating on how to revise the 1993 document, which was still insufficiently specific to medical industry needs and had some gaps because of evolving technology.

However, a larger concern of the post-1996 committee was that the general guidance about how one should design a display, for example, was perhaps less important than a broader approach that would define an optimal human factors design process — especially since this process could vary from device to device. So the committee began work on a separate document that was intended to be a national standard for the human factors design process. That document is currently out for final balloting, and is expected to be approved by July 1, 2001. [Editor's note: The document has since been published as ANSI/AAMI HE74:2001, *Human Factors Design Process for Medical Devices*.] Over the last year and a half, the committee has concurrently begun a parallel effort to revise and expand the classical "how-to" human factors design guidelines that are in HE48. Our current plan is to do this as a Web site, and in fact we very much need manufacturer support and encouragement to be able to deliver on this opportunity to provide good user interface design guidance. [Editor: As of Spring 2004, the committee was in the process of drafting a multiple-chapter "encyclopedia" on the best human factors practices in medical device design. A decision whether or not to deliver the content through a Web site was unresolved.]

I should have mentioned earlier that the AAMI human factors committee includes, in almost equal numbers, representatives from industry, clinicians, and others with interest or expertise in human factors and medical device design, including FDA representatives and human factors consultants.

Wiklund: Could you clarify one of the comments you made, which was that the last version of the standard was still considered less than ideal in terms of how well it is suited to medical devices? Perhaps you could retrace the history of why, even after a second revision, it still might not speak to medical devices as effectively as we'd like it to.

Weinger: I think the big problem, frankly, is that especially back in 1993 — and even now — we just didn't have a lot of medical device-specific design guidance available. Even though individual device companies have a lot of knowledge and experience (although how much of it was documented is hard to say), this information was not public. The material that was available to the committee prior to the 1993 document consisted primarily of published standards from other domains, especially the military. And so the committee lifted heavily from military design guidance standards, and, together with some material from the NRC and other published design documents, tried to modify them as best they could for the medical industry. However, it was recognized at the time — and certainly since — that some of those modifications were more successful than others. In particular, the human-computer interface sections were not modified sufficiently to address the needs of medical device manufacturers with respect to building actual devices, particularly for critical-care applications.

MD&DI: Why did the committee initially focus on design process issues rather than principles of good design? What are the core elements of AAMI's recommended process?

Wiklund: What I can perhaps do is personalize the question. As a consultant, I'm asked from time to time to take a look at a medical device and render a judgment regarding its usability and safety by virtue of the quality of its user interface. Now, that's a really hard job to do. Occasionally there might be some low-lying fruit that you can pick — that is, obvious cosmetic shortcomings in the design, the nature of the labeling, the size of characters in a display, things that you can readily identify by inspection and application of known principles of good design. However, it's generally very difficult to make more overarching judgments about the usability of a device just by looking at it. Moreover, as a designer, you may come up with a design that you think would pass any litmus test in terms of good design practices, but, until you validate it in the context of a usability test, you can't be sure that you have developed a good design.

The AAMI work and the FDA's guidance do stress good design processes, because we would all probably agree that such an emphasis represents our best hope for producing a high-quality user interface. As a practical objective, it's difficult to create perfection right off the bat by virtue of outstanding design talent being brought to a task. A more workable objective is to create an iterative process of researching users' needs and preferences, turning those into design goals, developing a design concept that reflects those goals as well as good design practices, then going ahead and modeling a design and having people interact with it and seeing how things go — and then repeating the process. You might liken it to the way you wash your hair: you wet, lather, rinse, and repeat. One could say the same thing about cleansing a medical device design of any kind of human factors shortcoming. The objective is to get end-users involved in the process of expressing their needs and preferences up front, and then evaluating the product by having them put their hands and minds on it and seeing how things go when they try to perform tasks. That's probably the most reliable way of producing a design that will perform well.

Hasler: One of the reasons we really focus on design process issues is that — despite the fact that people often want to just pick up some sort of a generic "cookbook" document and look for the exact "recipe" they want — there's simply too much variation in the user interface of medical devices for an encyclopedic guidance to work (in the absence of process guidance and advice on how to apply specific guidance selectively). In other words, if we're focusing on a ventilator or an infusion device, we could come up with great guidelines, but when it's a matter of the whole industry, an approach emphasizing good processes is initially the best way to proceed.

MD&DI: What is the status of international efforts to promote human factors in medical device design?

Carstensen: The International Electrotechnical Commission (IEC) is in the process of updating its big document, IEC 60601-1, which covers general requirements for the safety of electromedical equipment. As part of that undertaking, about a year ago they initiated efforts to develop a new collateral standard that, once in place, will become part of IEC 60601-1. Its number is IEC 60601-6; there are five other collateral standards, covering areas such as EMC testing. The first committee draft (CD) is scheduled for distribution to national committees for hearing and comment in February 2001, although the target date for publishing the final document is not until the fall of 2004 [Editor's note: As of Spring 2004, the document was still pending publication]. That sounds like a long time, but the good news is that, historically, companies will get wind of what's going on and procure copies of the first and second CDs and respond to them. They'll react in anticipation of a standard coming down the track, and derive much of the good effects well before the publication date of 2004.

The international standard — basically an international human factors engineering guideline — is based on the AAMI documents. But the IEC document itself probably doesn't occupy more than about 10 pages, plus an informative annex that tells you how to go about doing the job. That informative annex will be the newly revised AAMI human factors design process standard. The intent is to achieve global harmonization at the outset, as opposed to what we usually do, which is to have an international version of a standard and various domestic standards, and then get together years later and sort of argue about the differences and try to settle on something that is reasonably harmonious. This time, we're making sure it's harmonious from the beginning.

In addition, ISO Technical Committee 210 on quality systems has expressed an interest in joining the IEC working group that's developing the international version of the AAMI standard, so as to put out a joint ISO/IEC version of the standard. What that would do is allow us to expand the scope beyond electromedical devices to include all medical equipment.

MD&DI: Rod, as a human factors specialist working at a large company, what is your view of the new regulations? What are the greatest challenges you face in responding to them? What about cost pressures? Finally, are there differences in the way the regulations affect how you develop products for domestic versus foreign markets?

Hasler: Regarding human factors concerns in the medical device industry, companies can be divided into two camps. The camp I come from recognizes the importance of human factors at least as long ago as the early 1990s. At that time, we implemented a customer-focused process to define an IV infusion system, and quickly discovered that the feature most desired by the customer was ease of use. This drove us to see the importance of human factors practices, and how good human factors could benefit us. So my introduction to human factors was really on the marketing side — how to make better-selling products that are easy for customers to use.

And I think that's probably where you're seeing the companies that jumped into the discipline of human factors early on — they were really utilizing it for the ease of use, and to drive a better product to the customer. Those who didn't recognize that are a little bit behind as far as converting.

I think that most of the larger companies followed this same route, and typically have long-standing human factors programs. Many smaller companies are still in something of a catch-up mode; they're trying to understand exactly what is required and how they can implement it. But I believe that this regulation has a very strong upside for the entire medical device industry — it will really improve the industry as a whole, as far as reducing design errors.

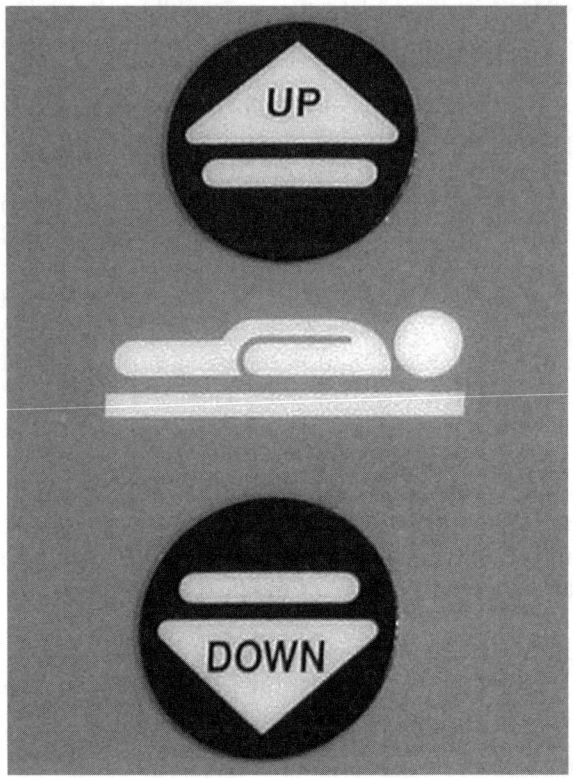

FIGURE 4.3
Labeling controls with symbols (icons) and text, such as found on this hospital bed control, help address the needs of people who do not speak the selected native language and those who have low literacy. Photo courtesy of Emerson Hospital (Concord, MA).

MD&DI: Do you notice any differences in the emphasis on human factors in products destined for the U.S. market versus the overseas market?

Hasler: What you see much less of in Europe is human factors used as part of a marketing strategy or approach. Regarding domestic and foreign markets, however, one of the problems in the device industry is that we tend to develop products that are oriented toward and designed for a specific customer in a specific country, but are then released to other countries with no changes. Whereas even though the actual clinical application may remain the same, there are often differences on a country-by-country basis in how the users react to the design and employ the device. So the biggest concern I have on a global front concerns releasing a product that was designed for one market into multiple markets (see Figure 4.3).

MD&DI: How do the new rules affect the marketing of devices that were developed before the human factors regulations were adopted? What happens with products that represent slight modifications to older products that may not have incorporated good human factors design principles?

Wiklund: I'd be happy to answer this question from a consultant's point of view. I think this is going to be a great source of anxiety in the future for those companies that are not getting clear signals as to their vulnerability in terms of selling any product that hasn't benefited from a good human factors design process. Because many companies will be introducing products that represent slight variations of previous versions, one could argue that they should conduct a thorough human factors evaluation of the modified design — which might infer getting customer feedback in the context of usability tests, and so forth. Of course, a company that has marketed a product for a long time — a product that was originally approved by the FDA — might ask itself whether it really needs to go through all of that effort after making only minor changes to the product.

Compounding this whole issue is the fact that, once regulations are in place and people become more aware of them, a company that doesn't follow good human factors processes could be accused of not applying due diligence in pursuing state-of-the-art practice. In other words, you raise the possibility of legal liability exposure if a firm fails to follow the new standard. My guess is that companies that carry out minor modifications to existing products will at least want to conduct a usability test to confirm that the new changes are in fact good changes. They'll want to make sure that they haven't inadvertently introduced other kinds of problems, or somehow corrupted the preexisting design in a way that could lead to user error. So at a minimum, I think that companies taking a conservative and careful approach will likely begin doing more usability testing than they would have before these regulations were in place.

Hasler: What I'm seeing in the industry reflects very much what Mike has just described. It can be quite confusing deciding how to handle a product that you've been producing for, say, 20 years once you recognize that a minor feature needs to be changed. According to all previous methods of evaluation, you would have gone ahead and made the change for any additional units sold. Now, however, once you start dealing, for example, with the user interface, you may realize that other aspects of the device may not meet the present standard and may need to be changed. Although a company certainly wants to support its customers, you're now faced with a full-blown project — a whole rework — of something that really isn't the product line you want to move into the future. In short, it is very difficult to understand how the regulations should be applied to older products.

MD&DI: What are the views of the FDA on this issue?

Sawyer: Any changes being made in product design should be run through a company's design control procedures. This applies to changes during the development of a brand new product or modifications to an existing one. Regarding human factors, the question of existing devices is one that manufacturers occasionally have asked us about. In the case of so-called evolutionary product development, many small modifications may have been made over an extended period, and there seem to be two questions: How big a change is necessary before human factors evaluations are required, and how do you account for every design change made over a number of years? First, since small changes in hardware or software design can affect the way a device is used, an analysis should be done to decide whether a change is trivial with regard to the user interface. Depending on the nature of the change, a human factors test may be necessary, as Mike suggested. Second, we realize that, 5 or 10 years ago, many manufacturers were not doing substantial human factors evaluations, and there may be no data on early design modifications, or even on the original design. But in making a change today, a company certainly can examine its complaint files, which provide a kind of track record, or baseline, with respect to safety.

MD&DI: What is the function of the design history file as it relates to the new regulations? Can you give a quick overview of what the FDA is looking for in terms of documentation?

Sawyer: A design history file can exist in various formats, as long as the company can produce it for our field investigators. If you look at our regulation, several areas are stressed regarding *what* is documented. Design inputs, or requirements, are important, and especially relevant to human factors are descriptions of the user population, working environment, potential hazards, and basic design concept. Verification data will pertain to inspecting, analyzing, and testing a device against such requirements. In human factors, this can involve anything from paper exercises like task analyses and walk-throughs to full usability tests with, for example, computer simulations. Validation addresses a broader question — will the device work in a real-world situation? Human factors validation testing is usually done on production-level models. The tests are simulations, and operating conditions should be as realistic as possible. On the other hand, although clinical trials sometimes yield some useful human factors information, because they involve actual patients, highly trained device users, and substantial manufacturer support, they often don't produce good and representative human factors data, and there are obvious limitations with regard to patient safety. In any case, as with any other design discipline, human factors efforts should be well documented.

Wiklund: In addition to some of the analytical results just mentioned, I would think that the design history file would include some of the classic products of human factors studies, such as reports from user focus groups, summaries of conceptual inquiries, on-site interviews with users, and so on. It might include a usability test plan and a report of usability test findings.

If we back up and talk about actually producing a design, the design history file might include usability goal statements — the goals created to underscore the design effort and keep the design team focused on what it wants to accomplish.

Sawyer: I agree, and this raises an important issue. Information from early usability studies and concept stages that may precede the actual formalization of the project are not required by the FDA. However, it makes a lot of sense and can work to a company's advantage to include data from pre-project or predevelopment efforts.

Wiklund: My recommendation to companies is to take some of their market research resources and create a close collaboration with human factors professionals, so that some of these traditional research activities can be given a new spin or expanded to address some of the human factors issues that concern the FDA. Many companies do a lot of this kind of work, but perhaps without the heavy human factors focus that is now warranted. So for many, it may not be a great cultural change in how they approach things, but rather simply an expansion and full embracing of the human factors requirements.

MD&DI: For companies seeking assistance, where can they find human factors specialists?

Wiklund: It's a great time to be in the human factors business, predominantly because the dot-com sector has soaked up a lot of human factors specialists. Human factors professionals are trained in graduate programs at many institutions around the country, so by contacting the Human Factors and Ergonomics Society, you can get a listing of where these people are training, and potentially recruit people from there.

In terms of finding human factors specialists who have more experience in the medical arena, that's not a huge population — though I expect many more people to gravitate toward the medical industry as it embraces human factors and its needs grow. I don't have a good road map for finding experienced people. Generally, they're working in companies and participating in the medical systems section of the Human Factors Society. You can obviously contact human factors consultants. You can also turn to the FDA, I understand, and they'll help you in terms of explaining what their goals and objectives are regarding the regulations.

But in terms of getting people to do the hands-on work, many companies will have to draw on the capabilities of people who are perhaps peripheral to the human factors field but are ready to invest themselves more substantially in practicing human factors. This might include personnel involved in tech writing; it might be those involved in industrial design-related activities; it might be people leading software development efforts. These are the folks who are going to have to become students of the human factors process and design principles. I don't think anybody has the patent rights — whether they're formally trained or not — to doing good human factors work. Obviously, I'm biased toward thinking that human factors is a profession that should be practiced by professionals. But recognizing that there will be a shortage, my sense is that people who may not be formally trained in human factors but are experienced in related disciplines should be able to do a reasonable job and make a difference.

MD&DI: Do companies typically think they need to hire human factors specialists to address these questions, or are they confident that individuals with different backgrounds can fulfill some of the functions we've mentioned?

Hasler: I think that both types of individuals add value to a product development process. Both have their pros and cons. Typically, a person who has considerable time with a company has some clinical experience and a solid understanding of the product being developed and of the needs of its users. I would agree that it may not be critical to have a degree in human factors, but I think that some formal training or course work should be required. There is certainly some excellent literature available for the study of human factors. However, some people look at it and say, "Well, that's common sense," and my experience over the years has been that "common sense" is not as common sensical as you might wish. So, I would definitely recommend some training.

Smaller companies or start-ups can do supplemental training or hire a consultant to review their work, perhaps designating an individual to be the human factors "point person" in working with the consultant. The key for the company is to get the human factors input early. Too many firms find themselves with a product at the very end of the design process, and they're asking themselves not is it okay from a human factors point of view, but is it acceptable? The time to apply human factors is at the very beginning, almost before the engineers put anything on paper.

Wiklund: There's a lot of evidence showing that any amount of money spent on human factors — especially early in the process — pays major dividends down the line. Books have been written that track the payoff from usability investment as ranging anywhere from a 3:1 return to upwards of 100:1. The benefits can include avoiding future liability claims and getting the product to market faster, since you don't encounter usability problems late in development and because the product will likely proceed through the regulatory process more smoothly if it reflects good human factors. Among other benefits are reduced customer service expenses and more effective sales presentations leading to improved sales. So in addition to being good professional practice, a company's investment in human factors — whether it be hiring a person in-house or using consultants — is going to pay off for them, in my opinion.

Hasler: I agree completely. First, your product development process is smoother and faster. Second, good human factors can be marketed and sold, because ease of use really shines when customers take the product in their hands. They might not even know just why a well-designed product is so special, but they realize it's special. Finally, those flaws that you caught early on will not be showing up in the field and you won't have field actions or potential product recalls to deal with.

MD&DI: Does the FDA believe that the new regulations are having their intended effect? Are they, in essence, paying off? Do you have any advice for our readers and the industry on the importance of good design in medical devices?

Sawyer: If you're talking about clear-cut evidence, it's a difficult call, in that the design controls really haven't been in effect for very long. Probably the most concrete evidence that we see is in premarket submissions when we consult our Office of Device Evaluation, and indeed we've seen some products that have had some really excellent design efforts behind them. And although it's not typical, I saw one product for which the company claimed to have put a million dollars into their human factors design process. I don't know whether it's true or not, but they certainly had a very interesting, well-designed device and they had done a lot of work on it.

So certainly there are some companies that are paying more attention to human factors, and of course I've already talked about the study we've done and the consultants who are finding more and more business out there. Overall, however, there's still an awful lot of variability. We see submissions with very little evidence of human factors work, and it shows up in the design. And then there are many cases that are sort of in between — when a manufacturer submits a product for approval saying, "Well, we tried to do a little human factors but can you tell us more," and so on, which initiates an ongoing dialogue. In general, I think we're optimistic, though the variability remains, and it's difficult to make simple before-and-after comparisons at this point in time.

Carstensen: What we're seeing is certainly encouraging, even though we only get a limited picture. However, taken as a whole, the industry has a ways to go. Our mission is to help firms get there as quickly and as painlessly as possible, so they and their customers can enjoy the benefits of good human factors design.

In a sense, our task should be an easy one. If we can convince the industry that competent human factors efforts pay off in terms of bottom-line business, the whole idea should sell itself, and that's our goal. We're going to continue to educate, to get the message out, and to persuade the industry that this is in its own self-interest. I firmly believe that such an attitude will be more effective than the alternative — to sit here with the big FDA stick threatening to beat industry over the head if it fails to "comply" with the regulations. That kind of approach merely results in companies putting window dressing on things and trying to convince the FDA that they are doing a good job with human factors when in fact they're doing a superficial job. We want to get them to do it for real, so it does pay off, so it truly is effective.

MD&DI: Do you think that message is resonating with the industry?

Carstensen: We hope it is. To the extent that we speak to the industry — through articles and conference presentations and so on — we always try to sell the benefits of a strong human factors process on its own merits. But the impact of that message can be hard for us to judge. Have the captains of industry, the people really making the management decisions, really gotten that message? I don't know. There's no easy way for us to measure that.

Hasler: From my vantage point, the message is getting out there. It isn't moving en masse just yet, but it definitely is gaining momentum, and I can't imagine what would slow it down.

Carstensen: We're all probably seeing about the same effect.

Wiklund: It's obviously very, very difficult to count nonadverse events. The sum of our efforts in good human factors engineering is to avoid what we could refer to as deleterious outcomes: if we do our job well, we'll see people using products on a daily basis without mishap. It may not be something that's going to grab headlines — for example, that so many infusion pumps were used effectively on February 1 of the year 2001. But given the great deal of alarm right now about the amount of user error related to medical devices and its effect on healthcare, there's certainly going to be considerable attention paid to this whole issue, and a full embracing of human factors will start to be a big part of the solution. Once we succeed in reducing user error and start achieving day after day of good outcomes, at that point — like airplanes getting safely where they need to go — there may be no news, but no news will be good news.

On the notion of human factors paying off, I think it's certainly paying off for the companies that have invested. The companies that have invested in good human factors are doing a pretty good job of burying the competition. It was mentioned earlier that studies demonstrate the fact that usability tends to float to the top in terms of a design priority. That's true of all the research we've done regarding dozens of different kinds of medical devices. Usability is always rated very high, if not the highest, among the 10 or 12 most important attributes. So the marketplace will have a strong effect in reinforcing good human factors practice. Speaking as a person who has participated on a jury for the Medical Design Excellence Awards, I've noted that some of the best products nominated for awards make a big case about the quality of their human factors design efforts — really showcasing that as evidence that they in fact do have a design that warrants recognition. This is one more indication that an awareness of the importance of human factors is really taking hold.

KEY POINTS

- In the mid-1970s, the Association for the Advancement of Medical Instrumentation (AAMI) set up a human factors committee to develop guidance for human factors in medical equipment. This initiative grew out of an effort to develop a standard for anesthesia gas machines that incorporated a lot of human factors-related content.
- An FDA study of device recalls in 1990 indicated that about 44% of manufactured recalls were due to design problems, giving the FDA the leverage to introduce design controls into the Safe Medical Devices Act of 1990.
- When you're talking about medical devices — which serve a life-critical function — there is an inherent justification for a very strong focus on human factors to help achieve important design objectives, especially safety.
- You can get users involved in the design process, but if you simply conduct focus groups you may end up with a less-than-optimal outcome. So, another element of a successful human factors design process is to conduct usability tests.
- In the FDA's view, there are a lot of companies out there that still don't understand what's needed in terms of a comprehensive human factors program.
- It is difficult to make overarching judgments about the usability of a device by inspection. Until you validate a design in the context of a usability test, you can't be sure that you have developed a good one.
- Because small changes to an existing design can affect the way a device is used, an analysis should be done to decide whether a change is trivial with regard to the user interface. Depending on the nature of the change, a human factors test may be necessary, according to the FDA.
- A design history file may include some of the classic products of human factors studies, such as reports from user focus groups, summaries of conceptual inquiries, on-site interviews with users, and so on. It might also include a usability test plan and a report of usability test findings.

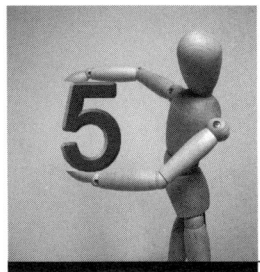

User-Centered Medical Product Development and the Problem of Egocentrism

Stephen B. Wilcox

As a product developer achieves a deeper understanding of his or her product area, it can become more difficult to understand the product user's point of view. How can this be overcome?

Theoretically, most medical product designers today serve the needs of a global marketplace in which seeing things from the customer's or user's point of view is the key to success. However, the very endeavor of designing products creates the potential for an egocentric subculture that is very different from the user's culture (see Figure 5.1). As a result, designers and engineers frequently fall into the trap of designing products for themselves and their professional colleagues, rather than for the real users.

The great irony is that more experience and knowledge can actually work against seeing things from the user's point of view. As an industrial designer, engineer, or marketer gains experience with a product category, he or she begins to use a specialized language (i.e., jargon) and to see the product through a set of distorted lenses. He or she sees a product as, for example:

- Fitting into a niche defined by its price point
- Having a target manufacturing cost
- Being assembled by means of a particular process
- Requiring certain types of maintenance
- Incorporating certain specific functions
- Being backward-compatible to the company's existing products
- Incorporating a particular software operating system

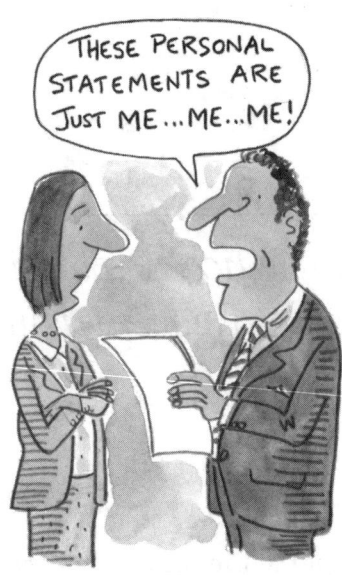

FIGURE 5.1
The problem of egocentrism.

The acquisition of such knowledge is the currency by which product developers are often evaluated within their corporate subculture. Experts in a given product area, as they meet to develop the product, or for that matter, as they discuss products over lunch, begin to talk in a shorthand about the products they are working on. Those who don't know the specialized lingo and who don't share the corporate "lore" about how products are used are treated with condescension, if not disdain. This creates a powerful motivation for product developers to create designs that please and impress their colleagues, rather than the intended users. After all, they see their colleagues every day and may seldom or never actually meet representative product users. Indeed, many companies discourage contact between the developers and the customers, leaving those kinds of interaction to people in marketing and sales.

In reality, most actual product users, i.e., clinical professionals or patients, have limited knowledge or interest in a majority of those things that capture the interest of product developers. For example, a nephrologist may be intensely interested in a hemodialysis machine's overall capabilities, but have only passing interest in the nuances of its microfluidics. An electrophysiologist may have an enormous interest in the clinical criteria for shock delivery in an implanted defibrillator, but little or no interest in the specific engineering algorithms that allow the device to operate according to those clinical criteria.

Thus, when the user, such as a physician or nurse working in a critical-care environment, does not properly maintain a device, or uses it the wrong way, or fails to appreciate it, the developers have a tendency to blame the user rather than the product. Likewise, far too many products display information that in form or content is of greater interest to the engineers who designed the algorithms than to the user. In fact, some products, in effect, force the clinician to think like an engineer rather than to focus on the clinical issues that are their primary interest. Or, products contain more functions than users need or want because the corporate subculture has standards to be met regardless of whether or not users can tell the difference. Or, products have elaborate functionality that goes unused because the corporate subculture values the engineering prowess to create such functionality, whether or not it serves a real purpose. We think that such logic explains why some advanced medical devices have embedded features that few caregivers have ever used or even noticed.

Those involved in product-design efforts can improve user satisfaction by trying to see and act more like a user. In the field of medical technology design, this means assuming the perspective of the caregiver or the patient. Such a change of perspective might have led earlier, for example, to MRI machines that feature an airy architecture in place of machine designs that place patients in a cramped space that triggers claustrophobia (see Figure 5.2).

There seems to be a general belief that people do things in particular ways because they see things in particular ways. While this is certainly true, the reverse is also true: people see things in particular ways *because* they do things in particular ways. Thus, the person in a wheelchair sees the "pathway" in a fundamentally different way from the person not in a wheelchair, just as the skilled dart thrower sees the dartboard in a different way from the casual dart thrower, alcohol consumption notwithstanding. This suggests that you, as a product-design team member, can see the world from the user's point of view to the extent that you, in effect, become the user. This may mean buying and using a target product or it may mean spending significant amounts of time in the specialized use environment for a target product (see Figure 5.3).

Such methods are not foolproof (some people cannot seem to alter their viewpoint regardless of what they do), but they can provide significant insight. So, it might make sense for the patient-bed designer to spend a weekend in a hospital bed. Similarly, the external defibrillator designer might want to spend some time riding around in ambulances and helicopters at night to develop a better sense for the environmental challenges posed by the people who will use the defibrillator that she or he designs.

A more systematic approach is to use the research methods that come from cultural anthropology, or *ethnography*, which we discuss in the next chapter. The essence of cultural anthropology is to study a foreign culture and then to describe it in a way that nonmembers of that culture can understand and appreciate. This skill can be developed through practice, training, and the use of various techniques. Ethnographers learn to ask questions in ways that

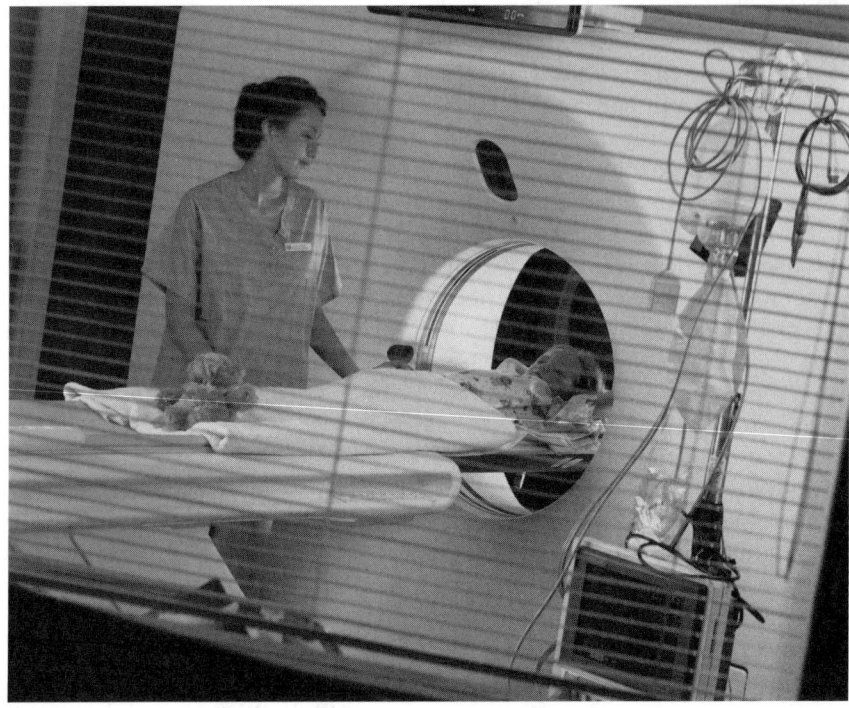

FIGURE 5.2
The newer style MRI systems protect patients from feeling claustrophobic; the older style MRI systems are more enclosed.

elicit people's unadulterated viewpoints, and they learn to observe behavior and analyze it in a way that is enlightening. A good ethnographer, or even someone with a natural talent for perceiving and extracting other people's points of view, can teach someone else these skills. It is useful, for example, to videotape interviews and observations and to have an ethnographer critique the researcher's style. Also, video can be a valuable tool for providing a type of "immersion" for those who were not able to place themselves in the relevant environment themselves.

Conclusion

It is possible to overcome the natural egocentrism that plagues product developers. However, it is not easy to overcome, which explains the influx of cultural anthropologists into the product development arena. But, even without the help of cultural anthropologists, the time that product developers can spend with real product users in real clinical environments can be of immense value in learning to see things from the user's point of view.

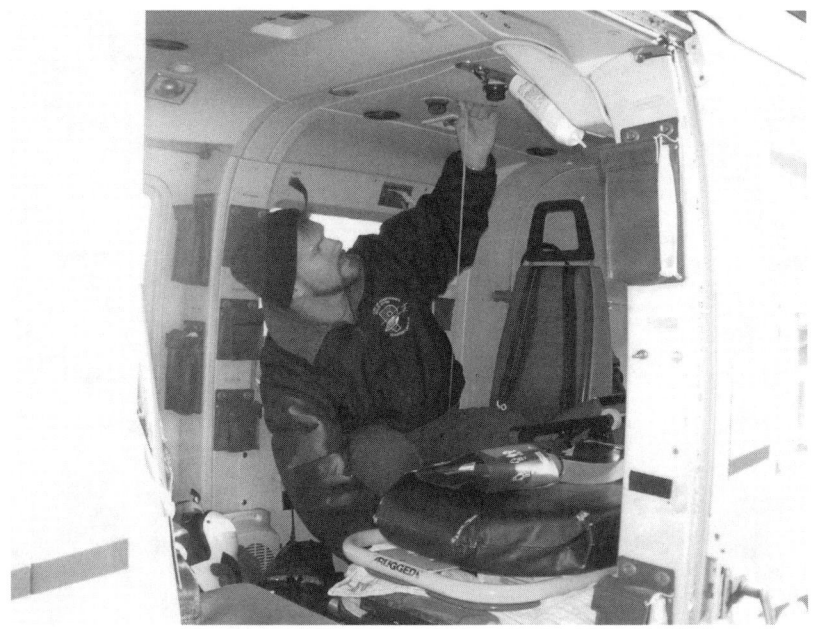

FIGURE 5.3
Helicopters present a special use environment.

Key Points

- A great irony of product development is that more knowledge and experience can cause a dramatic increase in the mismatch between the product developer's point of view and that of the product user.
- Product developers tend to use specialized language and to see products from the point of view of their own technical concerns, which are inevitably different from those of users.
- *Ethnographic* methods from cultural anthropology can help to overcome this natural "egocentrism."
- Even in the absence of ethnographic expertise, simply spending more time in the clinical environment can be of great value.

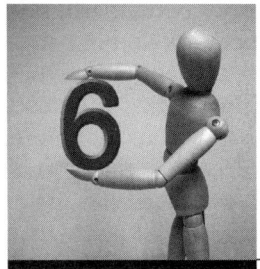

Ethnographic Methods for New Product Development

Stephen B. Wilcox

The use of ethnographic methods, from cultural anthropology, can provide tangible, workable information about devices — and the requirements of the people who use them.

Particularly with a user-centered approach to new product development, one of the central questions — if not *the* central question — is how do manufacturers determine what people want and need? Without a clear picture of what users need, it is impossible to channel corporate resources to yield the desired result. There is nothing more counterproductive and frustrating than generating solutions to the wrong problems — but such outcomes are difficult to avoid without good, solid information about what product users want and need.

How, then, does one go about this? In practice, companies often rely on what people say. Verbal behavior is the foundation of the overwhelming bulk of consumer research. Marketers make much of the difference between qualitative and quantitative research, but these terms describe variations on the same theme. Both are based solely on what people *say* — either in groups or individually, in person or over the phone, on paper or on the Internet. What such methods fail to focus on is what people *do* and how they do it.

When manufacturers and marketers rely solely on what users say, they fall victim to the fact that people often have difficulty describing what type of product they need or want. End-users typically cannot express their precise problem with a given device only by talking about it. This phenomenon occurs for several reasons.

One problem is that many important user issues are not particularly part of conscious awareness. If a device works correctly, operators do not necessarily notice how they hold the instrument or what exactly takes place when they use it. It is only when something goes wrong that they notice it. Indeed, as people become more expert with a task, they are *less* conscious, not more, of what they do. When learning a new procedure, a surgeon is likely to be highly aware of each hand movement, but after countless procedures, he or she is more likely to carry on a conversation about a recent golf game than to focus on the intricacies of a particular device. It is the same in learning to drive a car with a stick shift. At first, you notice every upshift and downshift, but then it becomes an unconscious act.

Furthermore, when answering questions about the past, people are subject to various errors. They conflate events that happened at different times; they remember events in such a way that they conform to what they expect; they are highly influenced by the way questions are asked. In short, people are a poor source of information about their past experiences.

Another problem is that people have all sorts of agendas that interfere with strict accuracy. They develop opinions about what interviewers want to hear and consciously or unconsciously tailor their statements to fit these opinions. They see themselves as possessing qualities that they do not really possess, so they answer questions for their "ideal" selves rather than their real selves. They are embarrassed to admit that they have problems with products because they fear those problems might reflect poorly on their abilities.

Also, to avoid sounding ignorant, people sometimes give answers to questions even when they have no idea what the correct answers actually are. Another issue is that people differ enormously in their ability to express themselves. Some people can paint a richly detailed picture with words, but many people cannot.

So, if there are inherent dangers in trusting what people say, why do product developers rely so heavily on exactly that? The balance of this chapter explores another option: ethnographic field research.

Ethnographic Field Research

Ethnographic research can augment — even supplant entirely — the traditional means of interviewing end-users about a device. As a methodology, it stems not from psychology (the source of virtually all of the traditional market research methods, such as surveys and focus groups), but from cultural anthropology, and so involves the study of people's behavior in the actual "environments of use" to generate insights about their needs. It means going to wherever people routinely use a given product, from operating

Ethnographic Methods for New Product Development 63

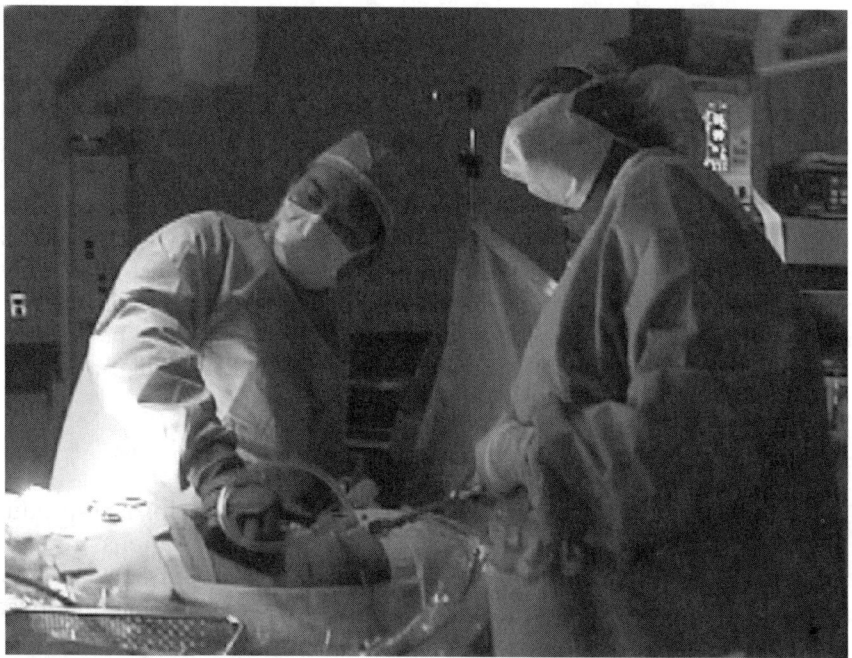

FIGURE 6.1
Ethnographic research in the OR is made easier by the fact that researchers wear scrubs.

theaters and radiology suites to waiting rooms, cafeterias, and even patients' homes (see Figure 6.1).

Ethnographic methods were originally developed as a way of coming to understand a completely different culture, whether it be the Trobriand Islanders of the South Pacific, or the Yanamano of South America. In studying such cultures, researchers could not assume any overlap with their own cultures or their own languages. Thus, they had to develop new methodologies, methodologies different from those that one would use to study people who are more similar to one's self.

So, part of the logic of applying ethnographic methods to new product development is that, if they can be used to understand aborigines or pygmies, they sure ought to allow us to understand the cardiac cath lab or the operating room. Furthermore, the great advantage of ethnographic methods is that they do not begin with the assumption that the researcher already understands what is going on, an assumption that can be the enemy of real understanding.

When conducting ethnographic field research, if a product is not yet available, researchers make every attempt to observe users working with something like it — a prototype, for instance, or a competitor's product. It is vital to observe behavior in the environments of use because each such environment is unique. Differences in use environments make it impossible to know, without seeing firsthand, what conditions most crucially shape the success or failure of a device.

If surgeons will be using a device in the operating room, researchers need to observe them using the product there, because nobody could artificially reproduce the sounds, distractions, and relationships that characterize that highly specific milieu.

The story is the same regardless of the environment. If people will use a device in their homes, then it is vital to learn how patients with the medical condition that the device treats actually behave with the product in their own homes. Their usual careful performance with log books, touch screen displays, and hypodermic needles may be compromised when they come home after a long day at work, or when they wake up in the middle of the night.

Firsthand Knowledge

Observing users in their natural habitat (see Figure 6.2) helps new-product developers understand the product's strengths and limitations from the user's point of view. But there are many additional benefits. By watching end-users interact with the device, researchers can see behaviors that reveal product performance attributes even when the users don't say a word.

Video Documentation

One way to make certain that the analysis is detailed and comprehensive is to document everything on videotape. Video documentation helps analysts take apart complex events and interactions that happen in rapid succession — such as special hand movements, gestures or facial expressions, offhand verbal statements, etc. — and study each one at a practical pace.

After viewing videotapes of user after user experiencing difficulty aligning two key components of a device (despite their insistence to interviewers that this was not a problem in the procedure), designers might decide not to include those components in the development program. Developers could also come away from the discovery process with a more realistic assessment of some common user complaints, and a better understanding of which issues need attention as opposed to those that don't reflect an underlying problem in product quality.

Richer Information

When compared with focus groups, surveys, and even one-to-one interviews, the discovery process of ethnographic research yields information that is typically more rich, vivid, and concrete. This is because working in a naturalistic context enables researchers to ask people questions while they use the product (or, at the very least, immediately before and after).

Ethnographic Methods for New Product Development 65

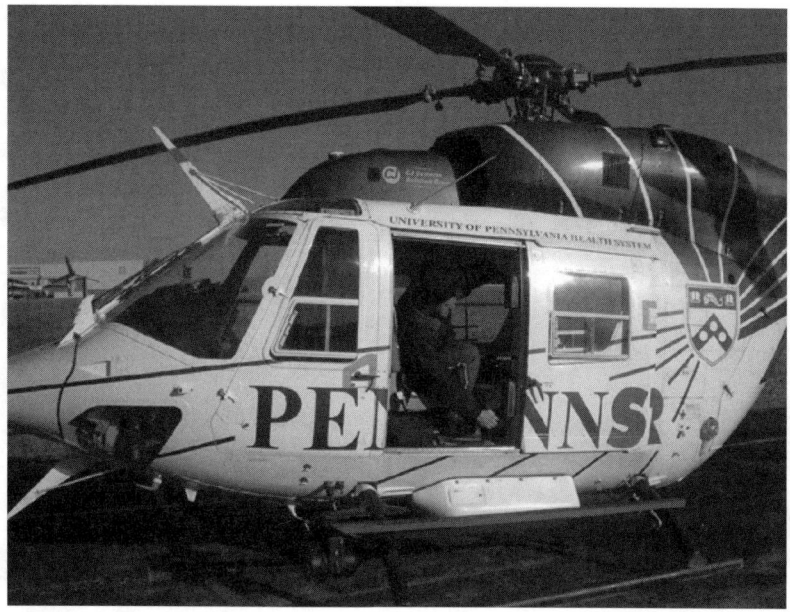

FIGURE 6.2
Medical products are used in a variety of environments; so is ethnographic research.

Why is this important? Timing and context have a huge impact on the responses to questions. In the case of design research, there are at least two big advantages to conducting interviews when people are using the product. The first is that they literally remember more because things just happened. The second is they tend to give more specific and useful answers.

People remember more while they interact with the device because the activity of using the product itself becomes a mnemonic system — it gives users a host of real-world, real-time cues to help them answer questions. Through the practice of "ask-and-watch," the interviewee is more likely to recall long-forgotten or disregarded concerns about the product than if he or she were asked about it outside the context of use.

By combining observational research with interviewing, researchers frequently hear comments such as, "Oh, I forgot to tell you about this problem," or "I guess I am having a little difficulty here. I never thought about it before — you just become so used to doing things."

The second advantage of on-site interviewing is that the observations people make tend to be more specific and useful than they would be if they had to think of them out of context — on the phone, say, or in a focus-group setting. For example, if researching a new type of self-administered therapy, product developers who visited patients' homes would discover a wealth of information (Figure 6.3). When asked out of context to discuss the kinds of mistakes they make when using a particular device, patients might volunteer very little information, at first. When they are observed actually using the

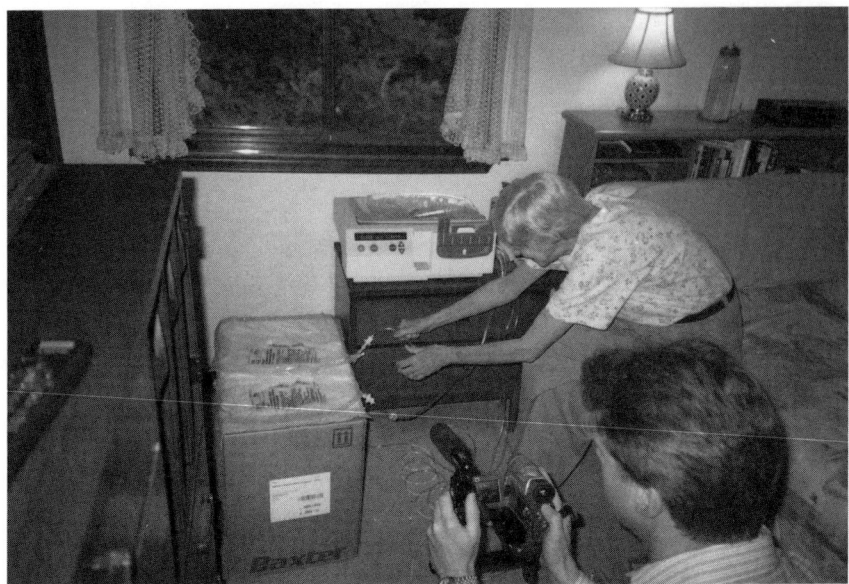

FIGURE 6.3
Ethnographic research for home-healthcare products can involve research in people's homes.

device, however, the patients tend to become more vocal and list the different errors they often make. Patients might point out tasks they were performing out of sequence, buttons they pushed by accident, and tubing connections they failed to secure when they were tired or ill.

Questions about the device might get the patient thinking, but actually using the device is what gets them talking.

Methodology: Understanding the Worldview

Conducting ethnographic field research is, of course, not quite as simple as just going into the field. If all that product developers needed to do was watch and take notes, everybody would be doing it. According to a study of successful new products over a decade, almost two-thirds of senior executives were disappointed with the results of their firms' new-product programs.[1]

To be repeatedly successful, fieldwork depends on adherence to a methodology. The approach under discussion relies upon the framework provided by ethnography. Literally meaning "writing about culture," the term and concept of *ethnography* describes the attempt to understand the beliefs, customs, and rituals of people in different types of societies (see Figure 6.4).

The main principle of successful ethnography is this: understand the other person's worldview. Doing so is not the same thing as merely listening to

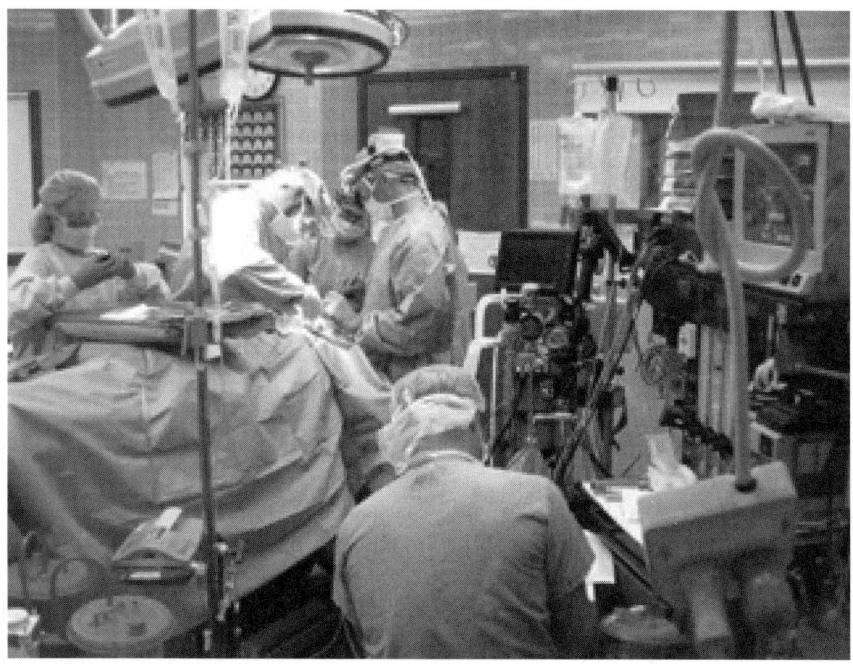

FIGURE 6.4
Anesthesia forms a separate culture in the OR.

his or her opinions. Understanding their worldview means discovering their values and norms, identifying their goals and expectations, and determining some of the basic ways they divide space and fill up their days.

Casting the net broadly in this way does not provide quick-and-dirty answers. But it can offer a measure of insurance that developers will not miss anything critical that could make or break the new product. Consider the modern pacemaker-defibrillator, a device that neatly straddles the professional worlds of the electrical engineer and the cardiologist, and whose widespread use has helped give rise to the hybrid discipline of electrophysiology. Electrical engineers have had a difficult time for years trying to develop a user interface for pacemaker programming that cardiologists will find easy to use. Why? Because to do it, the device manufacturers essentially need to learn how physicians think. They need to know, for instance, what day-to-day professional language cardiologists and electrophysiologists use, which diagnostic categories are most critical to them, and how they arrive at specific treatment plans.

To develop a user interface that physicians would find intuitive, and which would therefore greatly enhance its value to them, would require understanding their professional worldview in some detail. And yet the world of cardiologists and electrophysiologists is something to which few people, apart from the doctors themselves and others they work with closely, are privy (see Figure 6.4).

Rapport

The question then becomes — how does one gain access to such a unique and specialized world? The short answer is: by shadowing the people who live in it, by talking with them and observing them, and then by trying to understand their perceptions of the product.

This objective introduces a slew of new challenges, of course. First and foremost is the simple but often underestimated fact that people cannot be forced to tell researchers what they want to know. Short of some pressing utilitarian reason — such as the outright failure of a product — people simply will not share their real feelings, at least not to the level needed to provide a clear understanding of their personal situation, unless they have some authentic, interpersonal basis for interacting with the researcher.

Thus, a main ingredient in successful ethnographic work is rapport — developing relationships with people. These needn't be long-term relationships, of course, but short-term relationships characterized by basic expressions of trust and mutual goodwill.

Often, it is enough for informants to know and believe that researchers have a genuine interest in their personal situation, and in the difficulties and successes they experience with the product. But it also helps simply to spend time with them.

Though it sounds easy enough, researchers don't always follow this principle. A common mistake made while interviewing, for instance, is attempting to extract answers to "bad" questions — questions the data are proving to be on the wrong track. This is often a function of the need to generate statistics. But it makes no sense to amass answers that don't represent the end-users' true opinions. When people bend their answers to fit poorly-worded or misguided questions, researchers learn little of value to the product's development. Instead, an ethnographer takes a more flexible view of the interview guide or moderator's protocol, encouraging the person to talk about the product in his or her own words. Rather than doggedly following a predefined route, which can exhaust interviewees or put them on the defensive, the ethnographer is willing to talk around the subject, letting bits and pieces of relevant information gradually fall into place. In this way, the key questions nearly always get answered. In the course of informal give-and-take, some preplanned questions simply become obsolete, while other questions, inevitably, become better and more precise with an ever-improving knowledge of how informants think, speak, and act.

Why do so many market research practitioners ignore this natural trajectory? There are many reasons, but all boil down to essentially one theme: the unfair expectation that the interviewee is responsible for answering the researcher's analytical questions. Also, professionals impose pressure on themselves to be as productive as possible while conducting research, so they tend to push the process faster than it should go, saturating interviewees with questions so that no time is wasted. Obviously, this style of interviewing can distort the findings.

A related point is that informants can only provide so much. It is never their responsibility to provide a systematic analysis of their own behavior, nor, of course, to design products for manufacturers. Rather, their insights, comments, behaviors, and ideas are useful only as data — to be compared with other data and applied in an analysis based on a far wider sample of behavior and comments, and which is informed by a broader experience of problems associated with the product than individual informants are in a position to command.

Time as a Magnifying Glass

Ethnography relies on a combination of smaller sample sizes and longer interaction times with informants than is typical in market research. Spending time with informants is important, and it is one of the key factors that differentiates ethnography from other methodologies, such as surveys.

Time is critical; understanding what someone needs is a complex and time-consuming process. Just think how dimly most people understand their own needs with regard to many of the consumer products they use every day, from cell phones and tape recorders to dishwashers and vacuum cleaners. Understanding what others need is considerably more difficult.

So it often takes some time for informants in a research program to really understand what the researchers are after, reflect on their experience, and generate helpful information. The best research takes place over a day, or even over several days — working with a team of nurses, for example, or shadowing a cardiologist during her rounds.

On one hand, time helps establish good rapport. People tend to trust researchers more as they spend more time with them. As a result, informants begin to reveal more, both intentionally and inadvertently.

On the other hand, people need time to go beyond ideological responses. Strangers who have just met tend to relate to each other in terms of hackneyed stories and canned speeches about themselves, to which they seldom attach much value. They speak less as individuals, and more as types.

A similar phenomenon is evident with professionals in positions of high responsibility, such as physicians, chief nurses, and hospital administrators. In many situations, they tend to speak from their role as the member of a group, and with the group's ideology and interests in mind, rather than from their viewpoint as individuals with their own idiosyncratic opinions and feelings.

This is acceptable when all researchers want is official opinions — the kind of thing one might read in a medical journal or in a hospital newsletter. But it is not acceptable when researchers want practitioners to express their own opinions. And worst of all, if encouraged, group ideology will stifle the flow of authentic information.

For example, if an orthopedic surgeon in a focus group (or even in an anonymous survey) is questioned about the rate of infection at his or her hospital, he or she will likely provide the same numbers that could be read in a medical journal. But if a researcher asks that surgeon the same question at the end of a long day in which the researcher has participated in rounds, watched several surgeries, and heard the surgeon's explanations of surgical procedures, the odds are much better that the response will become clearer and more helpful, if not more honest.

So a good researcher will spend enough time to be able to recognize the informant's ideology, and to help him or her steer clear of it. The researcher will also be open to opportunities available in situations and spaces that offer less formality, such as the car on the way to the hospital, the office after the tape recorder is turned off, or the hallway during the minute or two after the interview. Relevant information often emerges from the interstices of a formal discussion, not from its official center.

Given time, not only may informants open up more, but they may bring to the surface of their own mind more of what they truly think and feel about a device. Everyone has had the feeling of some word or phrase being "just on the tip of the tongue." Some time later, the word or phrase surfaces out of nowhere. This is a common example of an important principle: the unconscious mind continues to work on a problem even when the conscious mind has abandoned it. In the same way, the quality of information tends to improve the longer an informant is permitted to ponder the question, meanwhile resuming his or her normal tasks.

Listen Closely

What do the users of a product talk about when they are using it? What terms and expressions do they employ? What names for things (and persons) have they invented?

Researchers who make the effort to learn about these things are well on their way to forming a map of their informants' worldviews, and, correspondingly, to developing a knowledge of key mental categories that shape their assessment of a given product.

Consider the following scenario: in a study of cardiac catheterization labs in the United States, a manufacturer was on the verge of producing an innovation that could move in one or more of several directions — improving patient safety, supporting medical recordkeeping, or decreasing costs all around. But to choose the optimal direction, the manufacturer needed to understand the dominant values in the cath lab.

Interviews suggested that the dominant concern in clinicians' minds was to improve patient safety. During procedure after procedure, however, researchers found that documentation needs drove much of the activity in the lab — even the performance times of the procedures themselves. After observing numerous procedures, researchers determined that documentation was a much more crucial factor than they had initially believed.

But to make this determination, they first had to understand the culture of the cath lab. That meant developing a knowledge of the division of labor (e.g., nurse as computer "driver"), of the unique pace (how long is too long to complete a given part of a procedure?), and, especially, of the relevant language.

The terms that clinicians used were sometimes medical jargon ("RV/LV pressures"), sometimes slang (such as "pulling settings" from a hemodynamics monitor), and sometimes a combination or contraction of medical and slang terms ("thermals" for thermodilutions).

The researchers observed procedures in a live cath lab to gain a clear understanding of how things worked. In the lab, the technologist, out of the sterile field in a viewing room, preserved the record of each step on her computer, meanwhile keeping an eye on some of the patient's hemodynamic information, such as the heart rate and blood pressure readings.

Examples like this drove home the importance of real-time recordkeeping during the cath lab procedures. Indeed, full documentation was important enough to force the doctor to actually halt his procedure, momentarily, to allow the technologist time to clear a paper jam and to enter patient data.

The language of the cath lab reflected this social reality: the technician was in a number of important ways the driver of the procedure. Chiefly, it was she who controlled the step-by-step documentation of each therapeutic maneuver.

Consider Context

Ethnographic research is holistic. It requires researchers to look beyond the immediate answers to their initial questions and to see the new product as part of the larger context of personnel, tasks, and incentives that its users confront on a daily basis.

In a study of behavior around office photocopiers, for example, anthropologist J. Blomberg discovered that office workers tended to define the term *mechanical breakdown* simply as any time the machine was unusable, not as when the mechanical components were physically damaged.[2] As one might imagine, machines that happened to be in offices with a helper, someone available to clear paper jams and handle other minor problems efficiently, were perceived as more reliable than machines of the same type in offices lacking such an employee.

This example is a good one of how context defines meaning. Had researchers been content merely to ask (as in a phone survey) how many times the machines in the office "broke down," they would have received a misleading impression.

From an anthropological perspective, such contextual definitions of device problems are wholly welcome and expected. Of course, product users often define *error*, *problem*, and *difficulty* differently than product developers — they live with the device every day.

Conclusion

Ethnographic field research is a crucial tool for user-centered medical product development. It is certainly not the only tool for determining what product users want and need, but it yields a depth and accuracy of results that are not available from any other approach. Of course, conducting ethnographic research can be more difficult in various ways than conducting more conventional research. However, the results are well worth the trouble.

Acknowledgment

Will Reese, of Design Science, co-authored an earlier version of this chapter.

Key Points

- Ethnographic field research provides a wealth and depth of information that is not possible using more conventional research methods.
- Ethnographic field research involves spending significant amounts of time in the real environment of use for a product.
- Observing carefully and interviewing in the context of use of a product produces information that is different from and sometimes contradicts that obtained by, for example, focus groups and surveys.
- Ethnographic research requires developing rapport with informants, listening carefully to everything that they say, and carefully considering the context in which observations and interviews take place.
- Videotaping is an important tool for ethnographic research.

References

1. Cooper, R.G., *New Products: The Key Factors in Success,* American Marketing Association, Chicago, 1990.
2. Blomberg, J., Social interaction and office communication: Effects on user evaluation of new technologies, in *Technology and the Transformation of White Collar Work,* Kraut, R., Ed., Lawrence Erlbaum Associates, Hillsdale, NJ, 1987, 195–210.

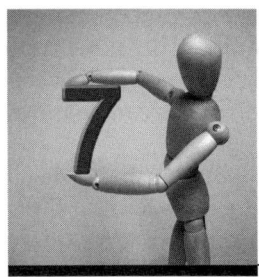

Time-Lapse Video Offers More Information in Less Time

Stephen B. Wilcox

Using time-lapse video compresses lengthy documentation, providing designers with both qualitative and quantitative data more quickly.

Addressing usability as part of the design of a medical product logically requires detailed study of relevant real-world tasks for which the product will be used. In order to study the tasks, it is necessary to observe them, and it helps enormously to videotape them for further review. However, the tasks in question are sometimes very lengthy. Videotaping and reviewing, say, six hours of open-heart surgery for each case can be a daunting and inefficient form of research.

This is where time-lapse video comes in. Time-lapse video entails taking samples rather than taping continuously. For example, a one-second sample every 10 seconds dramatically compresses the amount of video to review — of course, by a ratio of 1 to 10. When the tape is played back, the procedure unfolds like the old Disney films of blooming flowers. So, with a 1:10 time-lapse recording, a six-hour procedure can be reviewed in a little over a half hour. This time compression saves the reviewer's time, and it can allow patterns to be seen that are difficult to pick up without such time compression.

In addition to the advantages associated with reviewing a long procedure, time-lapse video provides distinct advantages at the recording end. With conventional videotaping, someone has to be there to change the tape, but with a time-lapse system, a multihour procedure can be recorded on a single tape. Although this may seem like a small consideration, it allows the observer to set up a video camera without the need to change tapes frequently. This means that acquiring video of several procedures can be much more feasible and less labor-intensive.

Another advantage is that time-lapse video documentation lends itself easily to quantitative analyses. Once a procedure is reduced to a set of finite video samples, each sample can be treated as a specific data point for quantitative analyses. For example, one might want to ask what percentage of the time a surgeon uses both hands or the percentage of time the physician's wrist is bent beyond a given number of degrees, or the percentage of time that a particular visual display is illuminated. These types of analyses can be performed with conventional video and a stopwatch. However, it is much easier and potentially more accurate to base such analyses on frequency counts of time-lapse samples, rather than to attempt to record the relative times directly. In other words, time-lapse video provides a manageable pool of data that makes quantitative analyses easier and more accurate.

The basic requirement for a time-lapse video system is that it contain a device for allowing one to set both the length of the video sample and the frequency of the samples. In practice, it takes some trial and error to set these parameters to be most effective for a given to-be-recorded procedure. The samples have to be long enough so that they contain dynamic events, if necessary, and the frequency of samples has to be such that nothing important is missed between samples.

It is imperative to determine settings that compress the procedure to a manageable length without losing crucial pieces of information. One approach is to determine the length of the final summary video and to work back from that figure. Fifteen minutes, for example, seems to be the tolerance level for many viewers. Typical settings might be a one-second duration with four samples per minute. Such settings result in a final tape length of four minutes per hour of the original procedure.

The system outlined in Figure 7.1 is one example of a method for achieving time-lapse video. It contains four pulse generators. Generator 1 creates a regular short pulse, which can be varied to alter the sample rate. This pulse stimulates generator 2, and a longer pulse, which turns the camera on. In the meantime, the second pulse stimulates generator 3, which can be varied to determine how long the camera will stay on. The end of the third pulse stimulates generator 4, which creates a pulse to turn the camera off. The camera remains off until generator 1 creates the next pulse to restart the cycle.

A useful addition for video study is a multiple-camera, split-screen system. Such a system increases the amount of information, providing an additional view of a procedure, or, in the case of minimally invasive procedures, a view of the "inside" and the outside simultaneously. This can be particularly useful when evaluating the user's needs for a complex device. Another advantage of a multiple-camera system is that it allows the viewer to see

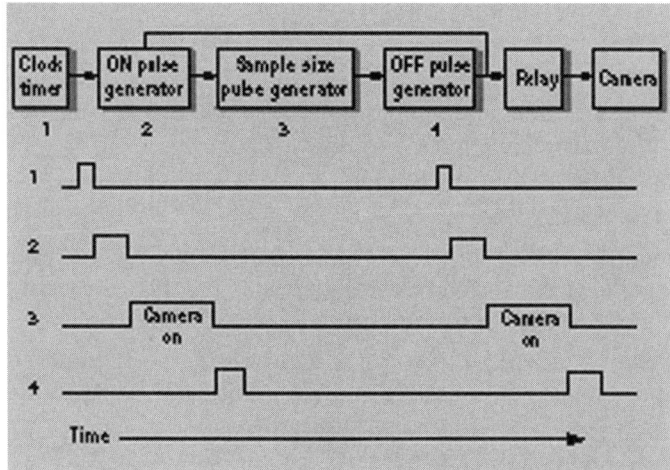

FIGURE 7.1
A time-lapse video controller system.

the tasks when one camera is blocked, which often seems to be the case under real-world conditions. Other useful advanced features are overhead shots for dynamic "plan views" and simultaneous feeds directly from scopes, to get a clean "inside" view and to see what the physician sees during a procedure.

Another useful tool is slow-motion video, which is the opposite of time-lapse. Where time-lapse is useful for compressing a long procedure, slow motion is useful for studying what happens too fast to be clearly seen — exactly what the hand postures are when firing a surgical stapler, for example, or the precise hand movements entailed in using a catheter. We have emphasized time-lapse here because it requires a bit of special technology, which slow-motion video does not (although the latter does require a system with high enough quality to allow clear frame-by-frame viewing). Both types of video, though, can significantly enhance one's ability to use observation as an effective tool for creating better medical products.

Conclusion

Video is a useful tool for determining how products are used under real-world circumstances or for testing of prototypes. Adding time-lapse capability to conventional video can provide convenience and functionality and, thus, allow one to conduct better product-related research. Other useful enhancements include multicamera systems and slow-motion video.

Key Points

- Time-lapse video is a technique for compressing a long procedure into a manageable length for analysis.
- Time-lapse video can also make video recording more efficient and less labor-intensive.
- Time-lapse video requires a system that allows for the adjustment of sample length and sample frequency; in practice, the right parameters need to be determined through pilot testing.
- Time-lapse video, by recording a procedure as a finite series of samples, makes quantitative analysis easier and more accurate.
- Related useful video tools include multicamera systems and slow-motion video.

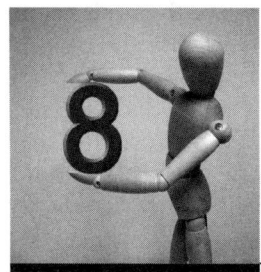

Finding and Using Data Regarding the Shape and Size of the User's Body

Stephen B. Wilcox

Tailoring the geometry of a product to the shape and size of a user's body can be more difficult than it may, at first, seem. There are a number of helpful new tools, however, to help.

Anthropometry is the study of the shape and size of the human body. The discipline has its roots in physical anthropology, where it has traditionally been used to make ethnic comparisons. However, at a certain point, the military discovered the value of anthropometry for determining the sizes of things used by soldiers — uniforms, helmets, cockpits, etc.[1] The military had the great advantage of a captive population to measure, so they have been able to perform large-scale anthropometric studies. For this reason, much of the anthropometric data that are available come from the military.

Documents That Contain Traditional Anthropometric Data

The compilation of anthropometric data that is probably used most often by product designers is that originally published in *The Measure of Man* (1960),[2] and periodically updated as *Humanscale 1/2/3* (1974),[3] *Humanscale 4/5/6* (1981),[4] *Humanscale 7/8/9* (1981),[5] *The Measure of Man and Woman* (1993),[6] and, most recently, in *The Measure of Man and Woman, Revised Edition* (2002).[7]

These documents are highly usable design tools that give the designer all sorts of information for tailoring products to people. They use the concept of the "percentile person" to provide average body dimensions as well as extremes (e.g., 1st and 99th percentiles).

However, it is often helpful or necessary to go back to the original data sets, since the summaries provided may not contain exactly what the designer needs for a given project. Some good sources of data include the following:

- Pheasant[8] is a great source for civilian anthropometric data. It provides separate data for a number of countries as well as the U.S., and it provides age-related data for the British population, which is reasonably approximate to that of the United States.
- Roebuck[9] provides a small amount of summary data from an anthropometric survey of civilians in the United States by the Department of Health and Human Services. It also contains a lot of good information about how to collect anthropometric data.
- *The Military Handbook: Anthropometry of U.S. Military Personnel*[10] contains the best compilation of military data, from a large number of military studies.
- Greiner[11] provides detailed anthropometric information specifically for the hand.
- White[12] is the source for detailed foot anthropometric information.
- *Anthropometry of Infants, Children, and Youths to Age 18 for Product Safety Design*[13] contains detailed anthropometric data for children.

Other Types of Information

Traditional anthropometry is one-dimensional. It provides the dimensions for various lengths and, as in the case of *The Measure of Man and Woman*, tries to link these dimensions into front views and side views. One thing that is missing, however, is a real 3-D picture of what the geometry of the body is. It is difficult to use the conventional anthropometric data to, for example, determine where the thumb will end up when wrapped around a given handle with a complex geometry.

This need is addressed by laser scanning, which is getting more and more sophisticated, and is now widely available. However, it has a number of limitations, the most important of which is that integrating data across individuals is extremely complex. But body scanning is gradually playing a larger role in design, a trend that should accelerate as the technology improves (see Figure 8.1 and Figure 8.2). In fact, there are some large-scale

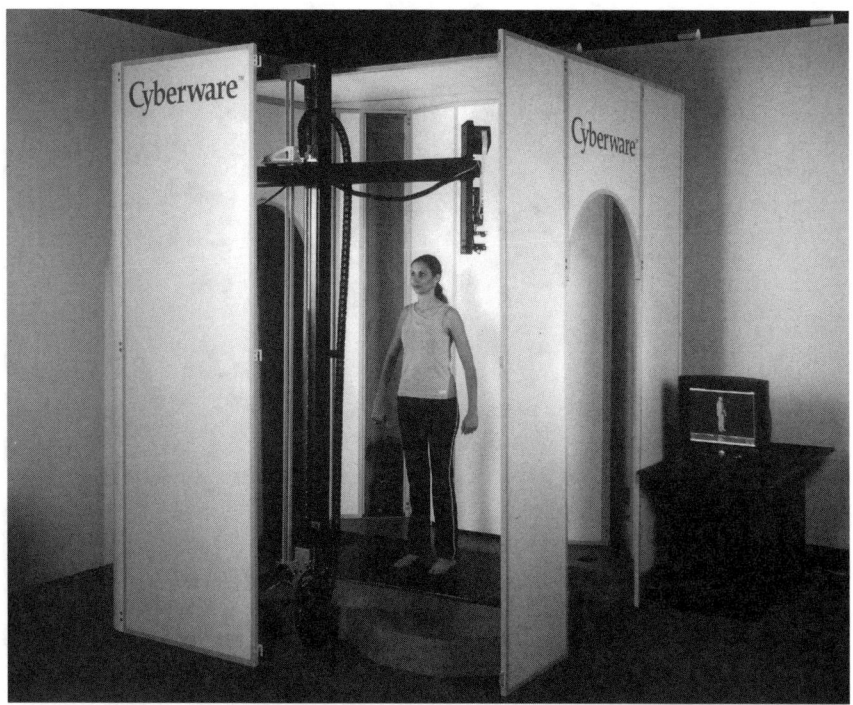

FIGURE 8.1
Full-body scanning system. Image courtesy of Cyberware.

3-D data sets that have recently become available, including the U.S. Defense Logistics Agency Apparel Research Network program and the Civilian American and European Surface Anthropometry Resource (CAESAR Survey).

CAESAR uses a 3-D surface anthropometric technology to capture "hundreds of thousands of points in 3-dimensions on the human body surface." The goal is to provide data that can be integrated into computer-aided design software packages.

With regard to body scanning, there are currently at least eight scanning systems available for use. The most common system relies on a "laser stripe" method; other methods include "patterned light projection" and "stereo photogrammetry" (see Jones and Rioux[14] and Daanen and van de Water[15]).

Human Modeling Software

Another approach to 3-D anthropometry is to create a virtual 3-D human. A great advantage is that the designer can do simple fitting tasks that would be extremely difficult using traditional anthropometric data (e.g., placing the

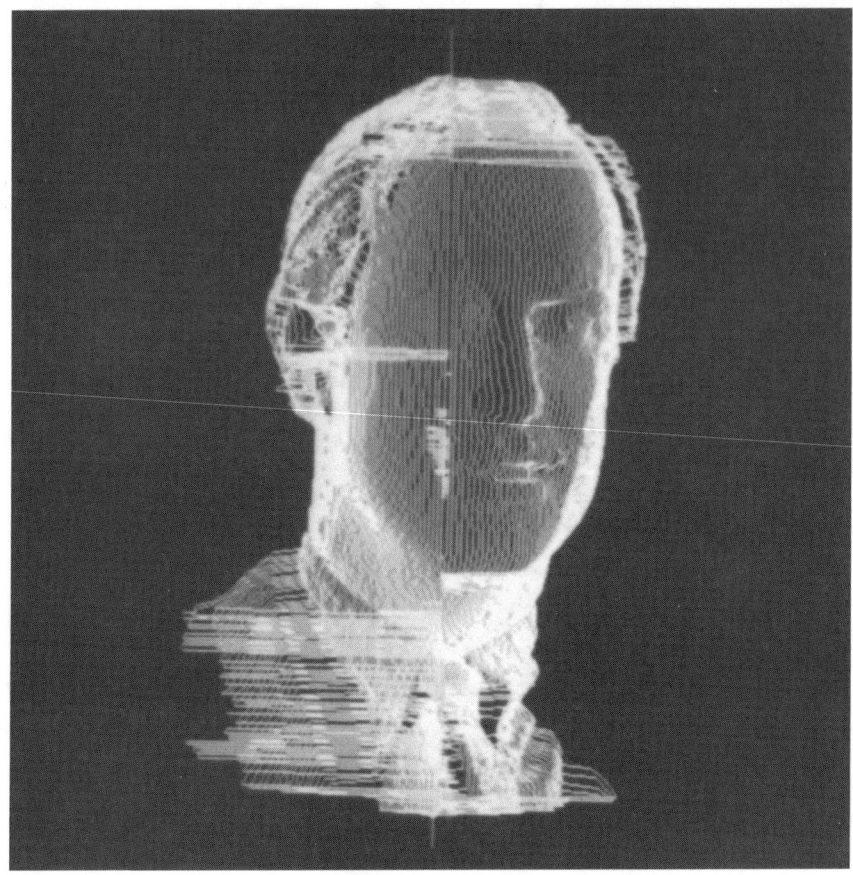

FIGURE 8.2
A scanned head. Image courtesy of Cyberware.

model onto a hospital bed or wrapping the fingers around a model and seeing where the finger controls need to be). There are three major systems of this type:

- *Jack* was originally developed at the University of Pennsylvania. It enables users to position digital humans of various sizes in virtual environments, assign them tasks, and analyze their performance. Jack can provide information about what "he" can see and reach, how comfortable he is, when and why he is getting hurt, and even when his strength is exceeded.
- *Safework* is another "mannequin" program. It does not have all of the functions available with Jack, but it has one fundamental difference — it departs from the "percentile" concept. The concept of the "1st and 99th percentile person," which is a standard way to think about the extremes of the population, is a reasonable first step or

shortcut. However, it has a fundamental problem — no real people are so extreme or so consistently extreme (cf., McConville and Robinette[16]). The extremes of the population actually differ in various ways. One person will be short and stout, another will be long-waisted, a third will have long legs, but short arms. Safework has addressed these issues by developing the concept of "boundary models," which represent actual people who are extreme in various ways, as opposed to the nonexistent "percentile person." Thus, Safework has incorporated correlational data (i.e., statistics that measure the relationship between different measurements) as well as the measurements themselves, so you can, for example, specify one dimension, say hand length, and get a picture of how people with that hand length differ in another dimension (say, arm length).

- RAMSIS is the other major human modeling program. It is used primarily in the automotive industry.

Other Anthropometric Software

One other approach to anthropometry is represented by PeopleSize. PeopleSize, created by Open Ergonomics, is a point-and-click software package that allows a user to click on a relative measurement and then select a nationality, age group, and percentile value. It is really, then, an electronic document, as opposed to an electronic model. It contains adult data from the U.K., U.S., China, Holland, France, Germany, Italy, and Japan. It also includes data on U.K. and U.S. infants (0–24 months) and children (2–17 years of age). Much of the data are from civilian sources, such as data obtained from the U.S. National Health and Nutrition Examination Survey.

User Testing

Regardless of what anthropometric tools one uses, though, it is always crucial to test a given design with actual people, that is, to conduct some form of usability testing. "Virtual" fitting studies can be performed with human modeling software, but the results still remain to some extent theoretical until one creates a mock-up and tests it with actual rather then virtual people. The challenge is to test it with the right people. One approach is to find individuals who are extreme in their dimensions (stature, for example, or hand size) to test as the limiting cases. Of course, these individuals may not be particularly representative of all people of their stature on their other dimensions, but this can at least provide a "sanity check" to assure that the design at least fits some people who we know are real examples of "1st or 99th percentile people." Furthermore, comfort and a "natural" feel can be hard to predict exclusively from data.

An adjunct to this approach is to build an in-house database of employee anthropometric data, so that the designer knows who to test when a given percentile is of interest.

It is a terrible mistake to rely exclusively on such testing. The need to go beyond such a "seat-of-the-pants" approach is, after all, the motivation for gathering anthropometric data in the first place. On the other hand, it is just as big a mistake to rely exclusively on the data without real-world verification.

Conclusion

In sum, anthropometric data are available from a number of sources, varying from simple documents with 2-D "percentile people" to very sophisticated simulation software. Whichever tools and databases the designer uses, however, should be supplemented by empirical testing of actual prototypes.

Key Points

- Data on the size and shape of the user's body are widely available.
- The traditional summary documents, such as *The Measure of Man and Woman*, are good quick references, but have limitations.
- Some newer simulation software packages, such as *Jack*, provide more sophisticated data and functionality.
- Whatever data are used should be supplemented by empirical testing with actual users.
- One technique is to create an anthropometry database of employees for quick prototype testing.

References

1. Hertzberg, H., Some contributions of applied physical anthropology to human engineering, *Annals of the New York Academy of Science*, 63, 616–629, 1995.
2. Dreyfus, H., *The Measure of Man*, Whitney Publications, New York, 1960.

3. Diffrient, N., Tilley, A., and Bardagjy, J., *Humanscale 1/2/3*, MIT Press, Cambridge, MA, 1974.
4. Diffrient, N., Tilley, A., and Harman, D., *Humanscale 4/5/6*, MIT Press, Cambridge, MA, 1981.
5. Diffrient, N., Tilley, A., and Harman, D., *Humanscale 7/8/9*, MIT Press, Cambridge, MA, 1981.
6. Tilley, A., *The Measure of Man and Woman*, Whitney Library of Design, New York, 1993.
7. Tilley, A., *The Measure of Man and Woman, Revised Edition*, John Wiley & Sons, New York, 2002.
8. Pheasant, S., *Bodyspace: Anthropometry, Ergonomics and the Design of Work, Second Edition*, Taylor & Francis, Bristol, U.K., 1996.
9. Roebuck, J., *Anthropometric Methods: Designing to Fit the Human Body*, Human Factors and Ergonomics Society, Santa Monica, CA, 1995.
10. *The Military Handbook: Anthropometry of U.S. Military Personnel*, Department of Defense, Washington, D.C., 1991.
11. Greiner, T., *Hand Anthropometry of U.S. Army Personnel*, Department of Defense, Washington, D.C., 1990.
12. White, R., *Comparative Anthropometry of the Foot*, Department of Defense, Washington, D.C., 1982.
13. *Anthropometry of Infants, Children, and Youths to Age 18 for Product Safety Design*, Society of Automotive Engineers, Warrendale, PA, undated.
14. Jones, P. and Rioux, M., Three-dimensional surface anthropometry: Applications to the human body, *Optics and Lasers in Engineering*, 28, 89–117, 1997.
15. Daanen, H. and van de Water, G., Whole body scanners, *Displays*, 19, 111–120, 1999.
16. McConville, J. and Robinette, K., An alternative to percentile models, *Transactions*, 90, 938–946, 1981.

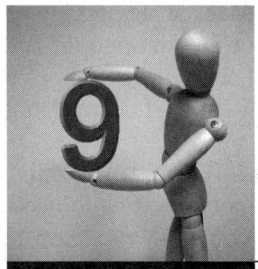

Can You Trust What People Say?

Stephen B. Wilcox

Medical product developers tend to rely heavily upon what their customers tell them. Unfortunately, there is significant evidence that what people say is a highly fallible guide to actual behavior.

As discussed elsewhere in this book, what people say provides only part of the story about user needs, and, in general, is a fallible source of information. Indeed, the fact that most new products fail provides at least indirect support for the proposition that the speech of customers cannot be fully trusted.

In this chapter, we summarize the evidence for the fallibility of verbal data and suggest some alternatives.

Fallibility of Verbal Data

The difficulty with finding definitive evidence from new-product development itself is that manufacturers and design firms seldom or never talk to the people who *do not* buy newly introduced products. If the product fails, it is impossible to tell whether the potential customers and users who were part of the product-development process provided inaccurate information, or if the failure was due to shortcomings having to do with some other factor, such as marketing or advertising strategies, manufacturing, distribution, or some sort of change in medical practices or trends.

85

Disquieting evidence comes from the work of A.W. Wicker.[1] He reviewed 48 studies that compared observed or recorded behavior to what people said they did, or would do, in a given situation. A few of the studies reported some correlation between speech and behavior; however, most correlations were insignificant.

There is also a large body of research (summarized in Loftus and Wells[2]) that demonstrates that people have great difficulty when it comes to accurately describing past events. That said, how can people be expected to accurately predict what they will do in imaginary circumstances?

The key implication is that traditional quantitative and qualitative market research methods should be augmented with other methods that do not rely so heavily on what people say. There is a strong movement in this direction. Methods relating to this movement fall into three categories — observation, methods for allowing nonverbal expression, and methods for obtaining better verbal information.

Observational Techniques

As we discuss elsewhere in this book, there is no substitute for field observation — watching people in their "natural habitats" such as ORs, procedure labs, ICUs, or patients' homes — for home-healthcare products. Watching what people do is nearly always surprising. More often than not, people's behavior contradicts, to some extent, what they say they do.

Observation can be overt, or covert, such as when the researcher poses as a tech or a patient. And, as we say in Chapter 6, video is a useful observational tool. However, the problem with cameras is that they may change people's behavior. Everything else being equal, hidden cameras are better, but they are seldom possible in a medical context. It is helpful to at least use a camera that is small and unobtrusive.

Particularly when videotaping patients, maintenance of privacy is a primary concern. Privacy may be upheld by masking patients' faces or by blurring the image just enough so you do not recognize the individuals or see various parts of their bodies, but you are still able to observe what they are doing.

Alteration of the speed of the video is also useful. Chapter 7 contains a discussion of time-lapse video, a tool for compressing long procedures. It can also be very useful to slow the image down to study the details of behavior that happen too rapidly to be seen clearly with the naked eye.

Another observational technique is *artifact analysis,* the study of the "residue" of behavior. Patterns of damage or wear, homemade devices, "cheat sheets," notes, etc., can give you empirical evidence of people's behavior not available from other sources.

Can You Trust What People Say?

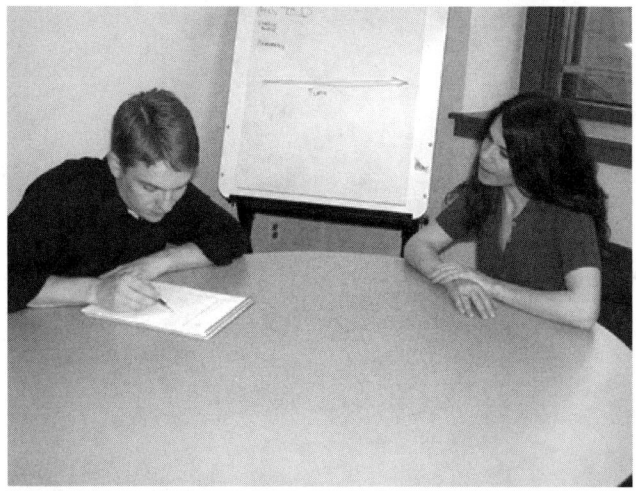

FIGURE 9.1
The "police sketch" method — illustrating users' ideas.

Nonverbal Expression Techniques

Another approach is to provide people with tools to express themselves nonverbally. People who can render can express themselves more fully than people who cannot. Since most physicians, nurses, and patients cannot render well, it can be useful to allow them to direct an illustrator to create their version of the "ideal product," or the product that solves a particular problem, or even a problem itself. In other words, the idea is for a member of the research team to serve as the "hands" of the potential product user to allow him to express himself or herself visually. This is sometimes called the "police sketch method," since it is similar to the method used by police to obtain a description of criminals (see Figure 9.1).

Alternatively, it can be useful to give product users categorization tasks. The way medical personnel categorize alternative products, activities, or prototypes can shed light on how they see things, beyond what they are able to express verbally.

Yet another method is to provide potential product users with "building blocks," using foam, Velcro, etc., or screen objects for software, so they can build their own products, illustrating their preferences (see Figure 9.2).

Finally, people can be given disposable cameras to document examples of issues that are important to them or examples of what is good or bad.

What all of these techniques have in common is that they provide people with ways of expressing themselves to supplement what they say. Some

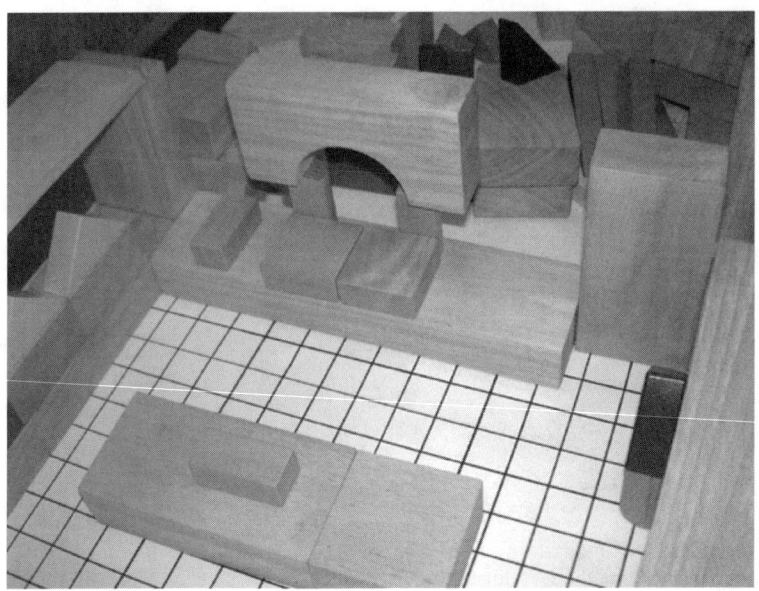

FIGURE 9.2
Model-building tasks.

people are good at "painting a word picture," but many are not. The techniques previously mentioned are particularly helpful for the latter.

Improved Verbal Techniques

Diary and workbook studies rely upon written responses, but they allow people to record information at the time it happens and in their "natural" environments. The schedule of information recording can be controlled by the researcher by contacting the participant via a device like a pager or a cell phone.

On-site interviews, of course, come along "for free" when conducting ethnographic field research, as discussed in Chapter 6. When interviews are conducted in the actual product-use environment, the user can show the researcher examples and can look to get more accurate information, rather than answering questions from memory.

Another method, the *Swift method*, originally developed by Phil Swift while he was Director of Design and Human Factors at Symbol Technologies, a Holtsville, NY-based manufacturer of bar-code scanners, is an interesting integration of design and research. Swift, who is now at Pitney Bowes, recognized the importance of creating models that systematically vary product parameters and of asking potential users which ones they prefer (see Figure 9.3). Though the Swift method relies on the users' stated preferences, it provides realistic rather than imaginary objects to which the users respond.

Can You Trust What People Say?

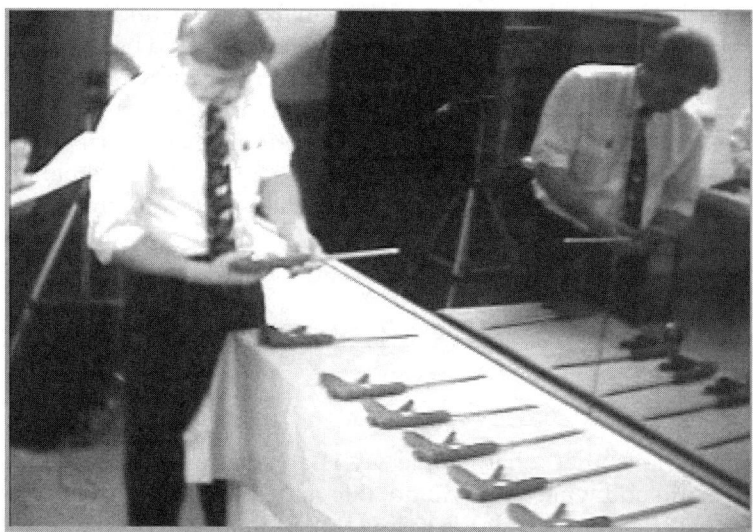

FIGURE 9.3
The Swift method — evaluation of alternative models that systematically vary on two dimensions at a time.

The aforementioned techniques are ways of reducing the error inherent in verbal data.

Some Real-World Examples

A common phenomenon with surgical instruments is the visceral rejection, by skilled surgeons, of any proposed instrument that has a radically different configuration from what the surgeons are used to. However, when using instruments, those same surgeons can demonstrate the superiority of the very instruments they say they cannot or will not use. In this sense, then, supplementing verbal data can be a key way of preserving innovative alternatives, as we discuss briefly in Chapter 11.

Another example comes from the nurses who use programmers for communicating with implanted pacemakers and defibrillators. When asked directly, they inevitably say that they are perfectly happy with the programmers they use and that it is easy to learn how to use them. However, careful observation reveals that novice nurses find it extremely difficult to learn how to use them, that errors are common, that nurses only make use of a very small percentage of the programmers' functionality, and that cardiologists, the expected "users," often have little or no idea how to use them, relying exclusively on printouts generated by the nurses. These are all symptoms of usability problems, which the nurses deny the existence of.

One final example also comes from pacemaker and defibrillator programmers. Cardiologists, when asked how programmers could be improved, said there is little room for improvement. However, when given some "tinker toy" tools and asked to create their ideal programmer, they came up with radical alternatives that differed dramatically from what is currently offered.

What these examples illustrate is that the adoption of nonverbal methods often (or even typically) lead one to different conclusions from those that result from verbal-only data.

Conclusion

It is simply false that what people say is a consistently accurate guide to what they do and what they will do. Life may be easier for the person who believes this fiction, but it leads to investment in products that do not meet user needs as well as they should. Fortunately, there are a number of methods that can be used to replace or supplement verbal data. These methods may not be as simple as purely verbal methods, but they can yield important results for achieving user-centered design.

Key Points

- Although there is a strong bias in product development toward heavy reliance on verbal data, there is a large body of evidence that verbal data is highly fallible.
- One alternative to verbal data is direct observation of behavior.
- Another alternative is to provide users with tools for visual communication (e.g., illustrations, images to categorize, physical "building blocks," or disposable cameras).
- Techniques for obtaining more valid verbal data include diary studies, on-site interviews, and the "Swift method," which asks users to evaluate alternative models or prototypes in which underlying dimensions systematically vary.
- Such methods may require some effort to restructure the research arsenal; however, they repay this effort by increasing the likelihood of understanding real, rather than imaginary, user needs.

References

1. Wicker, A.W., Attitudes versus actions: The relationship of verbal and overt behavioral responses to attitude objects, *Journal of Social Issues,* 25, 41–78, 1969.
2. Loftus, E. and Wells, G., *Eyewitness Testimony: Psychological Perspectives,* Cambridge University Press, New York, 1984.

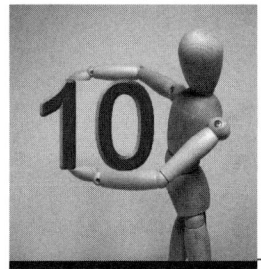

Eight Ways to Kill Innovation

Stephen B. Wilcox

Medical device manufacturers are supposed to thrive on change. Why, then, do so many of them make innovation difficult?

We've collectively spent a couple of decades now working with many types of medical device manufacturers on new product development. This experience has led us to two conclusions:

- Nothing is more important than innovation in the development of medical devices, particularly in trying to achieve user-centered design.
- The typical medical device manufacturer has managed to erect numerous barriers to product innovation.

How has this happened? To answer that question, let us begin with a bit of preaching to the choir about the value of innovation. Then we will discuss, in some detail, how manufacturers go about killing it.

Innovation Fuels New Product Success

Innovation is crucial for achieving good, usable products (see Figures 10.1–10.3). But more than that, you cannot make a living without it. Innovation is necessary to acquire a "monopoly," and without some sort of monopoly, you

93

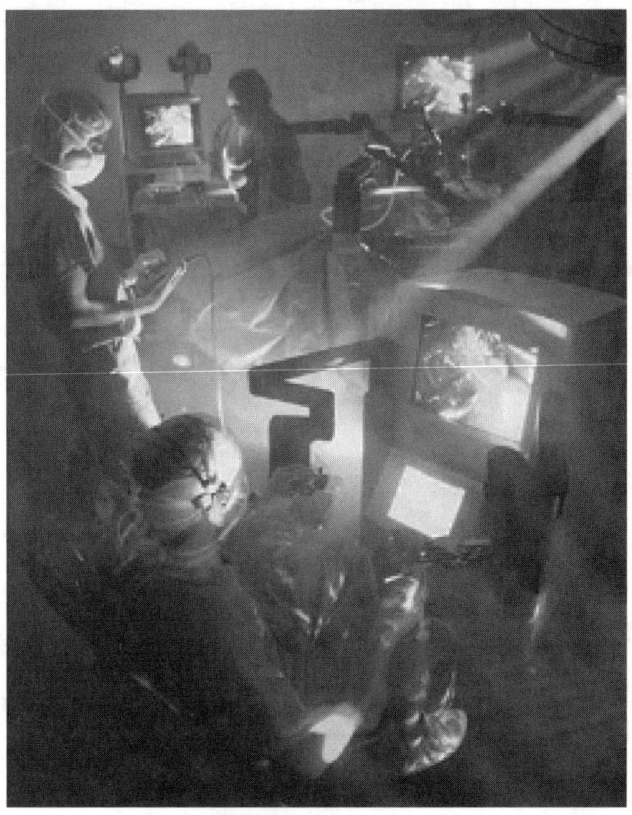

FIGURE 10.1 (See color insert following page 142)
The ZEUS™ Robotic Surgical System embodies innovation both in terms of product design and surgical technique. Image courtesy of NASA/JPL.

cannot be successful. The reason for this is simple. Unless you can sell something that only you have, customers will simply buy the cheapest alternative. This drives the prices down until there is no profit to be made by anybody. It is the classic "commodity syndrome."

So, again, you need some kind of monopoly. It may just be one little feature, or a special way of doing business, or even a geographic location that gives you a local monopoly. But you have to have something.

How do you get a monopoly? Innovation, of course. Without it, you are forced to copy someone else. All else being equal, the more innovative you are, and the more monopolies you have, the more control you will have of the marketplace. Who is it that must constantly play catch-up with their competitors, and who must cut their margins in order to sell products? Not innovators, or at least not savvy ones.

There is one other advantage of innovation. An innovative environment builds morale and helps your firm keep its best people, rather than letting them slip away to places where their ideas are nurtured rather than ignored.

Eight Ways to Kill Innovation

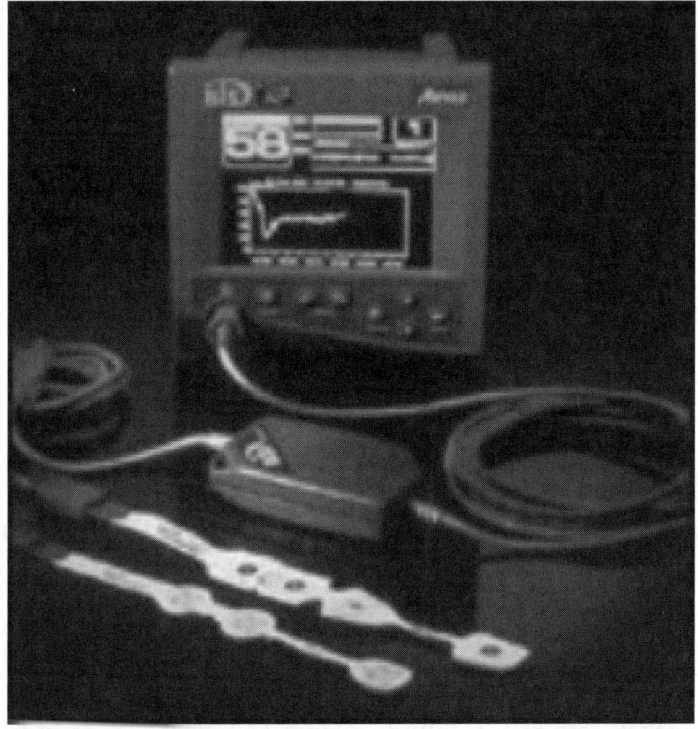

FIGURE 10.2
The A-2000 Bispectral Index (BIS) Consciousness Monitor challenges anesthesia providers to embrace a new means to manage the depth of anesthesia. Image courtesy of Aspect Medical Systems, Inc.

As we say, we expect this to be preaching to the choir. But if we all agree that innovation is good, and, from the point of view of this book, it is absolutely crucial for meeting user needs, why do so many companies go out of their way to kill it? There is no simple answer. But the ways companies crush innovation can be clearly described. Below, we present them as facetious advice on how to eliminate innovation.

Misapply QFD

The appeal of quality function deployment, or QFD, and its competitors and successors, such as Six Sigma is obvious. They hold out the promise of a systematic procedure that, if followed, will yield products with superior customer satisfaction relative to competitors. In QFD, you create a matrix in which customer requirements are listed. Then a given product alternative is rated according to the customer requirements.

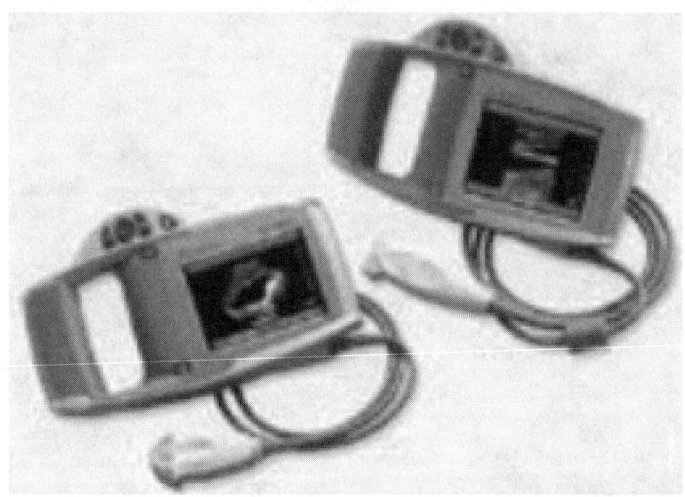

FIGURE 10.3
The iLook Personal Imaging Tool adds a new dimension of portability to ultrasound imaging. Image courtesy of SonoSite.

The great advantage of QFD for those who fear innovation is that it represents, in effect, the cannibalization of product design by quality control, a discipline that, despite its many advantages, has never been accused of being a fertile source of creativity.

Begun in Japan in the 1960s, QFD first emerged in the United States when it was applied in the automobile industry in the late 1970s and early 1980s. It provided just what was needed by the sagging automobile industry of that era. It was a means of finding small advantages in a mature marketplace. It allowed the car companies to find out what aspects of cars customers cared about, so that they could focus on and improve those aspects. The winner was the car that was just a little bit better than others in those characteristics that mattered most.

Thus, QFD was a terrific tool for that particular time and that particular market. But QFD may or may not be the right approach in a highly dynamic medical marketplace. Inevitably, customer requirements are identified based on existing products. New ideas are then evaluated in light of those requirements. New alternatives that do not fit existing criteria (and that customers may not even know they want) are at risk of being rejected early in the process.

In other words, QFD can help develop a successful family sedan. But can it help you find a new way of performing surgery, or a new type of imaging? Can it help you turn a problem upside down and see it in a new way? We have our doubts.

The application of QFD has two additional effects that can help crush innovation:

- It uses up a lot of resources identifying customer requirements and filling out the matrices. You won't have much time left for coming up with new ideas.
- It can enforce a linear way of thinking about product development that leaves little room for the type of unconstrained (anarchic?) thinking from which innovation flows. To come up with something really new, you sometimes need to escape all the constraints and generate wild ideas. QFD does not leave much room for that.

Is QFD a villain? No. As the heading of this section indicates, the problem is misapplying QFD. There are certainly ways of applying the technique in your company that will leave the ability to innovate intact. But if you want to kill innovation, make sure that you apply QFD as slavishly and crudely as possible. In other words, apply it just as it is often applied in the real world.

Treat Industrial Designers as "Stylists"

Innovation is very much a part of industrial design. Industrial designers tend to be creative, both by nature and training. Thus, they like to innovate, and they are good at it, particularly when they effectively balance their creative impulses with an egoless, empathetic attitude and deep understanding of the users' needs and preferences. However, this natural resource is often thrown away when they are treated as "stylists," brought in merely to place an attractive skin on a product that has already been designed by the engineering team. Designers are much more effective as true partners in the development process, rather than as stylists engaged to make the product look pretty, even though, of course, looks can be important to a product's success.

The designer-as-stylist model is much less common than it once was. But if you really want to stifle innovation, stick with it. Or, better yet, don't include industrial designers at all. Leave the styling and underlying design strategizing to the people who studied thermodynamics in college and hope for the best.

Put Time-to-Market above Everything Else

It is always safer to make a small change to an existing design rather than to come up with something new. You know the design will work and you know how to make it. A new approach is much less predictable. You can never be sure that you can produce the design at all, let alone that you can do so by the drop-dead date.

There is a natural psychological tendency to take the tried-and-true path. It is exaggerated when the reward structure favors time-to-market, since that path will always make it easier to meet your deadlines. What company is going to rescind bonuses when a product thrives for only a brief time in the marketplace before it is overcome by a more innovative solution?

Turn Tales of Product Failures into Corporate Lore

Every company has had some product failures, maybe even spectacular ones. Sometimes, those failures happen when the product is something radically different and will take some time to settle in with a conservative user population. This can then lead to the confident conclusion that the innovation in question is a loser. This belief is then passed on from one person to the next: "That idea doesn't work." "Customers don't want that type of product."

Of course, the conclusion may be correct. But can you be sure? There can be many reasons why a product fails. Not all of those reasons mean that the whole approach didn't make sense.

For example, when Apple Computer introduced the first major graphical operating system, in the Lisa, the product flopped. It would have been easy for the conclusion "graphical user interfaces do not fly" to become part of Apple's corporate lore. Instead, the company stuck with its system, concluding, presumably, that the Lisa died because of its price or for some other reason, not because of its innovative operating system. If you want to eliminate innovation, try not to exhibit the type of persistence that Apple demonstrated.

Punish Failure More Than You Reward Success

Here is another good way to stifle innovation. Make it clear to project managers that they will pay a huge price if their products are not successful. Also, make it clear that you will not be patient as a new product finds its place in the market. This works especially well if managers have no reason to expect to become corporate stars should they come up with a breakthrough success.

Design by Consensus

Requiring consensus, particularly with a large team, tends to stifle innovation. Someone will always object to anything that is really different. So to minimize innovation, keep your design teams as large as possible and keep them free of strong leaders with the discretion to buck the consensus. It also helps to subscribe strongly to the "not-invented-here" philosophy — to display extreme skepticism to any innovation that didn't come from your team.

Embrace Complexity

Caregivers have got to work at a fast pace to keep up with their workload. This leaves precious little time for them to learn to use new products and master advanced features. Accordingly, a truly innovative medical device might be one that has very little complexity, making it easy to learn to use and leaving few if any advanced features to master. So, to be sure that your new product does not break new ground in terms of its simple operation, be sure to load the new product with every possible feature found in competing devices and the advanced concepts lab. You are sure to win the "Features War" and keep the medical technologists busily employed planning refresher courses and responding to calls for assistance from staff who cannot make the "thing" do what they need it to do.

Do Simple Preference Tests of New Concepts with Existing Users

A syndrome with hard-to-use products is that people who do master them tend to like them. Mastering a difficult product provides a great deal of pride and satisfaction. It also serves to differentiate "pros" from lesser beings who cannot use the product. Thus, skilled users, such as extremely dexterous surgeons, do not want to hear about changing a poorly designed product because it would take away their competitive advantage.

Do you want to make sure that your new product will be exactly like the old one? Then test it with "thought leaders" who are highly skilled with existing products. By all means, do not do careful usability testing. You may find that the behavioral results can demonstrate the superiority of a new approach, despite what users say. You may also find that extended use reveals advantages of a new approach that are not immediately apparent. Furthermore, avoid testing with novice users, who may prefer a radical alternative, and who may find the new product much easier to use, not having gone through the learning curve with the existing product.

Stay Out of the Field

Spending time in hospitals and patients' homes and watching carefully how products are actually used is a rich source of new ideas. If you want to stave off innovation, then talk to people in groups outside of the use environment. It is much harder for them or for you to understand what the real issues are or to come up with really innovative alternatives.

Conclusion

Yes, it is easy for us to pontificate about innovation and its common causes of death. We are not making decisions that put millions of R&D dollars at risk. Fair enough. Economic risk certainly needs to be addressed, and quantitative methods need to be applied to assess and reduce it. However, there is also economic risk in not taking chances. As we have all seen, many new ideas that led to successful products came not from industry leaders but from start-ups, the products shown above being prime examples, as are Abiocore's artificial heart, or chemical sterilization originally developed by the then-start-up, Steris, or compact insulin pumps developed by Minimed.

Sure, you can eventually buy the start-ups. But which would you prefer — to pay top dollar for new ideas once they demonstrate their value in the marketplace, or to generate them within your own company? If you want to avoid innovation, you will know the answer.

Key Points

- Innovation is crucial for successful user-centered medical product development.
- Many companies, however, have (presumably unintentional) systems in place for discouraging innovation.

- Some specific ways to kill innovation include misapplying QFD or similar systems, restricting industrial designers' roles to that of stylists, emphasizing time-to-market above all else, punishing product failure more than rewarding product success, designing by consensus, embracing product complexity, relying exclusively on user preference testing, and avoiding studying how products are actually used in the field.

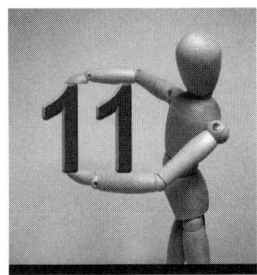

Developing Testable Product Simulations: Speed Is of the Essence

Stephen B. Wilcox

New technology allows for the creation of testable prototypes earlier in the product-development process. Earlier testable prototypes means better user-centered design.

User testing can be difficult for any product. A common source of frustration is the message that user testing would be futile early in the process because there is nothing to test. Then, later, when there is a working prototype to test, the message is that it is too late to make changes, that the design is frozen due to limited development budgets and a tight schedule — a classic Catch-22.

Is it possible to undertake user testing at an early stage of product development? In this chapter, we discuss methods for doing just that — simulating products early in the development process in order to enable user testing to be performed before more sophisticated look-like/works-like prototypes are available.

While we focus primarily on electronic products, the methods can often apply to nonelectronic products as well.

The Platform

The first step is to select the appropriate platform for the prototype. The purpose of the platform is to take some sort of input (either user input or

103

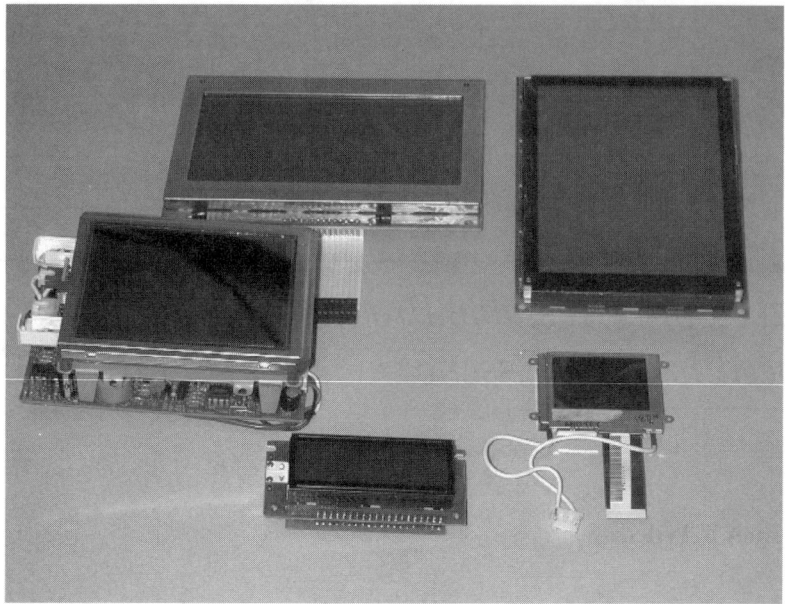

FIGURE 11.1
Some display options.

input from some sort of sensor) and to create various outputs as a response to the input. Possibilities for platforms include PCs, PDAs, or microcontrollers.

Windows and the Mac Operating Systems are relatively flexible environments for user interface prototyping. Generally speaking, if the final product will run on a Windows- or Palm-based computer, the same device should be used for the prototyping. Often, difficulties arise from using a prototype language that is slower than the language to be used in the final software development; such difficulties can be avoided by using a faster PC or PDA to make the speed more similar to that of the final product. However, there are cases when one would need to slow down a prototype to match the response time of the actual product. This is particularly true when prototyping a device that uploads and downloads information to a network — a step that can incur delays due to network response times.

The Display Device

For prototypes running on PCs, there are two ways to "talk" to displays: through the PC's video output, or via the serial or parallel port. These two methods require different types of displays (see Figure 11.1). Only serial displays are supported in a prototype running from a microcontroller.

Developing Testable Product Simulations: Speed Is of the Essence 105

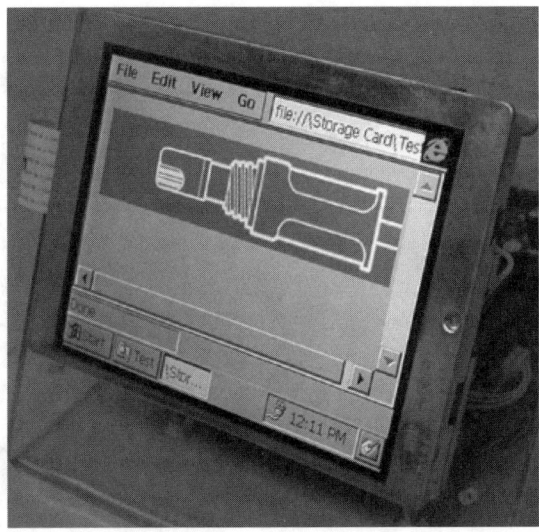

FIGURE 11.2
Testing of a prototype on the actual screen.

The display used for the user interface prototype should be as close as possible to the real device. Size, resolution, color, brightness, contrast, and viewing angle should be considered. Discrepancies between the prototype and the final product can result in usability or acceptability problems with the product that cannot be detected in the user testing. For example, a color scheme that works well on a conventional CRT may be perfectly dreadful on a color LCD display. Thus, it is always prudent to test screen designs on the actual displays (see Figure 11.2).

The Input Device

Input devices allow users to interact with electronic devices (see Figure 11.3). The most frequently used input devices are keyboards, keypads, buttons, mice, touch pads, touch screens, rotary controls, and joysticks. A simple approach to selecting the appropriate input device for the prototype is to list the types of input devices the final system can work with, then to choose the best option from this list. You will then need to select an input channel for the prototype (e.g., keyboard/mouse port, serial port, or parallel port).

As with the display, prototype parameters should be as close a match as possible to what is known about the final product. Triggering force, travel distance, size, button spacing, and types of tactile feedback are among the elements that should be considered. Of course, many of these parameters

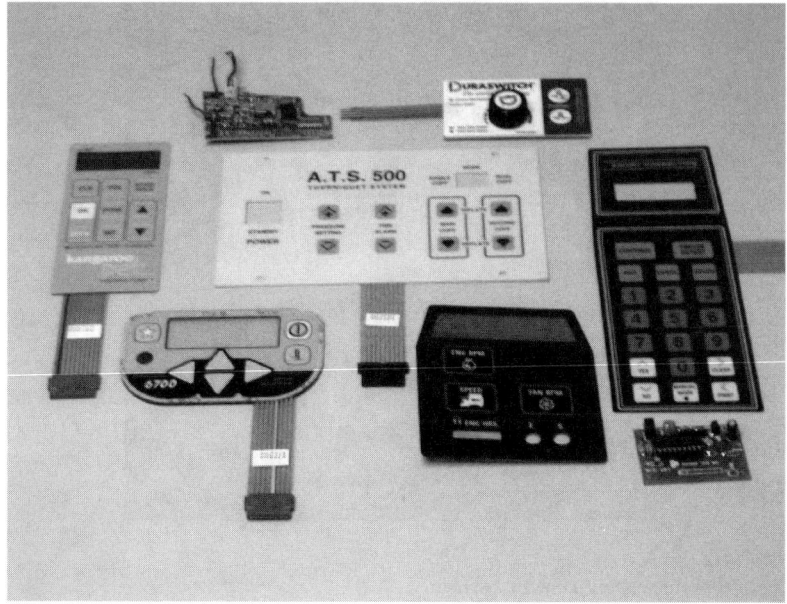

FIGURE 11.3
Input devices.

may not yet be resolved by the development team. However, it is important to make educated judgments about such features in order to reach the maximum level of realism possible.

Prototyping Software

There are a number of elements in prototyping software that will affect how well the user testing is able to mirror the real use of the product. Key criteria for the selection of prototyping software include the following:

- Short development time: The whole point of a testable prototype is to have it available as soon as possible. Thus, development time is a crucial factor for selecting user interface prototyping software.
- Easy modification: Creating a good product requires many changes during design concept development and preliminary usability testing. A good user interface prototyping application should allow changes to be made quickly and easily. There is nothing worse than having to stick with a bad interface because it is too much trouble to alter the prototype.

- Easy data input: To accurately evaluate the performance of a user interface design, the prototype should provide a "works-like" user input mechanism. The input should be accessible without requiring substantial additional hardware or programming effort.
- Easy text and graphics handling: To be able to display informative screen designs, the display should be able to handle different fonts in different sizes. Generally speaking, software development tools do not provide sophisticated graphics tools. Graphic design software, such as *Illustrator* or *Freehand*, should be used to create user interfaces that are similar to those that will be in the final product. This means that the prototyping software will need to accept common graphics file formats, such as *BMP, PICT, GIF,* and *JPEG*.
- Capability of handling lists of variables: Variables (parameters that are updated as changes occur) enable the developer to create detailed databases and other sophisticated systems.
- Sufficient mathematical functions: Math functions enable you to prototype devices that perform math calculations, such as a calculator.
- Sufficient timing functions: Timing functions are needed to prototype any electronic device that has a built-in timer or clock.

Software Options

Before making a decision about what prototyping and simulation software to use, it is important to know what functions are integral to the success of the final product and to the success of the user testing. You can then compare various software options based on your unique set of criteria. Macromedia *Director*, Microsoft *VisualBasic*, and Macromedia *Authorware* are among the most popular programs. Each of these tools meets the basic criteria listed above, but their relative advantages and disadvantages may make one or another better suited for different purposes.

Macromedia Director

At the beginning of its development, Macromedia Director was a time-based animation and presentation tool. However, it has been gradually developed into a complete programming environment, similar to VisualBasic or C++ (see Figure 11.4). Director is much slower than these alternatives, but the rapidly increasing processing power of PCs is making speed less and less important. Macromedia Director is capable of prototyping just about anything one can imagine in a fraction of the time required for a similar prototype in VisualBasic or C++. Changes and modifications are also easy to make. Macromedia Director runs on Windows or Mac OS.

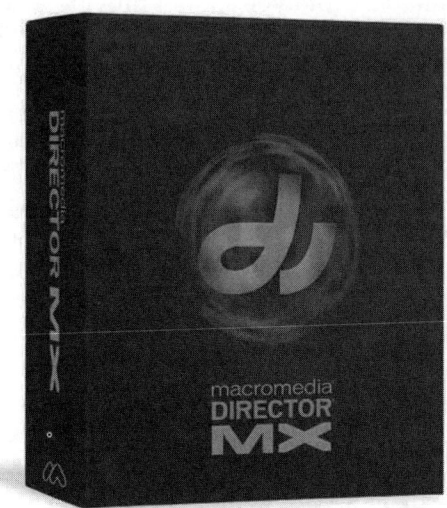

FIGURE 11.4
Macromedia Director is a flexible and fast software interface prototyping tool.

VisualBasic

Although VisualBasic was originally thought of as a prototyping tool, it is being used increasingly for software development. Since Macromedia Director does not run on Palmtop computers, VisualBasic may be a good choice for Palm or Windows CE-based interface prototyping. It is relatively easy to make changes and modifications in VisualBasic, but not as easy as with Director. The development time of VisualBasic is much shorter than for C and C++, but it runs much more slowly. VisualBasic runs on Windows-based PCs and PalmOS (through Palmtop software development tools), but not on Macs.

Macromedia Authorware

Macromedia Authorware is a good choice for nonprogrammers who are creating their own user interface prototypes. Users build user interface prototypes by placing icons on flow lines, much like creating a flow chart of the user interface. Authorware's development time can be even shorter than Director, and it is easy to make changes. However, because of the limitations of a visual programming tool, Authorware is much less flexible than both Director and VisualBasic. Authorware programs run on both PCs and Macs.

Developing Testable Product Simulations: Speed Is of the Essence 109

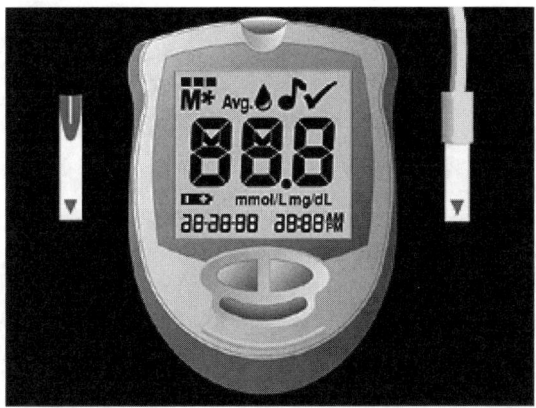

FIGURE 11.5
A screen simulation of hardware and the software interface.

Simulation Alternatives

With the aid of new technology, all sorts of quick prototypes are feasible, making it easier and easier to get user feedback while it is still early enough to make a difference. There are a few ways that all this can be put together. One obvious way to do prototyping is to simulate a software product on a PC. Other alternatives (shown above) include:

- Simulating hardware devices on a CRT screen (see Figure 11.5). Of course, much of the look and feel get lost, but the basic logic and understandability of a system can be tested when a "working" prototype is created via the computer screen that can be operated with the mouse. Increased realism can be added by using a touch screen.
- Adding buttons, keypads, or LCD screens to foamcore models, or other simple models, and tethering the result to a PC. A working prototype can be very quickly cobbled together this way (see Figure 11.6).
- Using off-the-shelf products to simulate products. We have used Palm Pilots with various types of input and various sorts of overlaid bezels to simulate a wide variety of handheld products.
- Embedding stamps, displays, and controls into rough models. Stamps are microprocessors without all of the bulk of full computers. They are very useful when you want to maintain a realistic form factor without tethering to a computer.

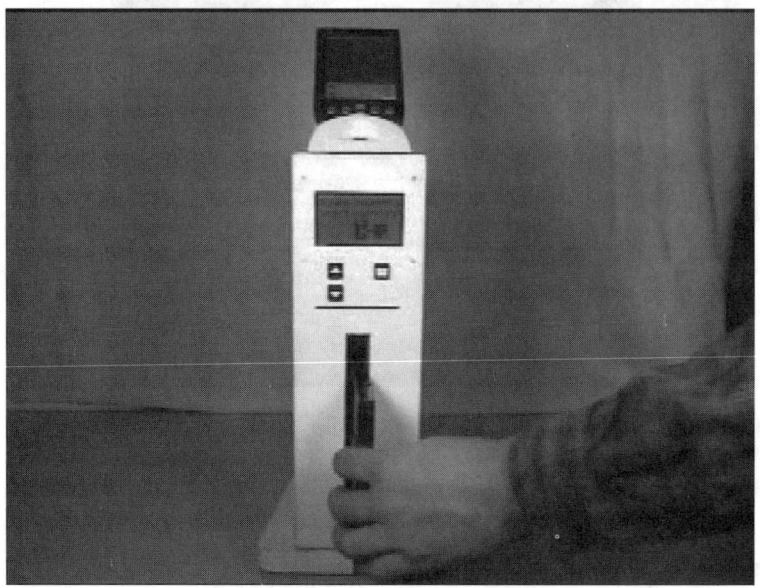

FIGURE 11.6
A low-fidelity hardware and software prototype.

Conclusion

Regardless of the type of simulation you decide to pursue or the tools you use to generate it, the key is to do user testing as soon as possible so you can get user feedback early enough to refine the design before it is too late. Today's technology makes user testing feasible early on. There is no excuse to wait until you have an Alpha model to test various aspects of your design. So don't put off until tomorrow what you can do today, because, among other things, "tomorrow" can translate into "never" in today's world, where time-to-market is crucial.

Acknowledgment

Li Yue, of Design Science, coauthored an earlier version of this chapter.

Key Points

- New technology is available for creating testable simulations very early in the product development process.
- Important decisions that have to be made are the choices of platform, of display, or input device, and of software simulation tools.
- The most crucial determinant of the choice of platforms, displays, and input devices is to keep them as close as possible to what is expected for the final product.
- Prototyping/simulation software includes Macromedia Director, VisualBasic and Macromedia Authorware.
- Prototyping options include simulating hardware devices on a CRT screen; adding real input devices, such as buttons and pointing devices; to a rough model and tethering it to a computer; altering off-the-shelf products, such as PDAs; or embedding microprocessors (stamps) into models.

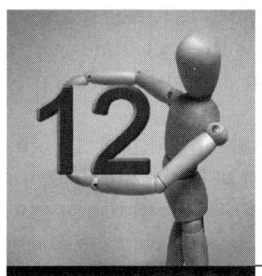

Patient Simulators Breathe Life into Product Testing

Michael E. Wiklund

Patient simulators enable device manufacturers to conduct realistic usability tests early in the development process, without placing patients at risk.

Late one evening in Chattanooga, a control-room operator scrambles to reestablish coolant flow to a nuclear reactor that threatens to overheat. On final approach to Atlanta's Hartsfield International Airport, a Boeing 757 pilot urgently advances the engines to full power to escape severe wind shear. And in Boston, an anesthesiologist works frenetically to lower the temperature of a patient experiencing malignant hyperthermia, a potentially fatal reaction to anesthesia.

How were these crises resolved? In all three cases, fast and effective action prevented disaster. But in reality, no one was at risk — because these emergencies occurred in advanced, computer-based simulators that could simply be reset, allowing simulation participants another chance to avert disaster.

Advanced simulators have been an integral part of control-room operator and pilot training programs for more than two decades. In fact, today's airline pilots are often certified to fly new types of aircraft based solely on their simulator training experience, training in real aircraft being cost prohibitive and arguably no more effective. By comparison, the use of simulators for medical training purposes is a more recent development, but one that is gaining in popularity.

Advanced simulation can overcome the limitations of the traditional training methods — such as classroom instruction and observation — used in

113

medicine. It allows learning by means of trial and error, in a risk-free manner. Adding to the credibility of this new training method is the fact that several teaching hospitals now include time spent working in a simulation facility as a residency rotation.

Medical device manufacturers who seek feedback on their product designs should regard the medical establishment's shift toward using simulators for training purposes as good news. Simulators give manufacturers the opportunity to see how prototypes perform in realistic use scenarios, without placing patients at risk. For example, a simulator makes it possible to test a prototype intravenous infusion pump's ease of operation without fear of overdosing a real patient.

During specified tasks, such as loading a tubing set into an infusion pump, one can introduce several kinds of ambient distractions and stressors, such as distracting comments by workmates, phone calls, paging system announcements, deliveries from the pharmacy, complaints of pain from the patient, a disconcerting drop in the patient's blood pressure or heart rate, and associated patient monitor alarms. These kind of environmental factors can make a large difference in the user's ability to concentrate on the task at hand, and can provoke use errors that may not arise in a laboratory setting.

Such testing may confirm the pump's operation as logical and intuitive, or it may expose design shortcomings that frustrate clinicians and cause them to make mistakes. Discovering and fixing such design shortcomings early in the development process — rather than after the product is already in clinical trials or in widespread use — has several payoffs for manufacturers:

- Avoidance of time-consuming redesign efforts, thereby reducing time-to-market
- Credible usability claims that benefit sales
- Reduced exposure to product liability suits
- Satisfying the FDA by approaching user-interface design in a manner consistent with the quality system regulation, which places strong emphasis on user testing

Realistic Testing

Typically, manufacturers use a combination of testing methods to validate their product designs. During the early stages of product development, a manufacturer may conduct a series of usability tests, which typically take place in a controlled laboratory setting. Testing is carried out in one room while unobtrusive observation takes place in an adjacent room via a one-way mirror and video equipment. Such tests focus solely on user-device interactions, albeit in a manner that is isolated from certain factors influencing human performance, such as the working environment, which could be congested and noisy, or interactions with other people who may present a distraction.

During a usability test, participants may freely explore how a device works as well as perform specific tasks, including those critical to patient safety. While performing tasks, test participants normally talk aloud while they work so that the test administrators can follow their thoughts, decisions, and actions and understand how these relate to the product design under evaluation. Such tests, which may include just a few days of hands-on product use by test participants, can be performed well ahead of the clinical trial while it is still relatively easy and inexpensive to make meaningful design changes.

Later in the development cycle, once operational devices are available, manufacturers typically conduct clinical trials over a period of several weeks or months. The focus of such trials is to evaluate a device's safety and efficacy in a real-world scenario with the obvious regulatory overtones. Clinical trials focus on usability in a less systematic way than in a usability test. Inevitably, it is difficult to conduct a complete usability evaluation of a device in clinical trials because some user scenarios rarely arise. Also, usability problems are reported anecdotally, which may result in inaccuracies, instead of being documented by trained observers as in the case of usability testing. Conducting usability tests in simulators provides the realism associated with clinical trials as well as greater control and freedom to introduce a wide range of user scenarios.

The Technology

One of the first modern simulators was constructed in 1986 at Stanford University. By the late 1990s, there were about 100 "full up" patient simulators in use worldwide, with the number of installations increasing rapidly, according to Dan Raemer, Ph.D., program coordinator at The Center for Medical Simulation, Inc. (CMS) in Cambridge, MA. It is estimated that there are hundreds more lower fidelity medical simulators used for training purposes that may employ a lower cost mannequin, simple video recording equipment (i.e., a camcorder), and a spare operating room, for example.

The majority of simulation facilities are concentrated in the United States on the East and West coasts, with several others scattered across the country and abroad. Most of the facilities are operated by teaching hospitals affiliated with academic institutions. CMS, for example, is a resource shared by several teaching hospitals in Boston, including the Beth Israel Deaconess Medical Center, Children's Hospital, Brigham and Women's Hospital, and Massachusetts General Hospital. It has trained more than 1000 clinicians since it opened and has been the site of several device usability research studies.

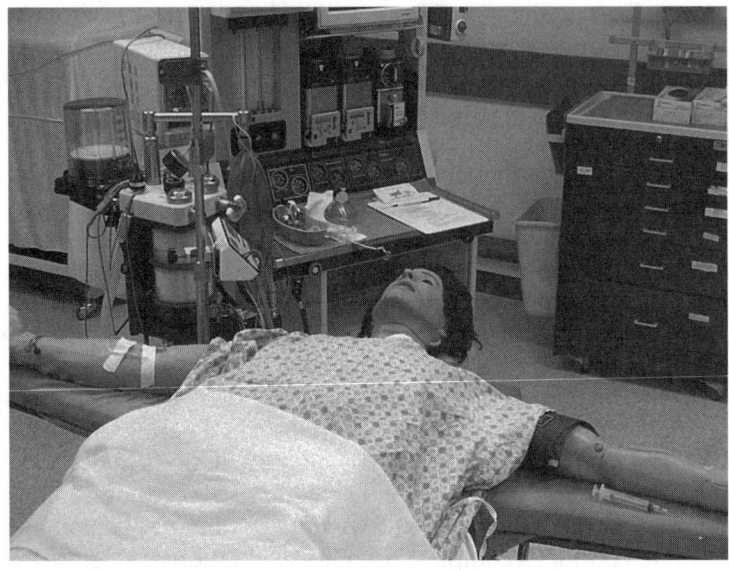

FIGURE 12.1
The patient mannequin moves, breathes, and reacts to stimuli, heightening the realism of the simulation. Photo courtesy of The Center for Medical Simulation, Inc.

Simulators comprise several core elements. The most visible is the patient mannequin (Figure 12.1), which resembles the mannequins used for cardiopulmonary resuscitation training, although much more advanced. For instance, patient mannequins used for simulation purposes produce breathing sounds as the electromechanical lungs inhale and exhale according to computer-based instructions. They have anatomically correct airways as well as a palpable pulse and heart rhythm that can be monitored on an electrocardiograph. Some mannequins have arms and legs that are capable of moving and swelling, and computer-controlled eyes that respond appropriately to various stimuli. Some even have gas analyzers that recognize the makeup of inhaled medications and cause the mannequin to respond accordingly.

The original Eagle Patient Simulator, developed by David Gaba, M.D. and others at Stanford University, connected to an interface cart that drove the mannequin's electromechanical functions. The cart also served as the interface for conventional monitoring equipment found in the operating room. For example, it provided a flow of physiological data to off-the-shelf pulse oximeters and invasive blood pressure monitors, further heightening the realism of the simulation. Stanford's simulator had a "split brain," consisting of two computers that operated simultaneously to control all aspects of the simulation. One computer ran the programs designed to simulate the human body, including its cardiovascular, pulmonary, metabolic, fluid and electrolyte balance, and thermal-regulation characteristics. The computer program's sophistication made it capable of accurately modeling the body's

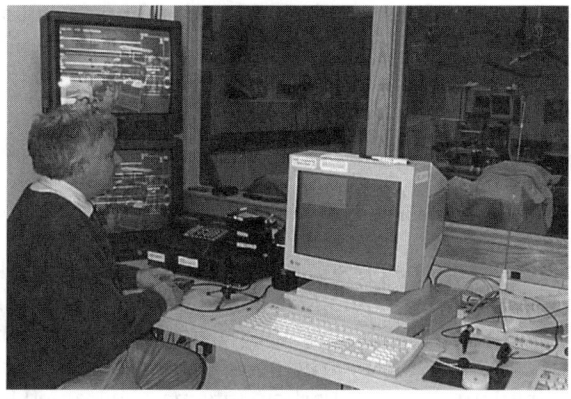

FIGURE 12.2
The patient mannequin and its simulated responses are controlled via keyboard and mouse commands. Photo courtesy of The Center for Medical Simulation, Inc.

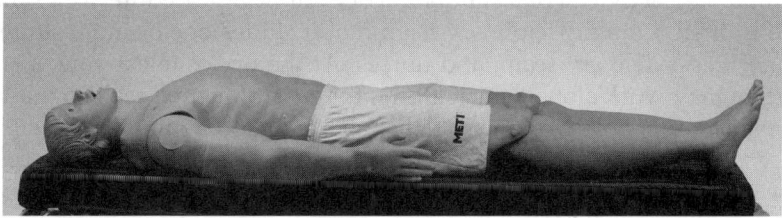

FIGURE 12.3
METI's Human Patient Simulator. Photo courtesy of Medical Education Technologies, Inc. ©METI 2004.

reaction to myriad physiological inputs, such as intravenous drug administration. The second computer ran the software that allowed the test administrator to control the simulation (see Figure 12.2). For example, it enabled the technicians to determine the patient's cardiovascular health and procedural events such as hypoxemia, anaphylaxis, or myocardial ischemia. Since its initial introduction, the simulator evolved technologically and functionally to present clinicians with an ever more compelling patient care experience. However, it is no longer marketed.

Today, there are two major players in the simulator market. One is Medical Education Technologies, Inc. (Sarasota, FL), which produces a patient simulator similar to the Eagle unit (see Figure 12.3). The company's Human Patient Simulator (HPS) is used at more than 70 institutions worldwide, including universities, hospitals, community colleges, technical schools, and military sites. METI claims that the simulator is so engrossing that students training on it have been brought to tears when the patient "dies." The other major player is Laerdal Medical Corporation (Wappingers Falls, NY), which markets SimMan®, which includes an advanced airway feature and allows the simulation of many different clinical interventions, such as blood pressure measurements at the arm.

Running a Simulation

Technically, it only takes one person to control a simulator via keyboard and mouse commands. However, another staff member is generally needed to orchestrate the simulation and coach the participants so the simulation proceeds productively. Additional participants can play supporting roles, such as charge and circulating nurses. Participants may be trained to facilitate the simulation, or they may assume roles that draw on their prior experiences and are designed to teach them to manage both complex medical situations that call for individual know-how and integrated teamwork.

The number of participants on the clinician side depends on the nature of the simulated activity. For a simulation of a surgical procedure, for example, there is often a multidisciplinary team that includes one or more surgeons, an anesthesia delivery team, and nurses. At the opposite extreme, a single clinician may work alone, which allows for environmental realism but lacks the realism of people working together as a team. Sometimes, if the simulation exercise has a technological research and development focus, one or more clinical engineers and manufacturer's representatives observe or participate in the simulation.

In keeping with a high-fidelity simulation, participants may follow a normal, preoperative routine, including scrubbing and donning gowns. To further increase the realism of the simulation, someone may play the role of the patient, conversing with clinicians prior to being wheeled into the operating room. A live conversation can still take place in the operating room between the patient mannequin and the clinician (presumably the anesthesiologist) up until induction and then again during recovery, by means of a speaker and microphone built into the mannequin.

The Environment

To achieve maximum realism, unused operating rooms are an excellent place to set up a patient simulator. However, the hospital setting presents logistical challenges — such as obtaining clearances for test participants and observers — that ultimately make it less tenable. For this reason, CMS is set up as a dedicated training facility that mimics an operating room in a conventional office building.

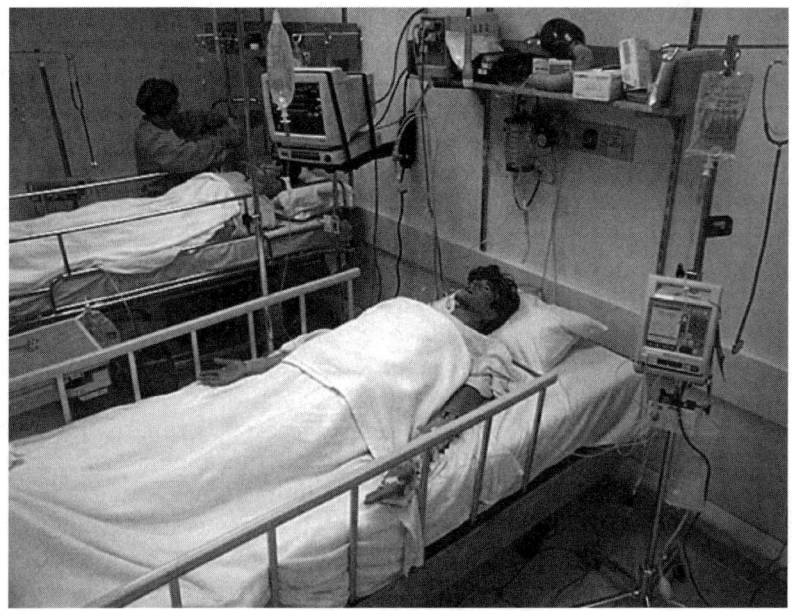

FIGURE 12.4
Simulated intensive care unit. Photo courtesy of The Center for Medical Simulation, Inc.

CMS's operating room is equipped with an operating table, appropriate lighting, a cadre of patient-monitoring and therapy devices, and attendant supplies, so that clinicians can work naturally. The simulated operating room is also equipped with one-way mirrors and video cameras for unobtrusive observation and documentation of simulator activities, including usability tests of medical devices. Rooms are set aside for technicians to run the simulator, for participants to prepare for mock surgery, and for observers and participants to discuss the proceedings.

While the majority of simulators are set up to mimic operating rooms, they are also used to simulate general and emergency medicine, and intensive-care settings and situations (See Figure 12.4). CMS reports that more than half of its simulation exercises are focused on acute-care situations, as opposed to anesthesia delivery alone.

The Costs

A state-of-the-art human simulator costs between $30,000 and $200,000, depending on whether or not it is capable of modeling a patient's physiological and pharmacological state and response to therapy. Facility modifications and support equipment, including audio and visual recording equipment, can cost an additional $200,000 or so, although more austere solutions are possible. Still, costs approaching half a million dollars or more are modest in comparison to the cost of medical facilities in general, particularly if the simulator costs are borne by large organizations that have an extensive, continuing need to train medical staff.

Such costs do place patient simulators out of reach of many medical device manufacturers. In fact, cost justification for building a simulator may continue to hinge on the training benefits to medical students, since many medical device companies are just beginning to embrace the need for user testing prior to clinical trials and have not earmarked the funds necessary for more advanced approaches. However, the FDA's push for companies to take a more user-centered design approach could lead to increased investments in such testing facilities.

While facilities such as CMS may appear to be set up primarily for training purposes, the staff is anxious to work with device manufacturers as well. "We have run a few usability studies for manufacturers at our facility, but we could and should be doing a lot more," says Raemer. "Considering how productive and comparatively economical the tests have been, I'm frankly surprised by the limited demand that we have experienced to date." CMS charges manufacturers a daily rate to use the facility, including the services of a technician — that is just slightly more than the daily rental cost of some focus-group facilities.

The Participant Experience

People who have participated in operating room simulations — occupying the "hot seat" — regard the experience as highly realistic. "People get geared up pretty quickly," Raemer says. "Within a few minutes, participants are taking things seriously. They get totally absorbed in the experience, to the point that it becomes nearly indistinguishable from reality." Although participating clinicians may initially tend to act somewhat reserved, this attitude typically changes quite quickly to a more relaxed behavior.

Raemer observes that a high degree of realism is essential to the thorough evaluation of medical devices: "People are going to behave differently under stressful and high-task-loading conditions. Whereas clinicians may be able to focus all of their attention on a device in a laboratory setting, they may be able to give the device only a fraction of that attention in an OR — real or simulated — when the patient is desaturating [experiencing a decline in the blood's oxygen level]."

Raemer compares these differing levels of attention to the experience of using a cellular phone in a car. "It's a lot easier trying to program numbers into a cellular phone when you are sitting in a parking lot, as opposed to while driving at high speed in heavy traffic. Analogously, the medical device that seemed so intuitive to operate in the laboratory may actually be confusing to operate in real-world conditions, for reasons you might not guess."

As an example, Raemer says he has watched innumerable test participants struggle to set up and operate a blood-warming device that seemed quite easy to use in an isolated environment, such as a test laboratory. He has also observed many simulator test participants experience difficulty locating a wrench used for adjusting the valves on gas bottles mounted to a particular anesthesia workstation, even though it is placed in a seemingly accessible position.

Raemer believes that not only is the hot-seat experience great for training medical personnel, but it can be equally beneficial for designer and engineer training. He allows that designers and engineers face limitations in terms of their clinical knowledge to the extent that they may require coaching; however, after their simulator experience, they are able to understand the user's perspective. For this reason, CMS has occasionally offered a course titled "Anesthesia for Amateurs."

A Clinician's Viewpoint

Matthew Weinger, M.D., formerly professor of anesthesiology at the University of California, San Diego, practiced at the Veterans Administration Medical Center (San Diego) and has a strong, professional interest in user-interface research and development. (He is currently at Vanderbilt University.) Weinger is co-chair of AAMI's human engineering committee, and spent approximately a year working with Gaba at Stanford's simulator. While in California, he had access to his own simulation facility at the San Diego Center for Patient Safety. In Weinger's view, "Simulators are an effective compromise or middle ground between laboratory testing and testing in the actual operating room or acute clinical-care environment."

Drawing a comparison with laboratory testing, he states that "the simulator enables significantly greater consideration of the context of performing tasks and interacting with other people. This may be especially important in the evaluation of devices that are complex, resource-intensive, and highly integrated with other devices and data sources. It is also important for devices that will replace well-established devices, or require tasks to be performed in a new or novel manner."

Regarding the selection of test participants, Weinger believes that simulators are too sophisticated to use nondomain experts as test subjects. As such, he advocates using surgeons in tests involving surgical devices, for example, as opposed to using people who may have extensive knowledge of surgery but have never used a scalpel. Nonetheless, Weinger acknowledges the value of involving nonclinicians in simulations to orient them to task demands and make them more empathetic designers.

Comparing it to a real clinical setting, Weinger says, "The simulator potentially may have greater availability, making scheduling easier; however, you still need experienced users who may be reluctant to participate without receiving renumeration, especially if they must forego regular clinical duties. This may result in an additional cost. The simulator can run the same scenario over and over — a real advantage over the clinical setting — thus it offers a more controlled environment. The simulator can also be used for worst-case scenario testing (e.g., crises or critical events). Generalization to the real clinical-use setting is much easier with the simulator than with laboratory tests, but it is still a bit of a leap — albeit a surmountable one."

What role should simulators play in medical device development efforts? Weinger thinks they can and should play a role, especially in devices that meet the criteria previously mentioned (i.e., complex, resource-intensive devices that are highly integrated with other devices and data sources, as well as devices that replace other well-established devices or require tasks to be performed in a new manner). However, he does not think that simulators can wholly replace testing in actual clinical-use environments. "There are too many complex, unanticipated factors," he says, "especially interpersonal interactions. So, I see simulators as a complementary, intermediate tool with specific and valuable uses, especially worst-case scenario testing. Their use may permit postponement of appreciable actual-use-environment testing to later in the development cycle; however, it will not reduce the need for extensive and continuous end-user input and involvement in the development process."

Weinger adds a cautionary note: "The cost [of a simulator for device testing] may be a big limitation for a manufacturer, unless the company already has its own simulator and trained personnel to run it. It may be more expensive than actual operating room testing, although a formal cost-effectiveness comparison has not been done. Another cost-related limitation is the need for clinical personnel to design and run the simulations."

Thus, Weinger views simulation-based product testing as clinician driven, whereas others may see clinicians as marginally involved, except when it comes to actual task performance in the simulator. The costs and benefits of both approaches are likely to be case dependent.

For Additional Information on Patient Simulators, Visit the Following Web Sites:

Note that the following Web sites were active as of this book's publication date. If they are no longer active, a search based on the keywords *medical simulation* or *patient simulator* should lead to useful information.

- Human factors requirements — www.fda.gov/cdrh/humfac/hufacimp.html
- The Center for Medical Simulation — www.harvardmedsim.org
- The Simulator Center at Stanford University — www.med.stanford.edu/school/Anesthesia/simcntr.html
- The Human Patient Simulator — www.meti.com/hps.html
- SimMan® Universal Patient Simulator — www.laerdal.com

Conclusion

In view of FDA regulations requiring the application of human factors engineering in design, the medical industry is just now embracing usability testing as a means to evaluate medical devices before they are brought to market. The change will be good for an industry noted for producing complex devices that can pose usability problems even for some of the most intelligent and highly trained individuals.

Some companies will approach usability testing in a minimalist manner, such as setting up a prototype device in an office and having prospective users run through a handful of tasks. This approach may very well produce useful findings, considering that a lot can be learned about a product when it's used intensively, in an isolated manner. However, many human factors experts would agree that test results can be distorted by such isolation. Accordingly, companies that are driven toward design excellence through usability testing should carefully consider the advantages of using a simulator.

The costs of a simulator are almost certain to be higher compared with laboratory-based or more minimalist testing approaches, but the benefits may be worth it, considering the potential competitive advantage arising from the resulting design improvements and associated marketing claims.

Companies should also consider the potential savings arising from finding subtle usability problems that manifest themselves only in realistic use, at a stage when it is still economical to correct them. Fixing such problems can be very expensive if detection is forestalled until clinical trials begin or—even worse—when the product comes to market.

Key Points

- Advanced simulation can overcome the limitations of the traditional training methods — such as classroom instruction and observation

- used in medicine. It allows learning by means of trial and error, in a risk-free manner.
- Simulators give manufacturers the opportunity to see how prototypes perform in realistic use scenarios, without placing patients at risk.
- Presently, there are about 100 "full up" patient simulators in use worldwide, but the number of installations is increasing rapidly.
- Conducting usability tests in simulators provides the realism associated with clinical trials as well as greater control and freedom to introduce a wide range of user scenarios.
- People who have participated in operating room simulations — occupying the "hot seat" — regard the experience as highly realistic.
- The most visible is the patient mannequin, which resembles the mannequins used for cardiopulmonary resuscitation training, although much more advanced. A patient mannequin may have lungs that expand and contract while producing realistic breathing sounds, an anatomically correct airway, a palpable pulse and heart rhythm that can be monitored on an electrocardiograph, arms and legs that are capable of moving and swelling, and computer-controlled eyes that respond appropriately to various stimuli.
- A simulator enables significantly greater consideration of the context of performing tasks and interacting with other people. This may be especially important in the evaluation of devices that are complex, resource-intensive, and highly integrated with other devices and data sources.

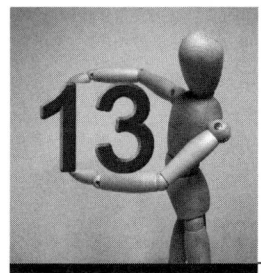

Return of the Renaissance Person: A Valuable Contributor to Medical Product Development

Stephen B. Wilcox

We live in an age of specialization. However, medical product development teams can greatly benefit from including people with expertise in multiple fields. Industrial design is one field that is inherently multidisciplinary in its approach.

It seems likely that the present period may go down in history as the Era of Specialization. We have gone from dry goods stores to separate stores for socks, refrigerator magnets, and bagels. You used to need a doctor. Now you need a specialist in arthroscopic knee surgery or an endocrinologist who specializes in type II diabetes.

In the case of medical product development, we have moved from designers and engineers to multidisciplinary teams of specialists representing more and more specialties. And, of course, in order to achieve user-centered design, it is crucial to include team members who are specialists in understanding the ultimate product users. But, to use our own discipline of human factors as an example, it appears to be branching into ethnographic human factors, biomechanical human factors, cognitive human factors, etc. What is driving this specialization is, among other things, the explosion of information, making it difficult for one person to know enough to be a successful generalist.

Don't get us wrong. Multidisciplinary team-based medical product development is immensely superior to its historical antecedents and at the core of user-centered design. We are by no means advocating going back to the bad old days of developing products without various forms of expertise or

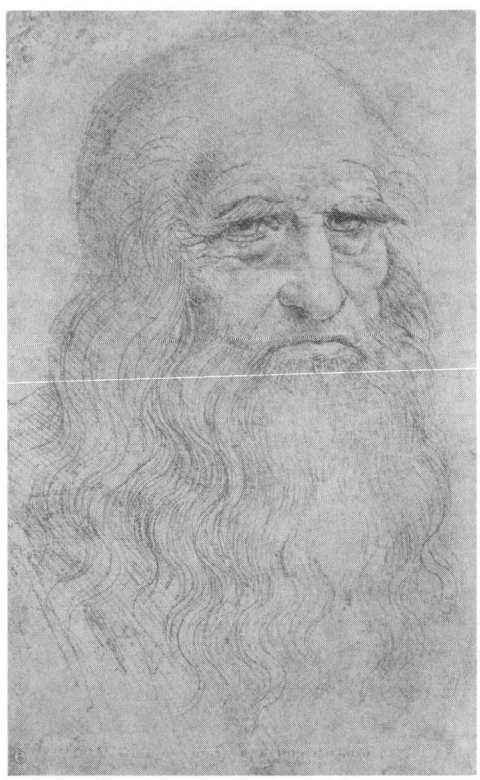

FIGURE 13.1
The original Renaissance Man.

developing products in a linear fashion, in which each discipline has control at a different stage of the process. But we fear that we have gone too far. Product development teams become more cumbersome as additional disciplines elbow their way to the table. As teams get larger, decisions get harder to make, jeopardizing the time-to-market advantage, a key reason for the multidisciplinary approach in the first place. Also, despite the value of added expertise, everything else being equal, the larger the decision-making body, the less intelligent its decisions. To summarize, we need to find a way of expanding the value of the interdisciplinary team as an approach to medical product design without imploding the whole process. The answer, we think, lies in the multidisciplinary person. What we need here is nothing less than a reversal of the trend toward specialization. We need that nearly extinct individual, the renaissance person, who is an expert in more than one discipline (see Figure 13.1).

Unfortunately, we can't see how anyone today can be a true renaissance person, in the sense of knowing a lot about a large number of disciplines. What *is* feasible, though, is to know a lot about at least two disciplines by training in an interdisciplinary program, conducting a concerted campaign of self-education, or training in two different disciplines. Some examples (taken largely from actual people we know) include:

- Business and industrial design, to produce design concepts that reflect a business strategy
- Mechanical engineering and industrial design, to constrain a design at the beginning by more sophisticated engineering considerations
- Graphic design and software engineering, to create attractive screen prototypes that are compatible with the constraints of the code
- Human factors and industrial design, to address the needs of users in a sophisticated way during the design process

These are just a few possibilities, of course. They indicate a way to get smaller teams and a more streamlined product development process: have individual members who can, so to speak, fill two slots.

And this miracle becomes possible as the continued acceleration of the information explosion — which led to specialization in the first place — changes what it means to be an expert. You no longer need to spend years developing specific skills or hours poring over all the journals in your discipline to keep up with the latest developments. Today, the body of knowledge in many fields is changing so rapidly that the young, rather than the old, are the repositories of knowledge, and there is just too much information to be able to keep up. Nowadays, then, to be an expert is to know how to quickly find the information you need, digest it efficiently, and put it to use effectively.

Whether or not co-training becomes more common, however, there is one discipline that appears to be ideally suited for operating in a user-centered, multidisciplinary world — industrial design. Industrial design has always been multidisciplinary by its very nature. The industrial designer is one person on a product development team who has to know something about virtually all of the other disciplines — enough marketing to communicate with the marketing people, enough engineering to keep from designing products that are not feasible, enough about human factors to be a credible advocate for the user. Thus, industrial design education includes some engineering, some marketing, some human factors, and so on. A real handicap in a world of specialists, the interdisciplinary nature of the industrial designer partially accounts, we suspect, for the fact that few CEOs of medical device companies have come from the industrial design studio.

However, in a multidisciplinary world, the industrial designer is uniquely positioned to play an important role. Who is better at, for example, integrating the concerns of marketing and engineering? Who is better at juggling cost vs. quality vs. safety vs. customer appeal vs. consistency among different products? Of course the industrial designer cannot accomplish these goals alone, but he or she can serve as a key integrator on a multidisciplinary team.

To summarize, industrial design is a key discipline for the development of medical products in today's world. However, for the designer to provide maximum value, he or she probably needs to do a better job than most at learning what needs to be learned, and product development teams probably need to do a better job than most at using the designer effectively.

Designers should, at a minimum, do a better job of learning basic quantitative and writing skills, so they can communicate better with other team members and corporate management. The typical designer has the special skill of communicating by creating visual images, but that is not usually enough. Designers should also make every effort to understand the underlying clinical issues in depth, how products are used in the real clinical environment, the dynamics of the marketplace, the complex intellectual property issues that the engineering team has to deal with, etc.

At the same time, medical product companies can use industrial designers more effectively if they integrate them more fully into the product development effort. The designer who is forced to simply execute a design already determined by the marketing or engineering team is a designer who is not providing adequate value. Industrial designers have a lot to contribute early in a program as the product is still being conceptualized. They are good at generating ideas, translating ideas into visual form, and at adapting technologies to the needs of product users. And, as we have said, in general, they are good at integrating information from a variety of disparate sources.

Conclusion

The second age of the renaissance person is at hand. Unless we want medical product development teams to require expanded facilities for their meetings, as we achieve user-centered design, it behooves medical product developers to supplement specialists with people who have expertise in multiple fields. The industrial designer, with his or her diverse training, can provide a special contribution in a multidisciplinary environment. However, it is important for both industrial designers and the organizations that employ them to adjust to the new requirements of integrated user-centered medical product development.

Key Points

- The need for several disciplines on user-centered medical product development teams creates a need for individuals with more than one form of expertise in order to reduce the size of the team.

- People who are co-trained in, for example, mechanical engineering and marketing, or mechanical engineering and human factors, or human factors and industrial design are particularly valuable as members of user-centered medical product development teams.
- In addition to specifically co-trained team members, industrial designers, whose training includes exposure to multiple disciplines, can help to provide the "glue" that integrates an interdisciplinary team.
- The most effective industrial designers are those who can communicate quantitatively and in writing as well as visually.
- The most effective use of industrial designers is to integrate them early into the development team.

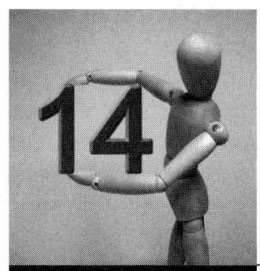

Patenting Software User Interfaces

Michael E. Wiklund

Supporters of patenting software user interfaces claim that the practice sparks creativity and contributes to the overall progress of the technology.

Patents are a testament to a company's technical prowess and artfulness, and the inventors named in a patent are typically proud of their achievements. In fact, many device manufacturers showcase their patents in a hallway or lobby display as one would an Academy Award. Patents also have a practical purpose, of course, placing proprietary technology and design solutions out of the competition's reach for many years or allowing for their use while generating substantial licensing fees for the patent holders.

Even those individuals who don't like the idea behind patents understand that they make perfect business sense. "I'm not a supporter of the ownership of ideas and the design solutions that emanate from them," says Christopher Goodrich, senior industrial designer at Datex–Ohmeda (Madison, WI), who nonetheless has experience with three software user interface patent applications for his company. "From the beginning of humankind, there's been an accumulation of knowledge, and to lay ownership of knowledge and its by-products doesn't seem right. However, companies gain a market advantage by owning the design solutions of their employees. It's an economic benefit for them."

Because patents are symbolically and financially quite valuable, many companies try to patent everything they can. Patent opportunities include various aspects of the software user interface, ranging from the software's general interaction style (often called its *look and feel*) to specific graphic elements such as icons.

Consumer software and product developers such as Microsoft Corp., Apple Computer, and Motorola have led the movement to patent the user interfaces, having been granted numerous patents with predictably jargon-filled titles, such as "task bar with start menu," "intuitive gesture-based graphical user interface," and "graphical user interface with icons having expandable descriptors." By comparison, medical companies that are accustomed to filing patents on hardware components (e.g., a new kind of pump or valve) have not taken full advantage of patent opportunities in the software domain. But the pattern appears to be changing. Joseph Rolla, a director at the U.S. Patent and Trademark Office (PTO), notes that "although the PTO has issued software-related patents for three decades, medical companies have become quite aggressive about pursuing patent protection for software user interfaces in only the past few years, particularly in the area of imaging."

Goodrich agrees that there has been a recent surge in medical-related software user interface patent applications. Having dealt with user interfaces for approximately 12 years, he has only recently been involved in their patenting. "It's a function of the medical product software as it matures in the marketplace," he explains, "and the usability of the user interface. As the number of companies entering the software arena increases, the products become quite similar. If there's one important aspect that distinguishes a product from another, and it's possible to protect that aspect, a patent can keep competitors from using it."

Form versus Function

Two types of patents pertain to software user interfaces. In essence, one type covers the form or appearance of a design and the other covers its functional features. Product developers may elect to apply for one or both types of patents to fully protect a particular user interface solution.

A *design patent* covers novel and nonobvious aspects of the user interface that can be considered graphical and ornamental in nature. Although the government uses the term *ornamental* to characterize visual design elements, there is actually no requirement that the design be attractive. However, there is a tacit assumption that design elements reflect a measure of artistic skill. Design patents typically cover user interface elements such as icons, type fonts, or the overall appearance of a particular screen. The patent protects the holder against other persons or companies creating a design that bears such close resemblance to the patented one, that a user may think that he or she is acquiring the original. Protection lasts 14 years from the date the patent is issued.

A *utility patent* covers the functional or useful aspects of the user interface, such as the overall organization and selection of menu options that comprise a process. This type of patent includes one or more claims that form the basis of protection against infringements. The patent holder's application is strengthened by claims that are as broad in scope as possible, as long as the claims are valid and do not infringe on those in other patents. A patent application can include up to 20 claims, although there are mechanisms to submit an even greater number.

As with a design patent, the utility aspects of the user interface must be original and nonobvious. Additionally, they must serve a useful and constructive purpose. Utility patents provide 20 years of protection, starting from the full patent application filing date. Because the PTO can take up to three years to grant a patent, the actual period of protection can be reduced to as little as 17 years.

According to Rolla, it is not difficult to establish the novelty of a particular user interface because most designs represent a unique combination of elements. However, one has to be alert to the existence of "prior art." For example, a company may develop a new medical device that employs a special pointing device, such as an isokinetic joystick, and seek patent protection because it is not found on any other medical device. However, if such a joystick was already in use in laptop computers, its existence would rule out a patent because the invention was not novel. A thorough review of related patents, Internet literature, existing software, textbooks, and published style guides for software user interfaces is the best means to ensure that a user interface is truly novel.

Nonobviousness is a more ambiguous matter that may present a greater hurdle to those seeking patent protection. To illustrate the concept of nonobviousness, Rolla gives a hypothetical example of a pivoting handle on a suitcase serving as inspiration for a pivoting handle on a briefcase. A patent application for such a briefcase handle would likely be rejected because it represents an obvious extension of the suitcase handle concept, albeit different in some respects.

Copyright protection automatically extends to written aspects of the user interface design, such as the text contained in an online help application or tutorial. Copyrights also cover the software code underlying a user interface, as it too is textual. The exception is software code that is not part of the originality one is hoping to protect but that is crucial to the basic functioning of the program. Copyrights on the text portions of a user interface design remain in effect for the extent of the author's lifetime plus 50 years — or 75 years if the work is owned by the author's employer.

A patent search helps establish a patent's scope (i.e., the extent to which one can make valid claims). Patent search specialists or members of a company's legal department can help identify and obtain copies of closely related patents. The related patents must be scrutinized to ensure that the new patent application will not infringe upon existing patents and to sort out which aspects of the new user interface are truly novel. This task should be relegated to the user interface developers most familiar with the design in question, as they are most qualified to evaluate the impact of claims made in related patents. Patent search consultants and attorneys can also facilitate the process.

"Sometimes the decision is clear-cut," says Goodrich. "For example, if your design is clearly in conflict with an existing patent, you stop. Other times, it may be fairly obvious that a slight change to your user interface will eliminate a conflict. But it's not always black-and-white." Applicants should be aware that if even one claim presents a problem, the entire product will infringe on the existing patent.

Can it be rewarding for an individual to create a potentially patentable idea for his or her company? Goodrich believes that most companies offer some type of incentive program to their employees — some giving incremental cash awards for a patent filing and issuance, or a lump sum, or a percentage of the product's sales.

The Patent Application

The application process can take between one and three years. Inventors or companies can get a head start on utility patents by filing a provisional application before the necessary work is completed for a full application. The major components of a provisional application are:

- A written description of the invention
- Any applicable drawings and associated descriptions
- The name(s) of the inventor(s)

A provisional application expires after 12 months and does not itself lead to a patent review. Rather, it is a placeholder for the full application, getting the application into the PTO's substantial queue before it is completed, thus cutting the overall waiting period. At times, it can take more than a year for a patent application to receive its initial action. Thus, submission of a provisional application could potentially reduce the waiting time for a full application review to as little as two months.

The delay in action is understandable when one considers that the PTO's staff receives hundreds of thousands of patent applications a year. Moreover, it takes an experienced examiner an average of three full working days to properly assess and render judgment on a single application.

A provisional application for a utility patent allows the term "patent pending" to be used in conjunction with a given invention. This status can give the patent holder a competitive advantage by discouraging competitors from producing similar designs. The exclusion of design patents from this benefit makes sense, considering that final appearance — as opposed to a fundamental process that may be subject to refinement — is the foundation of design patent applications.

Patenting Software User Interfaces

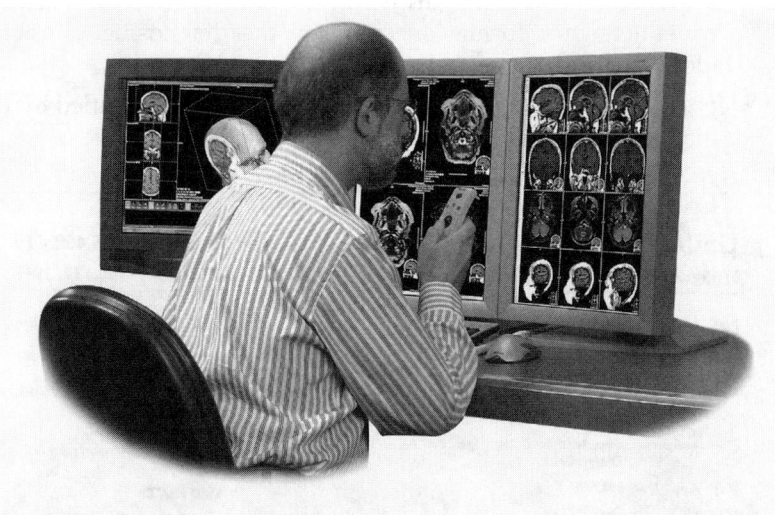

FIGURE 14.1
This database arranges images according to the reading radiologist's preferences. Photo courtesy of DR Systems, Inc.

A full or nonprovisional application includes a list of claims — the heart of the patent that may be the basis for infringement litigation. Goodrich defines a *claim* as a specific declaration regarding what is special about the item in question — "the meat of the product." Details of the unique features must be given in writing, which can be supplemented with line drawings or other illustrations. Since the claims tend to be the most difficult part of the application to prepare, Goodrich advises that any potentially patentable design be documented from the beginning of the product development process.

For example, in U.S. Pat. 5,452,416 filed by Dominator Radiology (DR Systems; San Diego, CA) in December 1992 and granted in September 1995, the company compiled 16 claims associated with the "organization, presentation, and manipulation of images" for the interface design of an MRI system (see Figure 14.1 and Figure 14.2). To illustrate the scope and tone of a claim, the text for claim 13 is presented below:

The computer display system of claim 1, wherein the respective fields of each diagnosing physician identifier specify:

- a mode of image series presentation
- a rectangular array format
- rectangular array dimensions
- the application means includes respective means for:
  - presenting an image series in a mode specified by a diagnosing physician identifer;

- presenting rectangular arrays in the first and second display containers in a format specified by the diagnosing physician identifier; and
- presenting the rectangular arrays in dimensions specified by the diagnosing physician identifier.

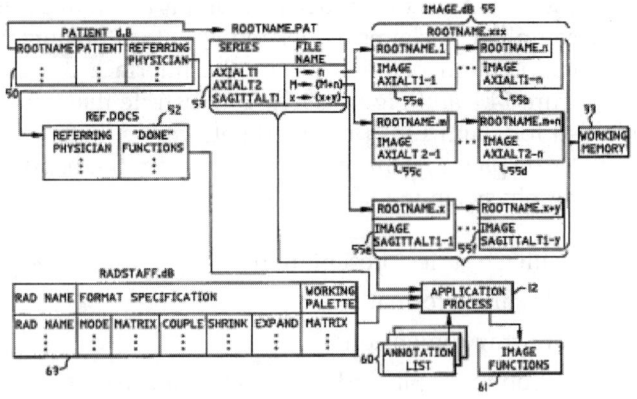

FIGURE 14.2
Selected documents relating to U.S. Pat. 5,452,416, filed by DR Systems, Inc. Drawings courtesy of DR Systems, Inc.; Images from the U.S. Patent and Trademark Office's Web site (www.uspto.gov/, as of April 2004).

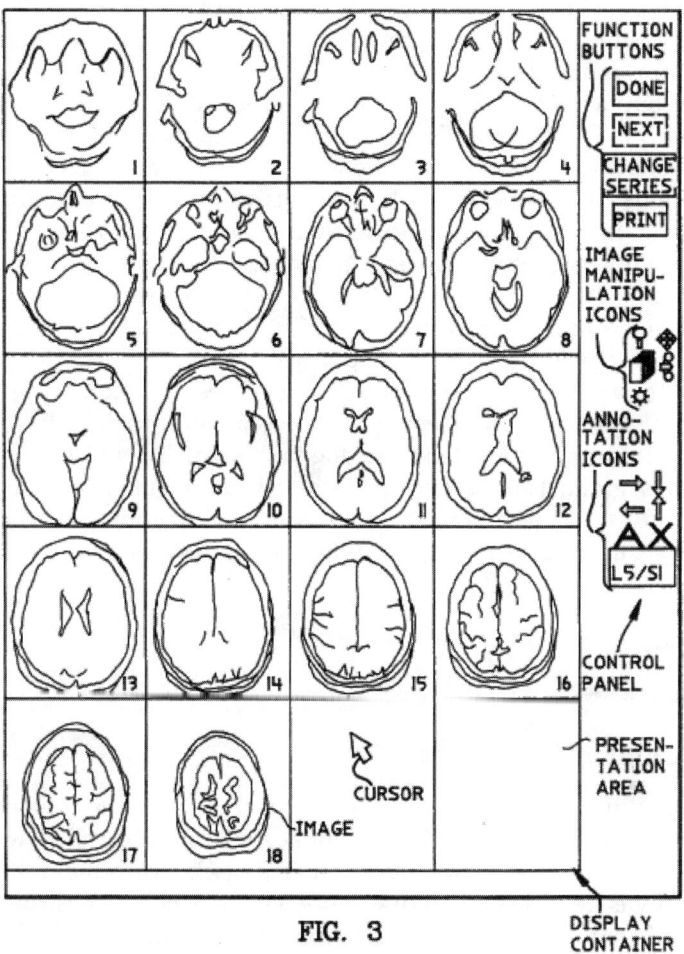

FIG. 3

FIGURE 14.2 (continued)

A number of patents can be viewed on a variety of Web sites.

Patent-Related Costs

Some patent application fees differ based on whether the patent entity — the inventor or the company that owns the invention — is classified as small or large (less than or more than 500 employees, respectively). Applicants must complete the appropriate form for small investor status, or the application will be treated as being from a large entity.

The basic filing fee for a full application is less than $1000, but additional PTO charges for services such as late filing or deadline extension fees can raise the application costs substantially. A schedule of such fees can be accessed on the patent office's Web site. However, the true cost of acquiring patent protection, including the patent search and attorney fees, can be tens of thousands of dollars. If the PTO rejects an initial application and the inventor or company chooses to resubmit the application with modified claims or with arguments against the cause of the initial rejection, the costs again escalate. It is rare for applications to go through more than two review cycles before a final acceptance or rejection is issued. However, if a patent receives a final rejection, one can appeal the PTO's decision in civil court and all the way to the Supreme Court, if necessary. According to Rolla, approximately 70% of all patent applications are eventually allowed. Maintenance fees for granted patents are due in the 3rd, 7th, and 11th years after the original grant. Failure to pay these fees can result in late fees or the expiration of the patent, with an attendant loss of protection. The maintenance fees can amount to several thousands of dollars over the life of the patent.

Avoid Common Mistakes

The most damaging mistake for a company seeking a patent is to start the application process too late. Patent applications must be filed within one year of the date on which an invention was disclosed to the public, or the opportunity is lost. This initial disclosure date may be much earlier than the first day of commercial availability if, for example, the product was used in trade show presentations or clinical trials.

Another potential problem is claims that are too broad. Claim writing is an art form, with the goal being to write the broadest possible claim — in order to gain the greatest level of protection by making duplication difficult — without overstepping the bounds of what can be considered novel and nonobvious. Accordingly, inventors or companies with sufficient time and resources can follow the tactic of submitting an initial, complete application with extremely broad claims, hoping that it will be approved. If the application is rejected because the claims are too broad, they can be modified or eliminated from the particular areas in question and the application resubmitted at a later time.

Getting Assistance

As stated previously, the PTO's Web site provides useful information about the patent process and associated costs. It also offers individualized assistance via its Patent Assistance Center, which is set up to help inventors and companies prepare effective patent applications and can provide contacts to patent examiners with relevant experience and responsibilities. However, the PTO is not in the position to provide legal advice.

Philosophical and Strategic Issues

Certainly, patenting a software user interface requires considerable work, time, and money. The decision to file for a patent may largely be a matter of personal or corporate philosophy or strategy. Proponents of patents view them as just rewards for the work and creativity that go into creating a new product. The bottom line is also important: securing a patent can translate into money. Supporters also believe that software patents fuel progress, forcing the competition to be more creative by coming up with yet another original idea rather than just copying prior work.

Opponents of patent protection for software user interfaces argue that patents have the potential to hinder product usability because they force others to use less efficient or effective software design solutions, to the detriment of end-users. Specifically, end-users would benefit more from software user interface consistency than from variety, which can make learning more difficult. Opponents also champion a view of the software community as mutually supportive, sharing the common goal of pushing the science of user interface design forward. In their view, patents represent an impediment to progress.

Medical device developers may find themselves agreeing with one side or the other on the desirability of software user interface patents, based on their position in the marketplace and the type of product they produce. But, regardless of a company's philosophy, it should consider a patent's relative value in relation to several mitigating factors, including:

- The likelihood that competitors would copy the design. Many companies value designing a product with a unique look and feel, akin to having their own corporate logo.
- The possible advantage of having a design mimicked, which might actually enhance a company's reputation as a design leader and increase market acceptance for a specific kind of user interface interaction scheme. If the original had no value, who would adopt it?

- The knowledge that the next generation of user interfaces was already being developed, which would leave mimics with an old-generation user interface in the near future.

Conclusion

Years ago, medical devices were a collection of hardware components that were stamped with a patent number. Now hospitals, clinics, doctors' offices, and even homes are inundated with medical devices that have a software user interface. The number of patent applications from device manufacturers for software user interfaces is likely to continue to increase because of the unique needs of the medical industry.

As Goodrich states, the clean environment of an operating room is not a practical place for a keyboard. "Our user interfaces must be created for items that are durable, portable, and that can be sterilized." The specific requirements of the health-care setting provide an advantage for medical-related user interface software designers relative to the big computer companies that tend to cater more to the general public. However, one cannot be too cautious.

Accordingly, medical device companies need to take stock of their patent opportunities, if only to maintain their right to introduce new designs while lowering their risk of infringing on recent claims by other parties.

Key Points

- Patents place proprietary technology and design solutions out of the competition's reach for many years or allowing for their use while generating substantial licensing fees for the patent holders.
- Medical companies that are accustomed to filing patents on hardware components (e.g., a new kind of pump or valve) have not taken full advantage of patent opportunities in the software domain.
- A design patent covers novel and nonobvious aspects of the user interface that can be considered graphical and ornamental in nature. Design patents typically cover user interface elements such as icons, type fonts, or the overall appearance of a particular screen. Protection lasts 14 years from the date the patent is issued.
- A utility patent covers the functional or useful aspects of the user interface, such as the overall organization and selection of menu

options that comprise a process. A patent application can include up to 20 claims, although there are mechanisms to submit an even greater number. Utility patents provide 20 years of protection, starting from the full patent application filing date.

- The application process can take between one and three years.
- For a company seeking a patent, the most damaging mistake is to start the application process too late. Patent applications must be filed within one year of the date on which an invention was disclosed to the public, or the opportunity is lost.
- Claim writing is an art form, with the goal being to write the broadest possible claim — in order to gain the greatest level of protection by making duplication difficult — without overstepping the bounds of what can be considered novel and nonobvious.

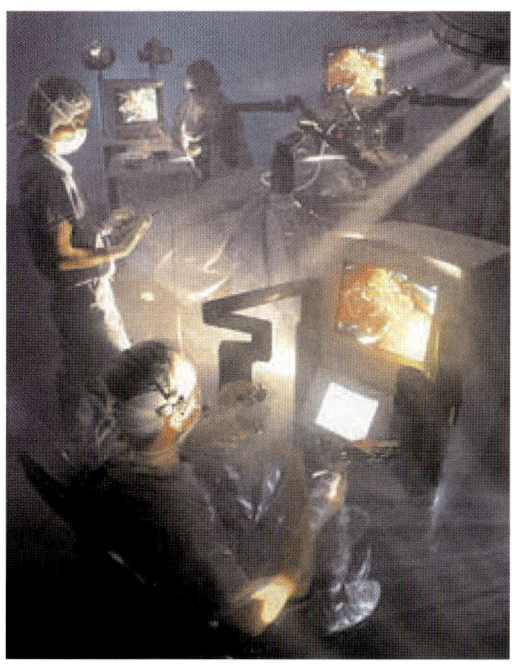

FIGURE 10.1
The ZEUS™ Robotic Surgical System embodies innovation both in terms of product design and surgical technique. Image courtesy of NASA/JPL.

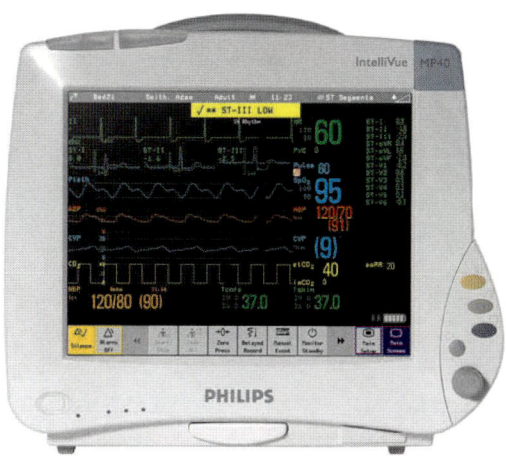

FIGURE 18.2
Philips Medical System's IntelliVue MP40 patient monitor annunciates alarms using large lights at top-left corner of the display and the important parameters are presented in large font so they are visible from a distance. Photo courtesy of Philips Medical Systems.

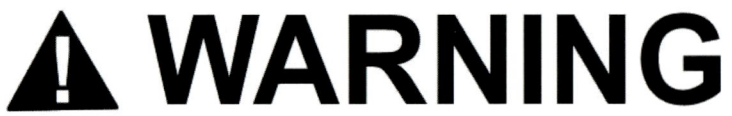

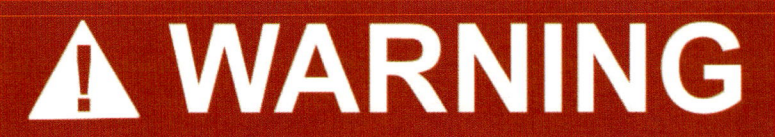

FIGURE 20.1
Warning message in black and white versus color.

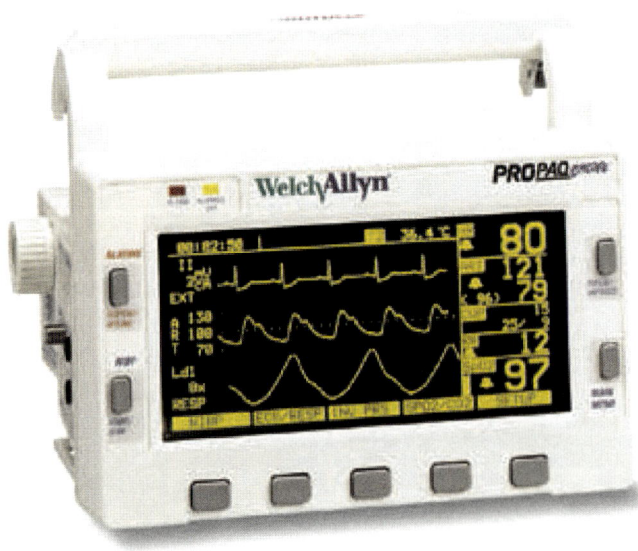

FIGURE 20.2
Patient monitor with a monochrome screen. Photo courtesy of Welch Allyn Inc.

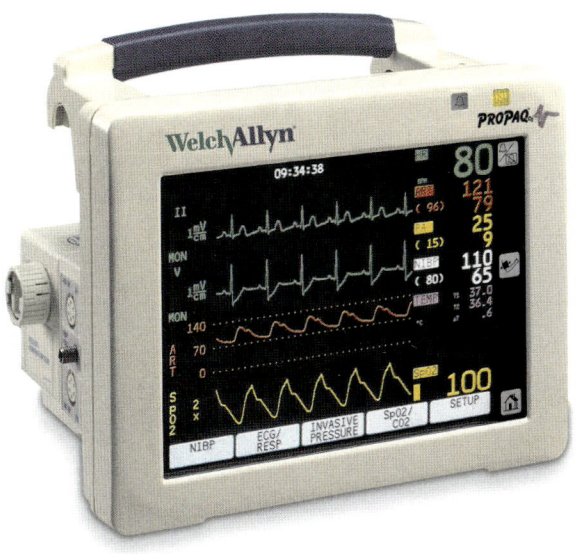

FIGURE 20.3
Patient monitor with a color screen. Photo courtesy of Welch Allyn Inc.

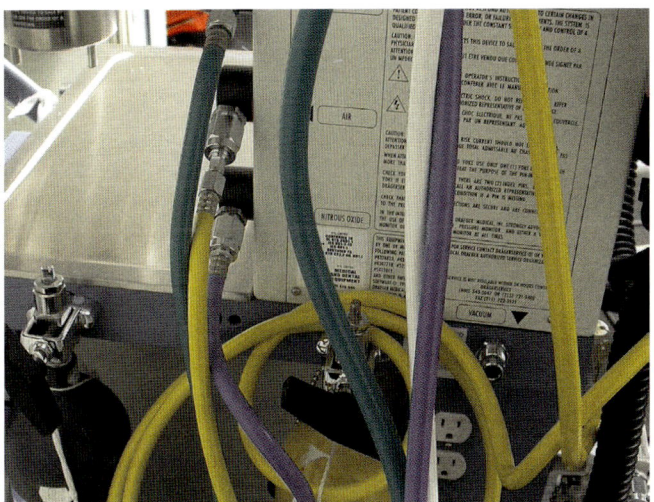

FIGURE 21.4
Gas lines running to the back of an anesthesia workstation are color coded. Photo courtesy of Emerson Hospital (Concord, MA).

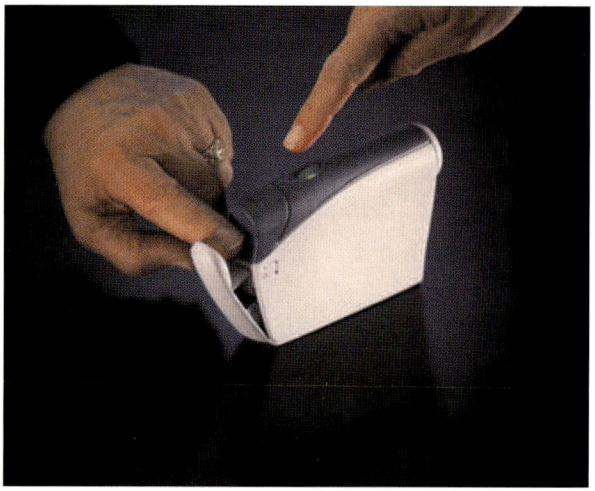

FIGURE 23.1
The Personal Lasette from Cell Robotics (Albuquerque) is designed for easy use by people with or without disabilities. Image courtesy of Cell Robotics International, Inc.

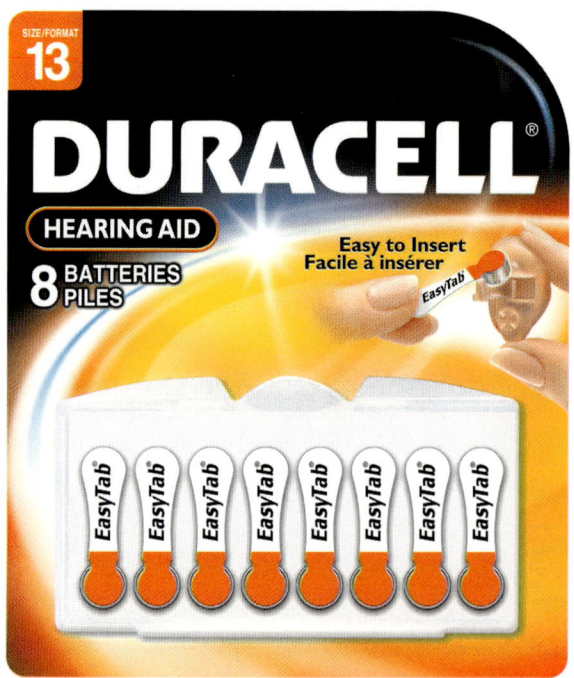

FIGURE 23.4
Duracell's EasyTab hearing-aid batteries make loading the battery much easier for

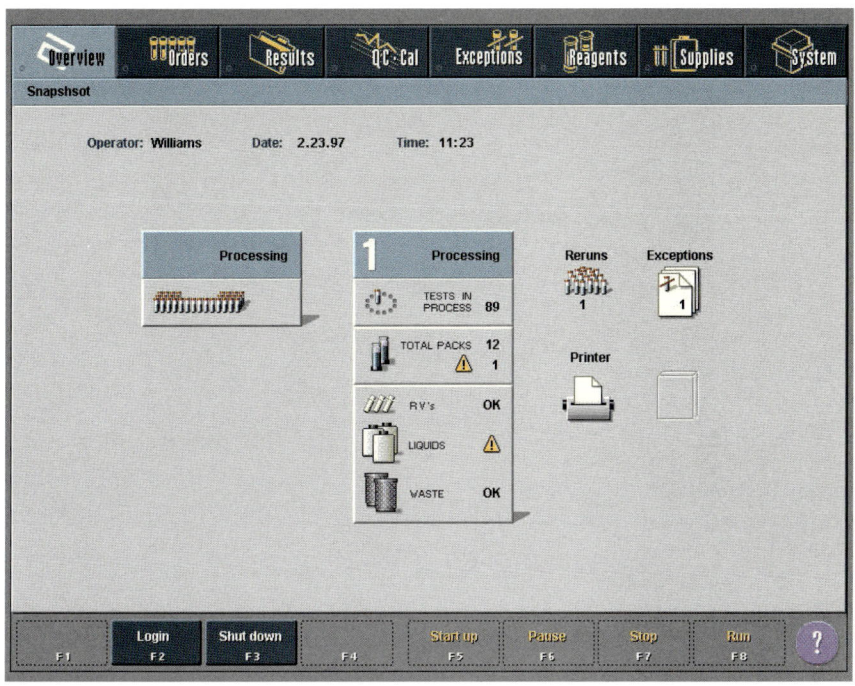
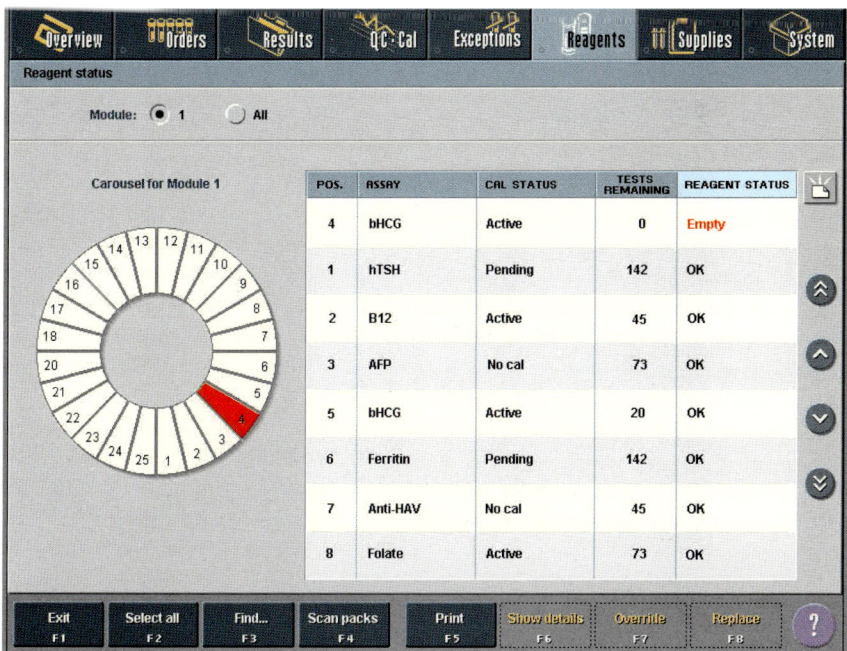

FIGURE 26.5
Sample touch-activated screens from Abbott's ARCHITECH£ anayzer.

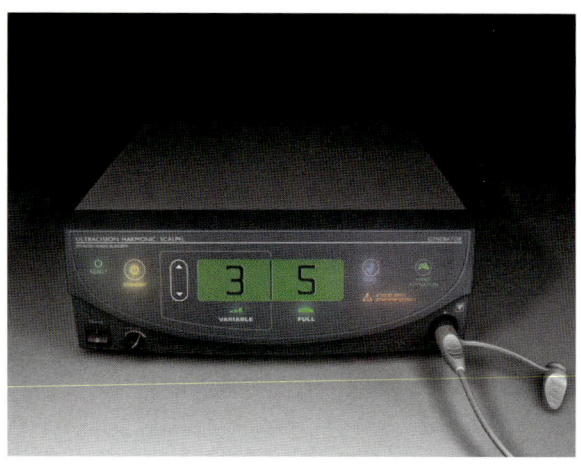

FIGURE 27.7
Generator for EES's Ultracision harmonic scalpel.

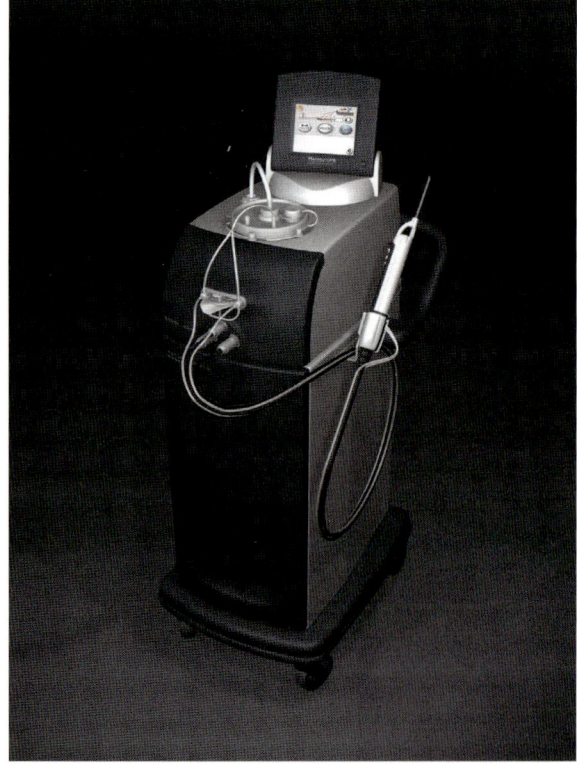

FIGURE 27.8
Mammotome breast biopsy system.

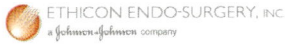
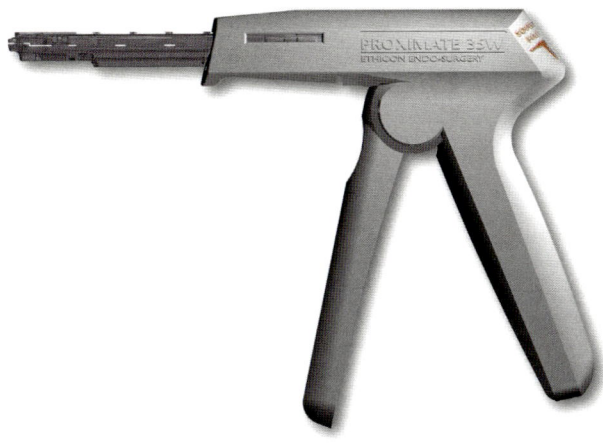

FIGURE 27.9
Surgical stapler.

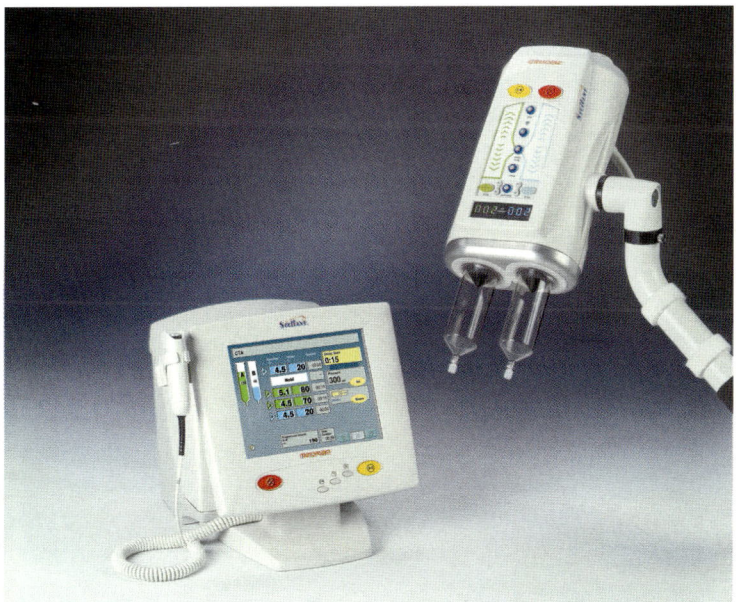

FIGURE 30.3
The Stellant CT Injection System — the injector to the left showing the disposable syringes at the top; the touch screen interface unit to the right.

Design Methods
and Guidance

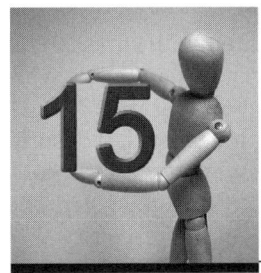

The Vision Statement for Product Design — In Your Mind's Eye

Michael E. Wiklund

What customers say they want, what designers think customers want, and what customers really want are often three different things. Sometimes customers overreach in detailing desired characteristics and describe a distorted caricature of their ideal product. The voice of the customer needs filtering — as does the voice of the developer, for that matter.

By involving customers at various stages of the design process, user-centered design can help to ensure that a final design meets customers' true needs and preferences. But it does not mean giving customers exactly what they ask for.

One filtering strategy is to capture design ideas, needs, and preferences in separate interviews with the development team and groups of customers, and then to use the input to write a vision statement for each of the two groups. Looking at the two vision statements enables a direct comparison between what the development team and what customers have in mind. The final step is to make rational trade-offs between the visions, giving due consideration to overarching business objectives. The result is a unified vision statement that can be used to guide the design effort.

The Origins of the Vision Statement

At the height of the total quality management (TQM) movement of the mid-1990s, corporations spent considerable time and money creating corporate vision statements. Often written in a spirit of partnership between managers and their staff, these statements were intended to communicate an organization's defining characteristics and ambitions in just a few words. The outcome was often cliché-sounding statements stuffed with superlatives that served as fodder for Dilbert cartoons. Yet, some vision statements were compelling and managed to place organizations on a winning path.

So, what does a TQM technique have to do with user interface (UI) design? Well, writing a unified vision statement is an effective way to place product design efforts on a winning path. Consider an architect's rough sketch of a new building. Such sketches set a basic design direction and are critical to winning a design contract. The rough sketch may depict a post-modern building, five stories tall, constructed of brick and glass, distinguished by a large courtyard. It provides a good sense of the structure's appearance and function, but it lacks the detail and resolution of trade-offs needed to begin construction. Similarly, the UI vision statement sets the direction for UI design, but lacks the details necessary to fabricate hardware, code software, or assure the usability and appeal of the final product. Meeting the latter objectives requires a full implementation of traditional industrial design and human factors engineering methods.

Regardless of the field in which it is used, the vision statement provides general guidance about what is to be achieved. Lacking this direction, the interaction requirements developed through task analysis or a designer's best judgment may dictate the product's design. This bottom-up approach may produce a polished design, but the design may be inappropriate, overly complex, or uninspired. Establishing a clear vision of what is desired before sweating the details promises a better design outcome.

The end goal of the UI visioning process is a unified vision statement that reflects the voice of both the developers and the customers.

Steps

An effective approach has four steps. Tips for taking each step follow.

Step 1: Learn about Needs

The first step is to learn about the needs and desires of the design team and prospective users. This is best done in a series of individual interviews or focus groups with the two groups. Brainstorming and other creative exercises can be used to help generate ideas. They may help nondesigners, in particular, communicate their ideas more effectively and discover unforeseen design opportunities.

Regarding a product's user interface, evocative questions could include:

- What should be the user's first impressions of the user interface?
- What tasks will users perform most frequently or urgently?

- What tasks are most critical to producing a positive use experience?
- Should the user interface represent an evolutionary or a revolutionary change from existing user interfaces?
- What is the existing user interface's most pleasing characteristic to an experienced user?
- What is the most displeasing characteristic?
- What should be the user's lasting impressions of the user interface?

Step 2: Write Two Vision Statements

The next step is to use what you've learned to write two vision statements: one expressing the designers' vision; the other expressing the customers' vision. To avoid cross-contamination or cross-fertilization of ideas, consider having a different person write each statement. Keep the vision statements short. Focus on general design aspects and include only those details that are imperative. (One page is sufficient for most projects.) Write the vision statement from the point of view of someone who (hypothetically) has used the product. Use active voice and present tense. If possible, ask research participants to review and comment on draft versions of the vision statements as a basis for final editing.

Step 3: Compare the Statements

The next step is to compare the vision statements to identify how they are and are not compatible. Listing attributes side by side in a table can facilitate the comparison. Then, discuss the statements with the design team, resolving differences in a structured manner. Sometimes, reaching an appropriate conclusion may require additional user research or analysis.

Step 4: Combine the Statements

The last step is to develop a unified vision statement that incorporates the strengths of the two points of view. This is the vision statement that will guide the balance of the UI design effort.

Sketching the Vision

In addition to a written vision statement, it may be useful to develop a sketch of the desired product. Use the same process to develop the sketch, first creating two sketches and then comparing them to produce a unified version.

Be careful not to make the sketch so detailed that it becomes overly prescriptive. Little effort should be spent on styling; rather, the focus should be conveying the general concept with just a few squiggles representing specific elements.

Using the Process: An Example

To illustrate the visioning process, consider the challenge of designing a wireless communication device intended for "sports-minded" adults. The consumer electronics market is already full of such products that not only provide cellular communications, but also provide the capability to browse the Internet, play games, and more.

You could begin the visioning process by recruiting potential consumers to participate in focus groups — say, two focus groups with 6 to 10 people in each. (More may be needed if one is concerned with regional and cultural differences.) At the same time, you could meet with the development team, including the product manager, the marketing manager, mechanical and electrical engineers, industrial designers, software developers, and others.

An excerpt from the development team's vision statement might read:

> Showcasing that the device incorporates many advanced functions, the main screen presents a scrolling list of menu options (in text). These options appear in order of the expected frequency of use, the first option would read [Phone].

An excerpt from the customers' vision statement for the same product might read:

> The main screen is dominated by a message (or symbol) indicating that the device is ready for use. To make a phone call, you just start dialing. You press a menu key to display an iconic menu showing the functions used most frequently. Selecting one of these icons takes you to an additional set of icons representing functions that are used less frequently.

Then, as described in step 3 above, develop a table to highlight differences between the two vision statements.

Next, come to consensus on areas where the vision statements differ to develop a unified vision statement. A unified statement combining the two earlier excerpts might read:

> The main screen is divided into two areas. One area uses large text (easily read from a distance) to indicate that the device is ready for use. The other area incorporates a scrolling set of icons depicting an expandable set of optional functions. Helpful prompts appear when you highlight one of the options.

TABLE 15.1
Comparison of the developers' and the users' vision statements.

Development Team's Vision Statement	Customers' Vision Statement
Provides access to functions at the top level via a scrolling list	Presents only the key function at the top level
Offers text-based menu options	Offers icon-based menu options
Requires user to select [Phone] to make a call.	Defaults to ready state, allowing you to start dialing a number right away.

Table 15.1 draws a comparison between the two original vision statements. Figure 15.1 presents illustrations of the original visions as well as the unified vision for the communication device.

FIGURE 15.1
Developers', users', and unified vision of a cellular phone's user interface.

Benefits of UI Vision Statements

Although the majority of design projects proceed without undertaking a visioning exercise, several benefits may be gained from developing a vision statement. The visioning process and vision statement may:

- Help the design team focus on opportunities for innovation and creativity at the start of a design project
- Bring structure to the process of deciding how the design team will and will not satisfy users' needs and preferences
- Help to ensure that the loudest or most persistent people on the design team do not unduly influence the design direction or decisions
- Improve communication among design team members
- Establish a common ground for conceptual design
- Encourage respect for and consideration of different perspectives and points of view

In short, conducting a visioning exercise early in the design process increases the chance of creating a great product that closely matches the original design goal, that meets the needs and desires of the customer, and that integrates the best features of several concepts into an integrated package.

Key Points

- By involving customers at various stages of the design process, user-centered design can help to ensure that a final design meets customers' true needs and preferences.
- The visioning process involves capturing design ideas, needs, and preferences in the course of separate interviews with the development team and groups of customers.
- The final step toward producing a unified vision statement is to make rational trade-offs between the developers' and customers' visions, giving due consideration to overarching business objectives.
- Conducting a visioning exercise early in the design process increases the chance of creating a great product that closely matches the original design goal, that meets the needs and desires of the customer, and that integrates the best features of several concepts into an integrated package.

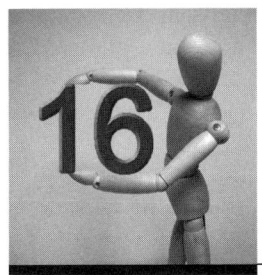

Making Medical Device Interfaces More User-Friendly

Michael E. Wiklund

It is not altogether uncommon for medical device companies to spend several months developing a preliminary user-interface design only to be dissatisfied with the result. Such firms can come to regard a product's user interface as its Achilles' heel, especially in cases where their competition has already brought a more user-friendly product to market. As a result, manufacturers may seek an objective third party such as a usability or human factors engineer, graphic designer, or marketing professional to enhance their product's usability and appeal without a major overhaul, given their schedule and budget limitations.

And it can be done. User-interface designs such as those associated with patient monitors, ventilators, blood chemistry analyzers, infusion pumps, and kidney dialysis machines often have superficial design problems that can negatively affect a device's usability and appeal but that are relatively easy to remedy. The following 10 solutions address such design issues.

Reduce Screen Density

A lot of medical device displays look overstuffed with information and controls so that very little empty space remains. Such space is important in a user interface, because it helps to separate information into related groups and provides a resting place for the user's eye. Overly dense-looking user interfaces can be initially intimidating to nurses, technicians, and physicians, making it difficult for them to pick out specific information at a glance. For such reasons, what the design engineer does not put on the screen can be as important as what he or she does put on it. To eliminate extraneous information, the user-interface designer can:

- Present secondary information on demand via pop-ups or relocate it to other screens
- Reduce the size of graphics associated with brand identity (i.e., logos and brand names)
- Use simpler graphics (e.g., replace 3-D icons with silhouette-styled ones)
- Use empty space instead of lines to separate content
- Reduce the amount of text by stating things more simply

Provide Navigation Cues and Options

Moving from one place to another in a medical device user interface, a navigator can sometimes become lost, much like someone traveling in an unfamiliar city that lacks road signs or has signs printed in a foreign language. Sometimes the problem results from the user's not knowing where he or she is in the user-interface structure.

For example, the end-user's goal may be to set the alarm limits associated with a monitored parameter such as arterial blood pressure, but instead he or she becomes lost in a complex hierarchy of setup options ranging from respiratory monitoring to reporting. At other times, the user may not understand how to move vertically or laterally within a structure because the methods of control are not apparent. A nurse, for example, may find the way to an alarm setup screen but not recognize how to go back a step or leave the screen after making alarm-limit adjustments.

Placing meaningful titles on every screen and subcomponent (e.g., message boxes and major elements) by means of a header — a contrasting horizontal bar that includes text — is helpful. Numbering the pages of an electronic document can also benefit the reader. For example, each page of an eight-page medical document could be marked "page 1 of 8," "page 2 of 8," and so on, for clarity.

Navigation options and controls, such as "Go to main menu," "Go back," "Previous," "Next," and "Help," should be grouped together in a single, consistent location so that users can easily return to a previous screen or undo an action without fear of getting lost or causing irreparable harm.

Centered	Left Justified
This is a sample of text that illustrates the appearance of centered text. This is a sample of text that illustrates the appearance of centered text.	This is a sample of text that illustrates the appearance of left-justified text. This is a sample of text that illustrates the appearance of left-justified text.

FIGURE 16.1
Effect of text justification on readability.

Ascribe to a Grid

Some medical device screens look like a checkerboard after it has been bumped — pieces all over the place instead of in an ordered arrangement. In rare instances, such disorderly looking screens may actually appear stylish or refreshingly informal. However, most screens look and work better when they serve a utilitarian purpose and when their screen elements are aligned.

Aligned elements seem less complex because they merge into a single, related set. Moreover, the human eye can generally find information more quickly when scanning a straight path rather than an irregular or discontinuous one. For this reason, experienced graphic artists tend to left-justify text instead of centering it. Centered text creates a *riverbank* effect that makes the eye work harder to locate where the next line of text begins (Figure 16.1).

Making the effort to fit on-screen elements into a grid will pay off in terms of visual appeal and perceived simplicity. Grid-based screens also tend to be easier to implement in computer code because the position of visual elements is predictable. Fitting these elements into a grid is fairly simple if the designer is working from scratch. However, converting an existing design that has no underlying grid structure into a more orderly arrangement is a bit more work.

When developing a grid structure, it helps to begin by defining the screen's dominant components and approximate space requirements. For example, one may choose to allot space for a title bar, menu area, body of content, and a prompt by dividing the screen vertically into four bands that are 1/16, 2/16, 12/16, and 1/16 the height of the screen, respectively. Similarly, one may want to divide the variable content area into field labels and data-input fields by sectioning the screen horizontally into bands that are 1/3 and 2/3 the width of the screen, respectively, with the wider vertical band being subdivided into three additional bands to provide for different-width fields. The visual appeal of such a grid is shown by folding a piece of paper and looking at the fold lines, or by drawing the layout using rectangles on a computer screen (Figure 16.2).

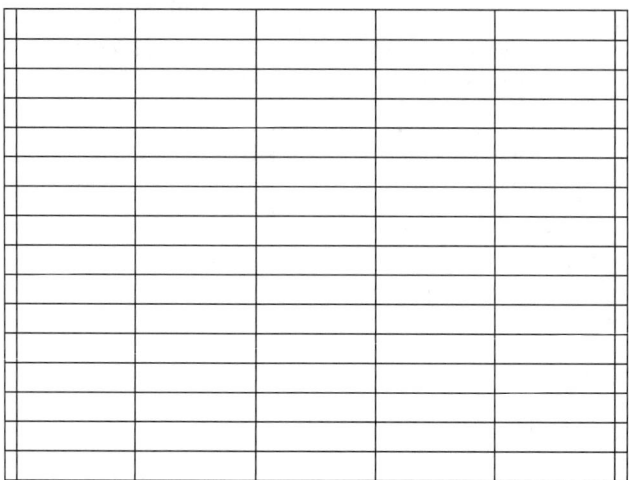

FIGURE 16.2
An on-screen grid system facilitates composition.

Keeping on-screen elements at a fixed distance (e.g., 10 pixels) from the grid lines can also provide visual appeal. In doing so, the designer creates margins around the grid lines. The resulting space (i.e., empty column) is a demarcation component that implies the grid and eliminates the need for actual grid lines that would add visual complexity to the overall composition. Taking things a step further, the margin width may also be used as a guide for spacing other composition elements, such as an ultrasound image and its caption.

Create Visual Balance

Visual balance or symmetry should be created, especially about the vertical axis. Visual elements should be arranged on either side of an assumed axis, so that each side has about the same amount of content as empty space. Such a balanced composition, whether it be an entire screen or a subcomponent (e.g., a message box), looks simple and whole — elements neither appear askew, nor seem to be missing. It is worth noting, however, that perfect symmetry may appear tedious, so one can be comfortable with the slight imbalances that are virtually inevitable.

Various methods can be employed to evaluate a composition's balance. Some people can judge balance at a glance, while others may want to squint at the on-screen composition or even use a highlighter pen on a screen printout to block out areas of content or empty space. Perceived imbalances may be remedied by reorganizing information, adjusting the gaps between labels and fields, relocating elements to other screens, or popping up elements only on request.

Limit the Number of Colors

Experienced designers suggest limiting the color palette of a user interface. The background and major on-screen components should be kept to between three and five colors including shades of gray, while one-of-a-kind and small-scale elements may feature additional hues. For the same reasons that an interior decorator chooses a color scheme for a room — a few harmonious colors that repeat themselves in the wallpaper, carpet, and couch upholstery, for example — a designer should select just a few congruous hues for the user interface.

A user-interface designer should also select colors carefully to be sure they are consistent with medical conventions. For example, red is commonly used to depict alarm information or to communicate arterial blood pressure values, and various secondary colors are associated with certain drugs and gases.

Simplify Typography

An efficient user interface is based on typographical rules that steer end-users toward the most important information first and make screen content easy to read. To achieve these results, a user-interface designer generally commits to a single font and just a few character sizes such as 12-, 18-, and 24-point type (Figure 16.3). While characters should vary in size, the sizes must not be so disparate as to create a tense visual contrast.

Another way to simplify typography is by eliminating excessive highlighting such as underlining, bolding, and italicizing. Because today's computer tools make it easy to highlight text in these ways, overuse can result. Usually, a single method such as bolding is enough to highlight information effectively when used in concert with different font sizes and extra line spaces.

Use Hierarchical Labels

Redundant labeling leads to congested screens that take a long time to scan. For instance, unnecessary indicators on a typical patient monitor — a unit

Font Size (points)	Sample Content
24	**Alarm**
18	Ventilation
12	Respiration Rate Volume Pressure

FIGURE 16.3
Hierarchy of font sizes.

that provides a summary of alarm limits associated with such patient parameters as heart rate and blood pressure —could be time-consuming and thus problematic for health-care professionals. Excess visual congestion can make it difficult for users to pick out even the most salient details. However, hierarchical labeling can save space and speed scanning by displaying such items as heart rate, respiratory rate, pulmonary arterial pressure, and arterial blood pressure more efficiently (Figure 16.4).

Use Simple Language

Medical device user interfaces are often characterized by overly complex words and phrases. Despite the fact that medical workers consistently state a preference for simple language, product designers often write in a technical manner that can be less than user-friendly. Today's designers are well advised to simplify their communications not only for health-care professionals but for the increasing number of patients and caretakers using devices at home who may not have extensive education or training.

User-interface designers should ask themselves this question: "How should this text be worded so that a bright youngster between 10 and 12 years old would understand it?" This question usually provokes ideas on how to word things more simply without dumbing down the user interface. Specific corrective measures include writing shorter sentences (½–2 lines) and paragraphs (2–3 sentences), breaking complex procedures into ordered steps, using meaningful headings and subheadings, and using consistent syntax.

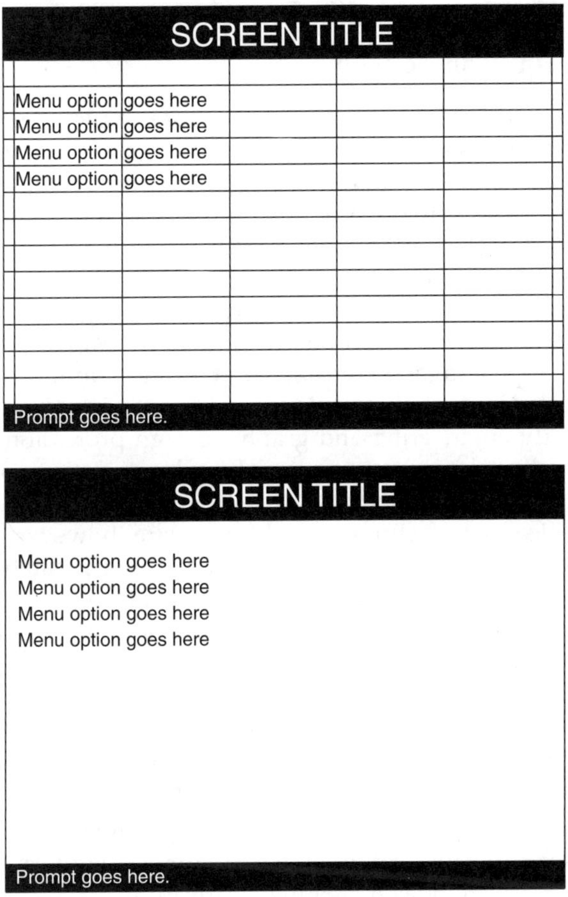

Making Medical Device Interfaces More User-Friendly 157

SCREEN TITLE			
Menu option goes here			
Menu option goes here			
Menu option goes here			
Menu option goes here			
Prompt goes here.			

SCREEN TITLE

Menu option goes here
Menu option goes here
Menu option goes here
Menu option goes here

Prompt goes here.

FIGURE 16.4
A template (above) helps designers produce clean-looking and consistent screens (below).

HR	Low	40	High	160
RR	Low	4	High	20
PA	Low	10	High	60
Art	Low	90	High	180

	Low	High
HR	40	160
RR	4	20
PA	10	60
Art	90	180

FIGURE 16.5
Redundant labeling on a typical patient monitor (top) can be time-consuming and problematic for health-care professionals to read. Instead, hierarchical labeling (bottom) can be used to save space and to speed scanning.

Refine and Harmonize Icons

Lately, a lot of medical devices, particularly those employing relatively large displays with high resolution (i.e., VGA or better), are presenting functional options — actions such as calibrating a device, setting alarms, or reading the user guide — in the form of icons. This shift within the medical industry to an iconographic user-interface style matches trends in the consumer and business software arenas.

Unfortunately, medical device manufacturers may find it difficult to match the major software developers in terms of their investment in icon quality. The icons that appear in most consumer and business applications are highly refined and tested by such firms as Microsoft, Apple, and Oracle, all of which employ usability engineering and graphic design professionals. Relatively speaking, a medical device company will have less time, money, and perhaps design talent to devote to icon design.

Medical device manufacturers should be aware, however, that a limited investment in icon quality may produce a disproportionately large payoff, provided that talented designers are involved and icon testing is performed. The following steps can be taken to maximize icon comprehension and give the icons a family resemblance to each other:

- Develop a limited set of icon elements that represent nouns (e.g., objects such as patient, syringe, or ECG strip), eliminating cases where several elements represent the same thing.
- Simplify the icon elements to eliminate potentially confusing and unnecessary details and accentuate the most significant aspects of the object or action, as if creating a caricature.
- Make similar-purpose icons the same overall size (build them from the same array of pixels, such as a 40-x-40–pixel rectangle).
- Perform user testing to ensure that no two icons are so similar that they will be confused with one another.
- Employ the same style for similar-purpose icons (i.e., two- versus three-dimensional, detailed versus silhouetted, monochromatic versus multicolored, fine-lined versus bold-lined, outlined versus filled-in, and so forth).
- Reinforce icons with text labels or "tool tips" that appear when the icon is selected or highlighted, for example.

Eliminate Inconsistencies

Design inconsistencies are especially toxic to user-interface appeal and usability and, for some medical devices, may compromise safety. For example, end-users may be confused or, at the very least, annoyed by the use of the color red to communicate both critical and noncritical data. Similarly, the use of different words like *enter*, *select*, *continue*, and *OK* to communicate the same basic function may confuse the end-user.

To prevent such design inconsistencies, a style guide should be created and maintained. Standard graphical user-interface (GUI) guides like Microsoft's User Interface Design Guidelines for Windows 95 are useful prototypes for style guides that are specific to medical devices. The reference does not have to start out as a refined document, but rather as an organized collection of notes and rules that ensure consistent design practice at the project's early stages. As a function of analyses and testing, the user-interface design eventually becomes more refined and the style guide is updated accordingly. Ultimately, the style guide can be integrated into final design specifications.

Conclusion

The success of most medical devices is closely linked to user-interface quality. This is particularly true in cases where there is substantial market competition and the associated technology has more or less matured, making user-interface quality a prominent factor in product differentiation. The safety of most medical devices is also closely linked to user-interface quality, because design shortcomings may lead directly or indirectly to use errors, with severe consequences that can include patient injury and death.

Medical device user-interface designers must aspire to excellence. Yet, experienced designers recognize that there is no such thing as a perfect user interface. Imperfections arise from many sources, including technological limitations, incomplete understanding of user needs, and aesthetic decisions that may not match everyone's preferences. As a result, designers must aim for an optimal rather than a perfect user interface. Looking beyond core design attributes such as a cohesive conceptual model, total user-interface quality is found in the details — the superficial elements like navigation cues that, when used most appropriately, can help to create a more user-friendly design. To this end, the aforementioned detoxification methods should enhance almost any medical device user interface in the works.

Key Points

- User-interface designs often have superficial design problems that can negatively affect a device's usability and appeal but that are relatively easy to remedy.

- Overly dense-looking user interfaces can be initially intimidating to nurses, technicians, and physicians as well as make it difficult for them to pick out specific information.
- When moving from one place to another in a medical device user interface, a navigator can sometimes become lost; to help, provide navigation cues and options such as a meaningful screen title.
- Ascribe to a grid. Most screens look and work better when they serve a utilitarian purpose and when their screen elements are aligned.
- Create visual balance. Perceived imbalances may be remedied by reorganizing information, adjusting the gaps between labels and fields, relocating elements to other screens, or popping up elements only on request.
- Experienced designers suggest limiting the color palette of a user interface.
- An efficient user interface is based on typographical rules that steer end-users toward the most important information first and make screen content easy to read.
- Hierarchical labeling can save space and speed scanning.
- Use simple language, worded so that a bright youngster between 10 and 12 years old would understand it.
- A limited investment in icon quality may produce a disproportionately large payoff.
- Design inconsistencies are especially toxic to user-interface appeal and usability.

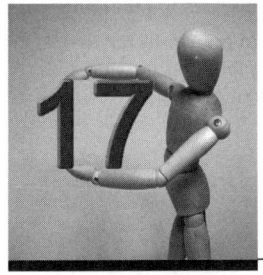

Controlling Complexity

Michael E. Wiklund

How to design user-friendly products.

Regarded as a "soft science," human factors engineering has few laws governing the nature of human-machine interaction. However, the discipline is rife with empirical data, design criteria, and rules of thumb that facilitate the development of user-friendly products. These resources can be quite helpful to designers working on complex products that could press users to the limits of their physical and mental abilities.

Generally, products get harder to use as their complexity increases (see Figure 17.1), presenting the users with more features and greater operational demands. For example, binoculars, syringes, stopwatches, and glucose meters tend to be easier to use than camcorders, patient monitors, document production centers, and magnetic resonance imaging scanners (see Figure 17.2). Users compensate for increased complexity by spending more time learning to use a product. Or, they may avoid using advanced features altogether, explaining why so few people choose to program a song sequence into their CD players or operate their automatic cameras in manual mode.

But, it is possible to buck the trend that puts consumers at odds with complicated products. Indeed, some feature-laden products remain easy to use. Consumers favor these kinds of products — devices that are powerful as well as user-friendly due to good human factors engineering. Important to manufacturers, such products tend to be a commercial success. When customers use them for the first time — perhaps in a retail showroom — they feel capable as well as impressed, which increases the likelihood of a sale. When consumers purchase and put the products to everyday use, they find they can accomplish tasks safely, efficiently, effectively, and with satisfaction. This results in goodwill toward the manufacturer, leading to repeat business and many other benefits.

Without Human Factors Engineering
Lacking an investment in human factors, usability tends to decrease as functional complexity increases.

With Human Factors Engineering
An investment in human factors helps to preserve usability as functional complexity increases.

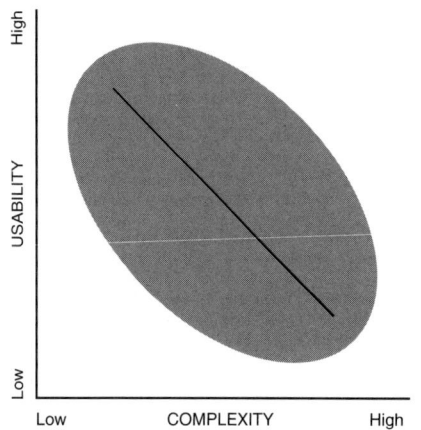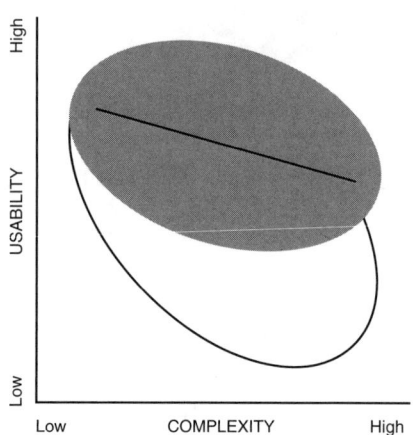

FIGURE 17.1
The relationship between medical device usability and functional complexity.

Good human factors engineering is partly a matter of following a user-centered design process. Initially, designers may conduct research on customer needs and preferences as a basis for forming design goals and initial concepts. Later on, designers may refine their design based on user feedback obtained in exercises such as a usability test. However, while extensive user involvement in the design process is important, so is resolving product complexities so the product demands are matched to the users' capabilities.

Design Tips

Here are some tips on resolving design complexities in order to produce user-friendly products. The tips are derived from established human factors engineering principles and applied design experience.

1. Bring the Important Features to the Surface

Many products reflect a minimalistic design philosophy — one that deliberately limits the number of surface-level displays and controls so the product looks "clean." This design approach tends to produce devices that look easy to use on first impression, but are not so easy to use on a continuing basis. Such products may force users to navigate their way through several software menus or press a cryptic series of buttons to produce the desired action. Bringing more features to the surface, especially those features used frequently and urgently, is likely to improve usability. A detailed task analysis will help designers determine which features should rise to the surface. As a compromise, designers pursuing a minimalistic aesthetic may be able to blend the extra controls and displays into the product's form in a pleasing manner.

2. Remove Unimportant Features from the Surface

In contrast to minimalism, some products overwhelm users with surface features. Such products, which may present the user with dozens of controls and ornate displays with flashing indications, tend to look powerful but intimidating. They also make it harder for users to figure out how to use the device, primarily because the important displays and controls are embedded in a noisy background of less important ones. Again, a task analysis will indicate which displays and controls should be placed on the product's surface. The rest can be removed from the surface, placed either in a lower level of the software interface (if there is one) or placed behind a hinged cover, for example.

3. Eliminate Extraneous Features

Designers often use the term "feature creep." The term refers to a tendency among manufacturers to add extra features to a product to make it more marketable. The problem with feature creep is that products become overly complex and intimidating. To avoid the problem, some designers maintain a philosophical commitment to keeping things simple and foregoing extraneous features that beef up specification sheets but offer consumers little real value. The 1990s was a decade in which all kinds of consumer electronic products exhibited feature creep, overwhelming users who sought products with basic capabilities. Fortunately, in the 2000s, there is a clear movement toward simpler products. So, manufacturers should take a critical look at a given product's feature set and see which features may be dismissed as more trouble for the users than they are worth.

4. Indicate Operational Status and Relevant Changes

Thanks to the availability of inexpensive microprocessors, products are getting smarter and more capable every year. For the sake of convenience and marketability, some are taking over functions normally assigned to users. This can reduce workload, enabling users to focus on other tasks. Unfortunately, such automation can leave users in the dark about a device's operational status — what is often referred to as a loss of situational awareness.

164 Designing Usability into Medical Products

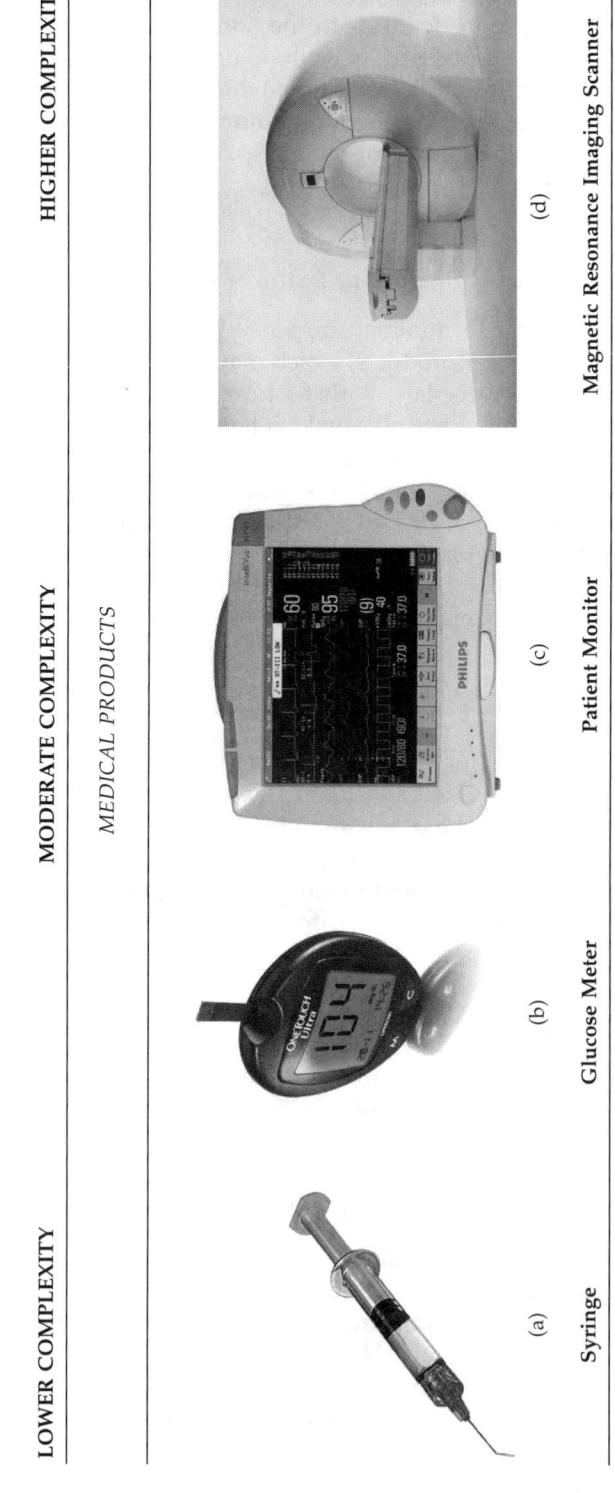

LOWER COMPLEXITY   MODERATE COMPLEXITY   HIGHER COMPLEXITY

MEDICAL PRODUCTS

(a) Syringe   (b) Glucose Meter   (c) Patient Monitor   (d) Magnetic Resonance Imaging Scanner

Controlling Complexity

CONSUMER AND BUSINESS PRODUCTS

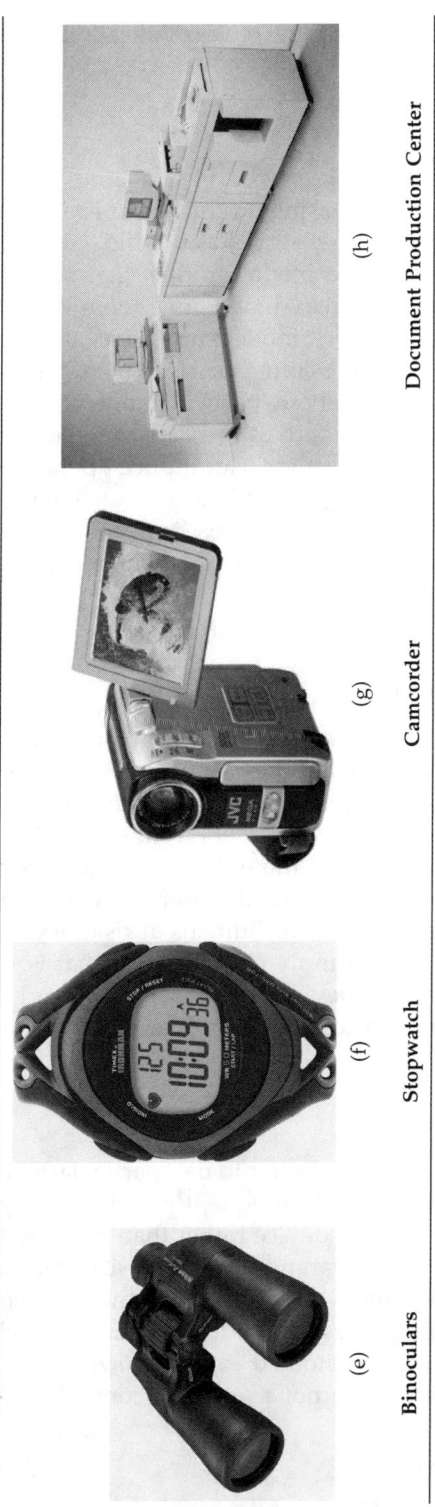

(e) Binoculars (f) Stopwatch (g) Camcorder (h) Document Production Center

Figure 17.2a: Photo courtesy of Ocularvision, Inc.
Figure 17.2b: Photo courtesy of LifeScan, Inc., a Johnson & Johnson company.
Figure 17.2c: Photo courtesy of Philips Medical Systems.
Figure 17.2d: Photo courtesy of Siemens Medical Solutions, Inc. USA.
Figure 17.2e: Photo courtesy of Nikon Sport Optics, Nikon Inc.
Figure 17.2f: Photo courtesy of Timex Corporation.
Figure 17.2g: Photo courtesy of Canon USA, Inc.
Figure 17.2h: Photo courtesy of Xerox Corporation.

FIGURE 17.2
Medical and consumer products distribute themselves across the complexity spectrum.

This problem can be addressed by providing a clear indication of a device's operation status and any changes.

5. Limit The Number Of Modes

A common means of dealing with increasing product complexity is to establish operational modes. A boombox that serves as a radio, CD player, and tape cassette player is an example of a modal product that uses one basic interface to control a variety of functions. An operating room ventilator that can be shifted from an adult and pediatric mode is another example. Regarding these and similar products, designers must take care not to burden users with too many things to remember about particular operational modes. Exceptions to a general pattern of use, such as pressing different controls to stop a function depending on the use mode, can induce operational error. Ideally, controls should serve a similar or identical functional purpose, regardless of the operational mode, so their purposes are not confused. Also, shifting from one mode to another should require a deliberate action or series of actions.

6. Incorporate Protective Mechanisms

As products become smarter, they can play a role in protecting against human error, or taking steps to mitigate the negative consequences of an error. For example, devices delivering medicine to patients, such as an infusion pump, can be programmed to prevent users from selecting a dangerously high dose or infusing two incompatible drugs. Or, devices can slow down or speed up their operations to match the user's operational pace. If something goes wrong, placing property or humans at risk, devices can be designed to correct the problem or simply shut down if that is the safest measure. In this manner, complex devices place some of the burden of preventing or dealing with emergencies on themselves, rather than the user.

7. Label the Important Features

Labels make a complex device easier and safer to use, particularly if the type of device is unfamiliar to users or used infrequently. In fact, designers are better off placing too many labels on a device rather than too few. All labels should follow consistent rules for appearance (e.g., font, size, and color) and placement. Labels should be slightly oversized to accommodate people with poor vision and facilitate reading in less than ideal conditions, such as dim lighting. Notably, Europeans are accustomed to iconic (symbolic) labels in place of words. While Americans are not averse to icons, they have less experience deciphering them.

Meanwhile, a manufacturer might want to use iconic labels for several possible reasons. First, iconic labels address the needs of a user population that speaks various languages as well as the needs of people who cannot read. Second, iconic labeling eliminates the need to produce and manage the distribution of language-specific models. Third, iconic labels often make products look more stylish and are arguably more modern or international. These compelling reasons to employ iconic labeling make it incumbent upon manufacturers to design icons that are easy to interpret or to develop language-specific products for generally monolingual markets.

8. Use Large Displays

Too many high-tech devices have diminutive displays that are hard to read and spread information across too many screens. The reason for the small displays may be limited real estate on the product's surface or component cost constraints. In such situations, it is tempting to crowd a lot of information onto a compact, inexpensive display, but the consequence is often reduced usability and appeal. Consumers usually prefer products that have relatively large, easy-to-read displays. Thus, product usability and appeal is somewhat proportional to display area. This rule of thumb suggests that manufacturers find a way to incorporate larger displays that allow for larger characters or symbols or allow for more information on a single screen. The cost of the larger display relative to the marketing benefits should make the investment worthwhile. And facing a trade-off, the first priority would be to use larger characters and symbols rather than compressing more information on a screen.

9. Avoid Coding Information

Consumers have little patience for learning codes and, even if they learn them, they do not remember them very well. It is nonintuitive and tedious to key "4," "1," and "Enter" as a means to tell a microwave oven to defrost chicken. Instead, employ interactive schemes that enable users to input simple commands in response to plainly worded prompts. For example, consumers could simply scroll through a list of frequently defrosted items and confirm the correct one (Chicken) by pressing a button.

10. Arrange Controls Logically

As the number of controls increases, it becomes more important to place them in logical order. The physical relationship between the controls and the features they affect is a critical consideration. Generally, controls should be placed next to related features or be placed in a pattern that mimics the features or reinforces functional relationships. Also, controls may be placed in an order that suits the expected order or frequency of use. Such arrangements make tasks proceed faster and mitigate use errors. Importantly, keep controls a sufficient distance away from open hazards, such as moving parts, but make sure they remain accessible when needed.

Conclusion

These tips should help designers wage their quiet battle to preserve product usability in the face of increasing product complexity. But, it is important to keep in mind the advice presented earlier regarding usability testing of prototypes. There is no substitute for bringing prospective users and product prototypes together in order to study their dynamic interactions. Normally, usability testing enables one to spot problems that may be corrected before product goes to market. In fact, regulators, such as the U.S. Food and Drug Administration expect manufacturers to conduct such tests of life-critical medical devices. Regulations not withstanding, usability testing identifies opportunities for the final refinement of a design developed based on good human factors engineering principles.

Key Points

- Generally, products get harder to use as their complexity increases, presenting the users with more features and greater operational demands.
- Designers who follow a user-centered design process can create a feature-laden product that is also easy to use.
- Strategies for controlling complexity include bringing the important features to the surface; removing unimportant features from the surface; eliminating extraneous features; indicating operational status and relevant changes; limiting the number of modes; incorporating protective mechanisms; labeling the important features; using large displays; avoiding coding information; and arranging controls logically.
- Designers should conduct usability tests to identify additional ways to reduce complexity.

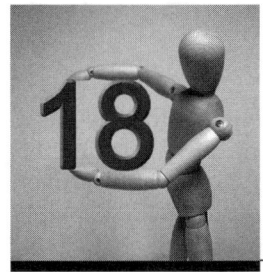

Eleven Keys to Designing Error-Resistant Medical Devices

Michael E. Wiklund

Manufacturers can help reduce use error in the clinical setting by integrating good human factors practices and user-friendly design into their medical devices.

Today, you may have made a mistake while operating a device. Perhaps you turned on the stove's back burner instead of the front one. Or did you switch on the car lights when you meant to turn off the windshield wipers? You may not remember. Such errors are part of daily life.

The reality is, people are not perfect, and neither are devices. Indeed, some people are especially prone to error. Similarly, the designs of some devices seem to invite errors in their use.

Most of the time, we can live with these deficiencies. But society expects more from medical workers and the devices they use. We expect doctors, for example, always to operate critical medical devices with skill and attention. Similarly, we expect those devices to be mechanically flawless, and to lessen the effects of any use errors that do occur. So when we hear the occasional news report of patient injury or death caused by a human mistake or device failure, we are shocked. Such mistakes are not supposed to happen in medical settings.

But, in fact, use error is quite common in the practice of medicine, as underscored by the 2000 Institute of Medicine report *To Err Is Human*.[1] Thinking realistically about medical care, we should not be surprised by its substantial rate of use error. Time pressures and fatigue are recognized as key factors leading to use error, and are abundant in the emergency room, intensive care unit, outpatient clinic, and most other health-care environments.

The Designer's Responsibility

Fortunately, medical device designers can play an active role in preventing, or at least mitigating, the effects of use error in medicine. Designers in other industries have succeeded in making nuclear power plants and airliners safer by designing their control centers to be less error-prone. For example, many of the controls built into aircraft cockpits are shape coded to avoid confusion when grasped by a pilot who is flying at night in heavy turbulence. The lever used to raise and lower the landing gear, for instance, is capped with a small wheel-shaped part, and the lever for positioning the flaps is topped with a little model flap. In a nuclear power plant control room, critical controls, such as the reactor-shutdown button, are surrounded by guards that prevent the buttons' accidental actuation — a use error that could cost the utility company several million dollars.

The medical industry has already made efforts to minimize the potential for use errors. For instance, over the past decade or so, manufacturers have worked closely with the U.S. government and national and international standards organizations to make anesthesia delivery safer. New technologies make possible the noninvasive monitoring of blood oxygen saturation and breath-by-breath carbon dioxide levels, and the alerting of caregivers when patients might be in danger. Anesthesia machines have been improved to guard against use errors of the past, such as mistakenly turning off the flow of oxygen to a patient, neglecting to restart the ventilator following intubation, or filling an anesthetic-agent vaporizer with the wrong fluid.

Such safety improvements have resulted from detailed risk analysis and abatement efforts involving the identification of possible failure modes and effects, and either eliminating the hazard or putting protections in place. Through its regulatory actions, the FDA has influenced manufacturers to make safety improvements as well, and companies have responded by applying good human factors practices at the device design stage.

Good Human Factors Practices

Attaching a miniature wheel to the tip of the landing gear lever to visually and tactilely reinforce the control's function is good human factors practice. The enhancement is no guarantee that a pilot will never mistake the landing-gear lever for another type of control, but it certainly reduces the chances. The same point holds true for various enhancements that can be made to anesthesia workstations, such as ensuring that oxygen valves on all machines turn in the same direction to increase flow.

Decades after the emergence of human factors engineering as a technical discipline and the establishment of good design practices, however, the number of medical devices with basic human factors shortcomings is substantial. Fortunately, the FDA has initiated regulations and enforcement mechanisms in the past few years that should help eliminate these human factors flaws. Manufacturers are now responsible for conducting human factors-related design studies, which include performing usability tests, to demonstrate to the agency that a device is suitable for use. A manufacturer who lacks evidence of device usability, which relates directly to safety, runs the risk of not receiving FDA approval to bring its product to market. Product designers are therefore seeking even more detailed guidance on accepted human factors processes and design principles.

Human factors guidance is already available from many sources outside of FDA documents. Traditionally, medical device designers have looked to military standards, guidelines published by the Association for the Advancement of Medical Instrumentation (AAMI),[2] and an assortment of human factors or ergonomics textbooks for information and instruction.

The sheer volume of guidance can sometimes be overwhelming, and detailed recommendations can be contradictory or mutually exclusive. To resolve these problems, AAMI is working toward producing a comprehensive, all-inclusive source of guidance within the next few years.

Experts already agree, however, that a handful of design practices are especially important for protecting against common use errors. Discussions among several human factors professionals and medical device regulators familiar with common device faults yielded the following guidelines. Though incomplete, the guidelines represent a reasonable starting point for thinking about designing an error-resistant medical device.

Guidelines for Design

Guard Critical Controls

Controls can be vulnerable to accidental and unauthorized actuation. As an example, a caregiver might accidentally bump up against a ventilator control and start or stop a critical function. The conventional solution is to guard the control so that its actuation requires a deliberate action, like pressing and holding the power-on key to turn the machine on or off.

Guards can take many forms. Push buttons can be recessed or surrounded by a raised collar (see Figure 18.1). Levers can incorporate interlocks, requiring the user to actuate a release mechanism before he or she can move the lever. Car makers recently adopted this approach to ensure that drivers apply the foot brake before moving an automatic transmission into drive. Some

FIGURE 18.1
An anesthesia workstation's oxygen flush button incorporates a collar to prevent accidental actuation. Photo courtesy of Emerson Hospital (Concord, MA).

devices that incorporate a software user interface, such as a patient-programmable analgesic pump, require the caregiver to enter a code or password before operating the device. This approach is an effective way to keep unauthorized individuals — particularly hospital visitors — from meddling with control settings.

Confirm Critical Actions

This design tip is closely related to guarding critical controls. The idea is to give users a chance to reconsider critical actions that are not easily reversed and to correct their mistakes. Software products often employ this strategy by requiring users to confirm a destructive action, such as deleting a file. Requiring confirmation lessens user frustration and the potential loss of an important document, although it might increase task time. In the case of medical devices, confirmation can also help prevent the loss of a file, such as a patient record, and it can prevent users from administering the wrong therapy if the user blunders and presses the wrong key. In fact, standards and regulations now mandate a two-step approach to particularly critical tasks.

Make Critical Information Legible and Readable

For the average medical device, all information is not created equal. Some information, such as blood pressure values or alarm messages, is vitally important and must be presented in a strictly reliable manner. There is no

Eleven Keys to Designing Error-Resistant Medical Devices 173

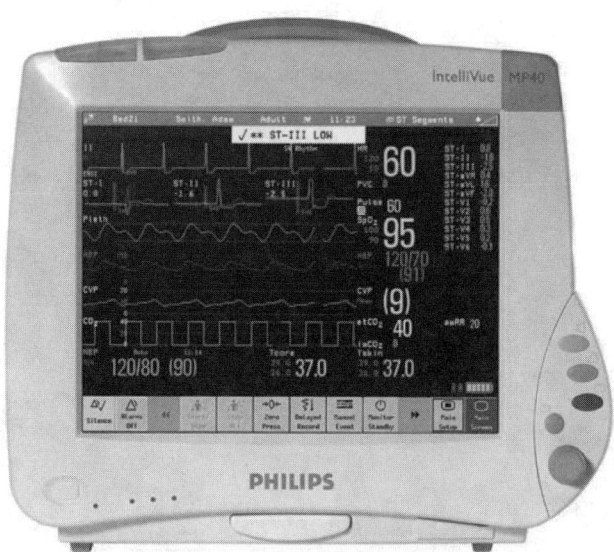

FIGURE 18.2 (See color insert following page 142)
Philips Medical Systems' IntelliVue MP40 patient monitor annunciates alarms using large lights at top-left corner of the display and the important parameters are presented in large font so they are visible from a distance. Photo courtesy of Philips Medical Systems.

room for error, such as mistaking a "7" for a "1" or an "8" for a "3," because such errors could lead to inappropriate therapy. Therefore, information legibility and readability is key.

One way to make data more accessible and visible is to make it very large (see Figure 18.2). That way, it is more likely to be legible even if it's presented on a smudged display that might also be reflecting glare at the time, or if it is read from a great distance. Another strategy is to ensure that displayed information contrasts sharply against its background; for example, use black characters on a white background, or the reverse. The display characters should also have an appropriate stroke height-to-width ratio so that numbers and letters are easy to discriminate.

Color-coding and segregating information is another method for helping data stand out against a potentially congested background. Finally, critical information should be placed on the surface of the device's user interface — on a control panel or top-level display, for example — rather than hidden behind a cover or in the depths of the display hierarchy.

Simplify and Ensure Proper Connections

Caregivers spend a considerable portion of their workday managing collections of cables, wires, and tubes that are often referred to as "spaghetti."

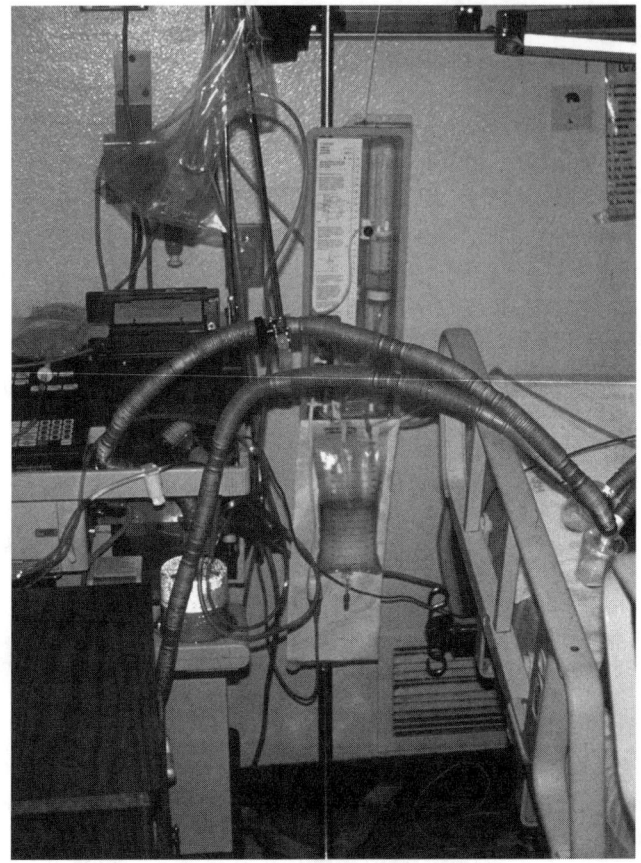

FIGURE 18.3
Collection of wires and tubes found at the bedside in a typical intensive care unit. Photo courtesy of University of Southern California, Department of Neurosurgery.

Precious minutes are spent sorting out lines, routing them from patient to device, locating the right ports, and making secure connections (see Figure 18.3 and Figure 18.4). Accordingly, anything a manufacturer can do to simplify these tasks and ease equipment setup is helpful. Moreover, manufacturers must consider the myriad ways in which poor cable, wire, and tube management can lead to serious errors. In two highly publicized and tragic incidents, for example, an infant respiratory monitor's ECG leads were improperly connected to a line power supply (one case involved an extension cord, the other a wall receptacle), and the monitored child was electrocuted.[3]

One protective measure to prevent accidents such as these is keying the connectors and associated ports, thereby making it physically impossible to insert the wrong cable or tube into a particular port. Visual and tactile cues, such as color- and shape-coded ports, provide additional protection by establishing associations, or mental dovetails (see Figure 18.5). All other types of equipment and receptacles that might be present in the use environment

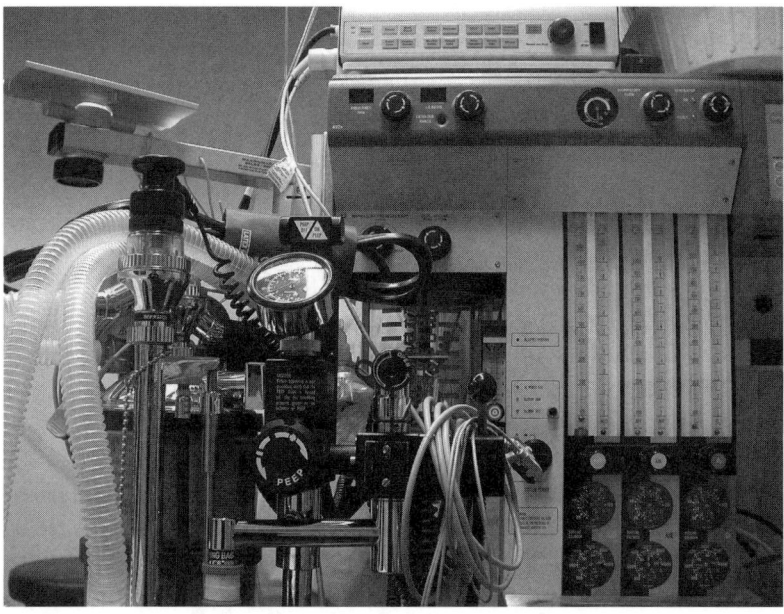

FIGURE 18.4
Collection of wires and tubes found at the front of an anesthesia workstation. Photo courtesy of Emerson Hospital (Concord, MA).

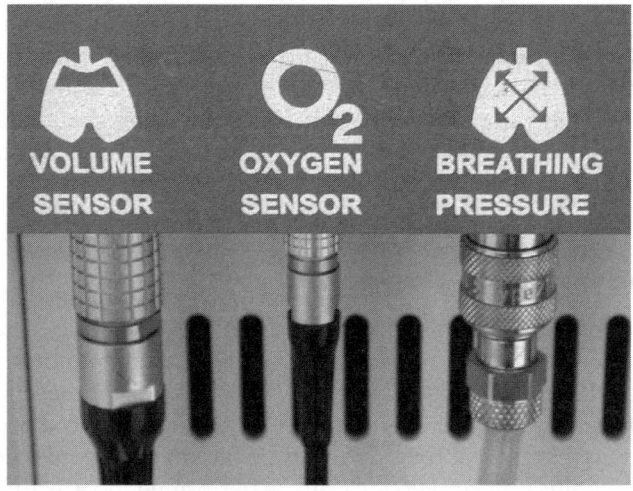

FIGURE 18.5
Proper connections are facilitated by symbol and text labels as well as connector shape coding. Photo courtesy of Emerson Hospital (Concord, MA).

also should be considered to ensure protection against improper connections. In the case of the children's apnea monitors, the leads could have been shaped and sized to prevent inadvertent insertion into a power receptacle.

Use Tactile Coding

Because caregivers must focus on several tasks at once, they are not always looking at a device while operating it. For example, an interventional cardiologist might be watching a television monitor for most of a case, manipulating surgical devices such as balloon catheters and dye-injection devices by feel, and possibly even operating them with a foot switch. Therefore, it is important to make devices and their associated controls recognizable by touch alone.

Tactile cues include the feel of a switch, the force required to actuate it, and the distance the switch travels. It is also possible to add audible cues, such as clicking and beeping sounds.

Prevent the Disabling of Life-Critical Alarms

The debate continues over permitting caregivers to disable the alarms built into life-critical devices. Proponents claim that caregivers need, and in fact demand, control over alarms so that beeping and flashing indicators will not cause distraction or produce a "cry-wolf" syndrome. Opponents claim that alarm systems perform a critical safety function that outweighs the nuisance factor. Both arguments are compelling; however, the arguably safest approach is to prevent the disabling of alarms while also making alarms smarter.

Some smart devices allow users to silence, but not disable, alarms for a predetermined period of time when a case is proceeding normally, but the conditions of the moment, e.g., apnea during anesthesia induction, would trigger an alarm. Because of the time limit, such alarms will still serve their purpose if a benign condition persists until it becomes dangerous. Turning alarms off altogether increases the chance that dangerous conditions will be undetected — an unacceptable, albeit rare, outcome.

Present Information in a Usable Form

Converting information from one form to another introduces the opportunity for error and makes additional work. Presenting information in an immediately usable form is preferred. Values should be presented in their appropriate units of measure. Otherwise, alarm or failure codes can be misinterpreted, and cryptic abbreviations or acronyms can be misinterpreted as well. Additionally, unit conversions can be performed incorrectly. To prevent these mishaps, users should be provided immediate or direct access to information in its final, most usable form.

The same rule applies to forming functional associations. It is more effective to place related information, such as waveforms and numerical values, within the same functional grouping rather than making users recall and integrate the information in their minds. Accordingly, designers should look for ways to take the cognitive workload out of information displays, without depriving users of valuable details.

Indicate and Limit the Number of Modes

Designers often introduce operational modes into devices in an attempt to simplify their operation. A ventilator used in a critical-care setting may incorporate pressure- or volume-controlled modes, for example, to initiate different therapeutic regimes. Other kinds of devices can have pediatric and adult modes. While operating modes can improve care and save work under normal circumstances, however, they also introduce the potential for operating in the wrong mode.

Consider the case in which a patient monitor was inadvertently left in demonstration mode and then used during actual patient care.[4] The doctors using the monitor reportedly detected a mismatch between their clinical observations and the data displayed on the monitor: the digital readout of the patient's blood pressure never varied from 120/70. Growing suspicious of the extremely stable data, the doctors finally noticed that the monitor was locked into "demo" mode, as indicated by a discrete message on the monitor's screen. The lesson to manufacturers is to conspicuously indicate a device's operational mode so that it is apparent at a glance. Limiting the number of modes to just a few that users can commit to memory is helpful. Besides, users usually prefer to operate devices in the familiar "standard" mode; they typically disregard more advanced modes.

Do Not Permit Settings to Change Automatically

Few things frustrate users as much as devices resetting themselves or unexpectedly changing their operational state without the user knowing. A change in operational state has reportedly occurred when devices have lost power or when their power supplies are changed. One consequence of an unwanted change — such as a return to default values — can be the suspension or alteration of an ongoing therapy that places patients at risk. Minimally, device displays should boldly indicate any changes that were not initiated by the user. Ideally, devices should give users full control of important settings under all conditions.

Reduce the Potential for Negative Transfer

Negative transfer occurs when a user applies her or his experience using one device to another one, even though the second device does not function the same as the first. This can be a problem when patterned behavior, i.e., rote task performance, leads to a negative outcome. Take, for example, the caregiver who is accustomed to changing the parameters on a therapeutic device by pressing arrow keys. A similar device requires the user to press arrow keys, then press a confirmation key. If the caregiver switched to the second device, he or she would be likely to enter the new value without confirming it. The consequence, attributable to negative transfer, would be that the device would still be set to the original parameter value.

The solution is to identify industry conventions or standards related to a particular device that is under development, as well as those of other devices used within the same care environment. Those conventions or standards should be followed, unless there is a compelling reason to diverge, in which case substantial divergence is preferable because it will reduce the chance of negative transfer. Minor differences might invite users to confuse the operation of the two devices.

Design in Automatic Checks

As microprocessors make devices smarter, adding software routines that detect possible use errors becomes more feasible. Some devices can alert users to unusual or potentially dangerous settings, such as a particularly high setting on an analgesic pump controlled by a patient. This error-prevention strategy can be thought of as an extension of a device's alarm system.

Conclusion

Together, these design guidelines and human factors practices form one part of an overall strategy that helps reduce the occurrence of device use errors. Intuitive, ergonomic, and smarter devices can help caregivers do their jobs better, which in turn leads to better patient outcomes and fewer mishaps.

Acknowledgments

The following human factors professionals provided input to this chapter: George Adleman (Siemens Medical Systems, Danvers, MA), John Gosbee (Veterans Health Administration, Ann Arbor, MI), Rod Hassler (ALARIS Medical Systems, San Diego, CA), Bill Muto (Abbott Laboratories, Irving, TX), Dick Sawyer (retired, FDA, Rockville, MD), and Eric Smith (American Institutes for Research, Concord, MA).

Key Points

- Some people are especially prone to making errors. Similarly, the designs of some devices seem to invite errors in their use.
- Use error is quite common in the practice of medicine, as underscored by the 2000 Institute of Medicine report *To Err Is Human*.
- Time pressures and fatigue are recognized as key factors leading to use error and are abundant in the emergency room, intensive care unit, outpatient clinic, and most other health-care environments.
- Medical device safety improvements have resulted from detailed risk analysis and abatement efforts involving the identification of possible failure modes and effects, and either eliminating the hazard or putting protections in place.
- Steps toward reducing the chance of use error include guarding critical controls; confirming critical actions; making critical information legible and readable; simplifying and ensuring proper connections; preventing the disabling of life-critical alarms; indicating and limiting the number of modes; not permitting settings to change automatically; reducing the potential for negative transfer; and designing in automatic checks.

References

1. Kohn, L., Corrigan, J., and Donaldson, M., Eds., *To Err Is Human: Building a Safer Health System*, Institute of Medicine National Academy Press, Washington, D.C., 2000.
2. Human factors design process for medical devices, ANSI/AAMI HE-74:2001, Association for the Advancement of Medical Instrumentation, Arlington, VA, 2001.
3. Katcher, M.L., Shapiro, M.M., and Guist, C., Severe injury and death associated with home infant cardiorespiratory monitors, *Pediatrics*, 78, 5, 775–779, 1986.
4. Ramundo, G.B. and Larach, D.R., A monitor with a mind of its own, *Anesthesiology*, 82, 1, 317–318, 1995.

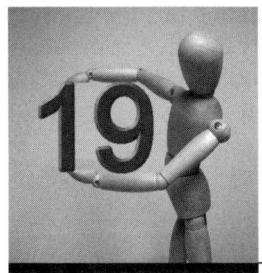

Designing a Global User Interface

Michael E. Wiklund

Manufacturers are loath to inventory several variants of a medical device, such as a ventilator or infusion pump, just because its user interface must incorporate local language or special features to meet the needs of a specific market. They would rather build a common version of the hardware than load it up with customized software that gives users the important sense that the user interface has been designed explicitly for them. This strategy can reduce tooling, production, and distribution costs substantially, usually outweighing any increase in software development and maintenance costs. However, it can also reduce a device's usability, especially its initial ease of use.

For example, generic or "global" hardware designs often replace text labels on a control panel with graphical symbols. In fact, European manufacturers who lack a large domestic market and sell to many nearby countries that speak different languages have motivated the International Electrotechnical Commission (IEC) to develop a set of standard symbols for medical devices that would serve this objective. However, usability tests of devices that incorporate graphical symbols in place of text often show that such devices are less intuitive to use. For example, when usability test participants encounter a symbol-laden product for the first time, they often end up guessing what a particular symbol means, unless the software provides some form of clarification. Many guesses are quite creative but off track. In real-life situations, such guessing may be required at a critical time when the clinician has little time to refer to the user manual or online help. The result could be errors or delays in equipment operation that compromise patient safety, result in property damage, or both. For this reason, manufacturers may regard the development of a global hardware design and user interface intuitiveness as mutually exclusive goals.

However, there are ways of addressing both goals in one design. Short of producing hardware variants, manufacturers can apply creative approaches to device labeling that make a product suitable for global marketing, while developing software solutions that are tailored to local needs.

Labeling Strategies

Eliminate Hardware Elements

One way to avoid placing language-dependent text labels on hardware is to shift controls from hardware to software. For example, older ECG monitors typically use dedicated knobs to choose among ECG signal sources (i.e., different leads). These knobs usually have labels above them, such as "ECG Lead." Now, many newer models provide the same control capability through software images or "virtual control panels" that include similar text labels. Instead of turning a knob several clicks, the user may use a trackball to highlight and select an object displayed on the computer screen.

Developing language-dependent software user interfaces does not pose the same logistical problems and costs for companies as does developing hardware variants. For starters, software variants on diskette are more easily managed than hardware assemblies since they are inexpensive to reproduce and ship. Also, text is a fundamental component of virtually all software user interfaces, so it has to be tailored to the user population anyway. But, a more compelling advantage to software vs. hardware modifications is that software variants do not require special tooling. For example, instead of producing a series of silk screens to place text on a membrane control panel, software programmers can simply change the names of variables in software code.

Companies that tailor software user interfaces to reflect local language can run into trouble if they do not anticipate the need for such tailoring in the original design. For example, German terms that appear on a software screen may require 40% more space than English terms. Accordingly, original screen layouts developed in English need to leave room for larger amounts of text.

Use Softkeys

A clever way to retain direct access controls and avoid the need to place text labels on hardware is to use "softkeys" that are common to automatic teller machines (ATMs). Typically, a softkey is a blank key placed on a control panel adjacent to a computer display. The function of the softkey depends on the current state of the device. Users determine the function of the key at the time by reading a label displayed on a computer screen, adjacent to the associated blank key. Depending on the capabilities of the display, the

Designing a Global User Interface 183

label may be textual or graphic. In essence, softkeys allow designers to label physical keys with language-specific text, without having to commit to specialized hardware.

Due to experience using ATMs, more people than ever before are accustomed to how softkeys work. Accordingly, people find devices that employ softkeys to be relatively intuitive to use. It is only when the number of softkeys gets large, say more than six, and the menu hierarchy grows to many layers that people start to have trouble using softkey-driven user interfaces. The major complaint is that people lose track of where they are in the user interface, primarily because screens tend to look alike. However, if the number of softkeys is limited to perhaps six or fewer, this should not be a problem.

Is it acceptable to include softkeys on a user interface that employs other menu navigation methods, such as arrowkeys or a rotary encoder that moves a highlight bar among menu choices? Generally, the combination of these elements should not create problems, as long as functions are assigned to the control mechanisms in a consistent manner and screen layouts remain balanced-looking. After all, everyone who drives a car is comfortable using a wheel to steer, foot pedals to modulate speed, and buttons to select radio stations.

Use Symbols with Care

Designers face a special challenge when symbols emerge as the only viable way to identify controls and associated user interface elements. Part of the challenge is designing an icon to communicate the associated meaning or message. The other part of the challenge is confirming that it communicates reliably.

Designing a good symbol is harder than it may seem, particularly if the symbol will represent an action (verb), as opposed to a recognizable object (noun). For example, it is easier to design a symbol for "patient" than it is to design one for "returning controls to default settings." As shown by this example, developing graphics to undo something that is already ambiguous is particularly difficult. Also, as we pass through a time of symbol proliferation (particularly in the software domain), developing graphically appealing, unique symbols is becoming more difficult. As such, symbol design is a task best left to talented designers who appreciate the nuances of graphical communication (see Figure 19.1 and Figure 19.2). Even then, symbology is best limited to cases where the message lends itself to graphical interpretation. Also, designers need to beware that some symbols, such as hand gestures, may convey the intended meaning in some cultures while having a different, if not insulting meaning in other cultures. Therefore, designers should consider working closely with representative customer to develop and test symbol sets. Some may go as far as to pair graphical designers with customers in what some term a participative design exercise. In such exercises, the customer can suggest possible symbols or elements of a compound

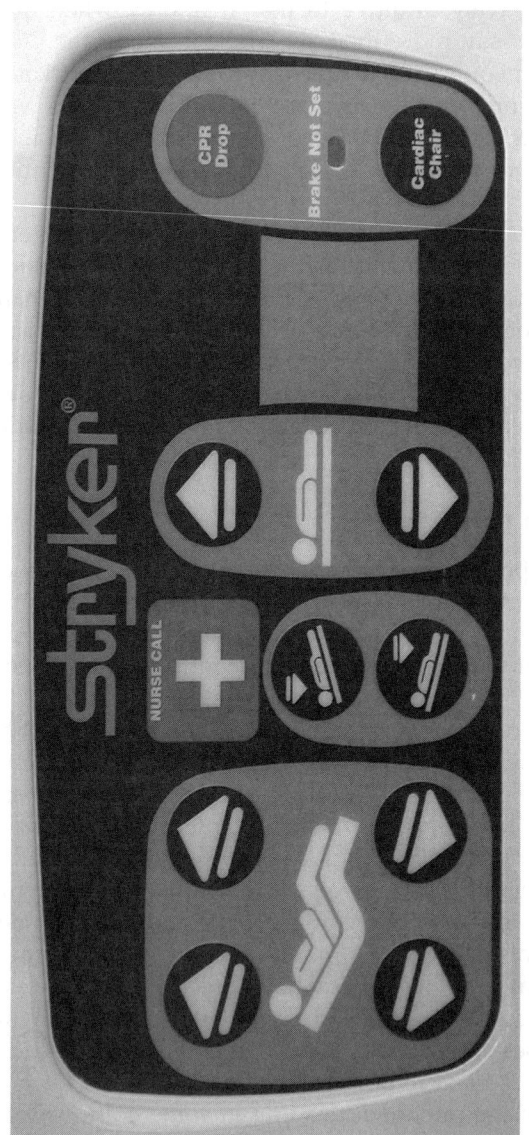

FIGURE 19.1
Diagnostic device uses icons to indicate control functions. Photo courtesy of Emerson Hospital (Concord, MA).

Designing a Global User Interface 185

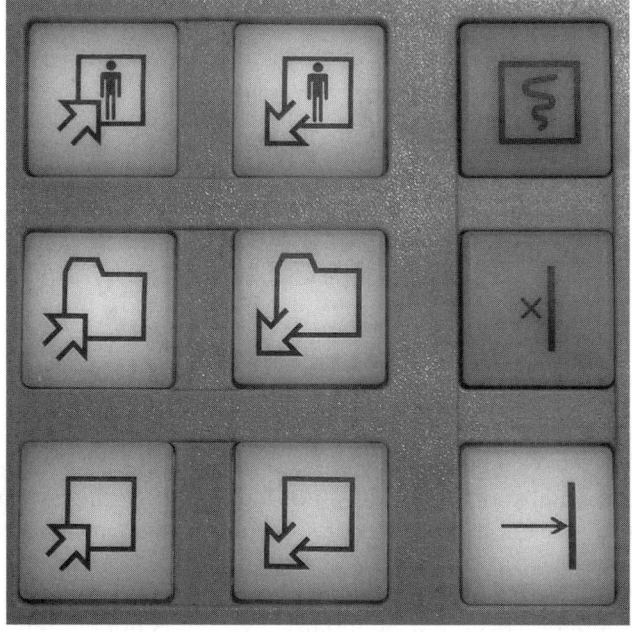

FIGURE 19.2
Hospital bed uses icons and text to indicate control functions. Photo courtesy of Emerson Hospital (Concord, MA).

symbol and the designer can render them in a professional manner for further assessment.

Regarding the reliability of symbols, the American National Standards Institute (ANSI) promulgates a symbol acceptance criteria of 85% correct for symbols incorporated into safety signs.[1] This criterion is tough to achieve. It may even be regarded as too stringent for most medical applications. Nonetheless, usability-conscious companies will strive to meet this criterion for products intended for use in the U.S. as well as abroad.

To test symbols, ANSI suggests showing one to a potential user only a short moment, then asking the person to say what they think it means. Objective investigators record the user's impressions and judge them according to predefined symbol definitions. A symbol interpreted correctly 85% of the time is regarded as acceptable, as long as there are no more than 5% critical confusions.

In the context of such acceptance testing, many companies will face the dilemma posed by "standard" symbols that do not meet the ANSI criterion. For example, the International Electrotechnical Commission has developed the symbol shown in Figure 19.3 to represent "Menu." One presumes pressing a button with this symbol on it (or displayed adjacent to the button) will evoke an on-screen menu. However, some people may not understand the meaning of this symbol on first impression. It may take a few times for people to learn the symbol's meaning, principally because the symbol is

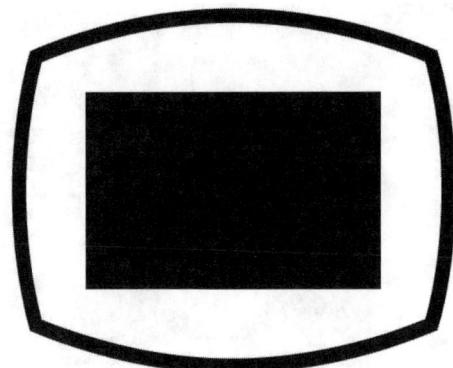

FIGURE 19.3
Symbol for "Menu." Graphic courtesy of International Electrotechnical Commission.

somewhat of an abstraction; it does not look precisely like a real menu. In such cases, designers may be tempted to design their own replacement to respond to criticism of the standard symbol. Of course, such a well-intentioned action can only frustrate the medical industry's goal of standardizing symbols. Therefore, even if a "standard" symbol is not entirely intuitive, it may be in the best long-term interest of a company to adopt standard symbols and let the users catch up.

Still, the most critical symbols may need to be reinforced with a language-specific text label. Figure 19.4 illustrates how imaging technicians have added English labels to two different panels to ensure the correct use of controls.

Develop Multilingual Labels

In many cities where more than one language is spoken, public signs and even restaurant menus are presented in two languages, such as French-English or Swedish-Finnish. Is this a solution for the labeling medical hardware? It may be worth considering if the majority of customers speak one of two languages, there are not too many things to double label, and there is the space to do it. After all, clinicians encounter such double labels on disposable medical products and the practice is widespread in the consumer electronics business. Also, a double label may satisfy the needs of a large proportion of the potential user population.

Applying a double labeling scheme, it would be important to differentiate the text for rapid acquisition of the native language term. For example, text could be printed in different colors (black-blue) and placed in a consistent orientation (top-bottom or left-right) to differentiate language.

Of course, double labeling adds to visual clutter and cannot be regarded as preferable to single-language labeling, unless one is certain a product will be used concurrently by people who speak different languages.

Designing a Global User Interface

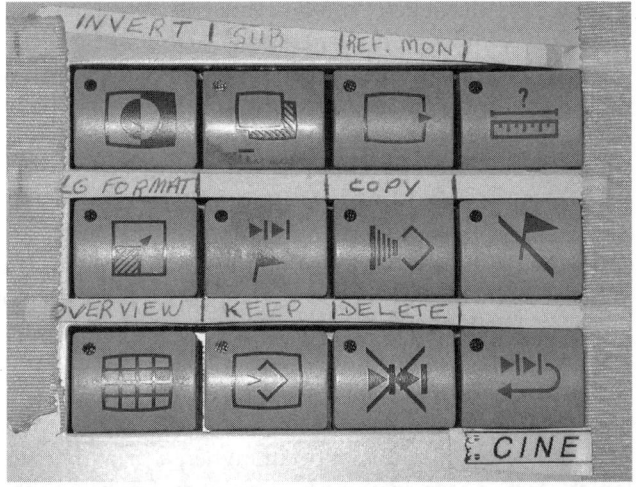

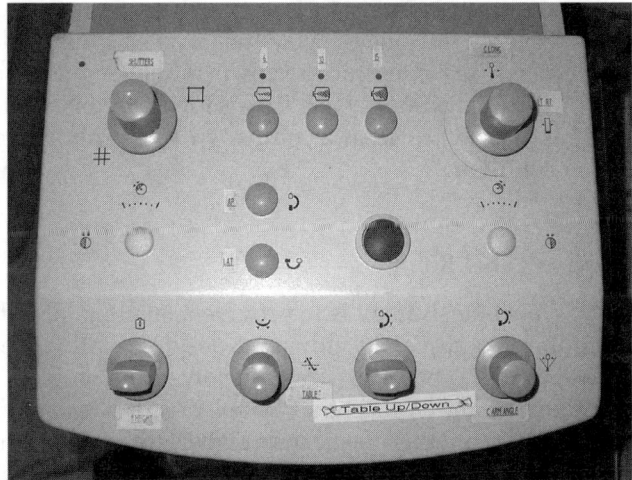

FIGURE 19.4
Handwritten labels have been added to an imaging machine's symbolically labeled controls to ensure correct use. Photos courtesy of Emerson Hospital (Concord, MA).

English-Only Labels

What about companies that market their products predominantly to English-speaking markets? Should they aim to produce a more global design, or assume that the limited number of non-English speaking users will "adjust?" It seems the answer to this question depends on the proportion of non-English users and the company's long-term goals. If the goal is to succeed in a local market, then maybe address the international market, it may be important to optimize the product for the local market first or "nationalize" the product. In this case, the smart move might be to commit to the major market's language for the sake of maximizing the intuitiveness of the product's user interface. However, designers may also want to access the level of compromise necessary to make the product suited to a global market from the beginning. Early usability testing will provide companies with a quantitative sense of the trade-offs.

How do foreign users cope with English products today? Apparently, without great trouble considering the predominant use of English in the worldwide medical community. In contrast to American clinicians, clinicians in foreign countries are typically multilingual and are likely to know English. However, some products may be used by people who do not have full command of the English language. They may resort to applying their own local labels, using adhesive tape and whatever else. Ultimately, this may be an acceptable outcome for the users. However, it may place a manufacturer at risk — perhaps leading to lawsuits — if the homemade labels lead to confusion and error. Another potential problem occurs when a primary user, such as an anesthesiologist, starts a case or procedure using an English-only device, then delegates monitoring responsibility to a nurse who may not be comfortable reading English. One can imagine the potential problems this could cause.

Manufacturers can ease communication by printing language-specific user manuals to go with English-only hardware. However, this strategy has its own costs and may be perceived as a company-driven solution, as opposed to a user-driven solution.

Provide a Custom Label Kit

Another creative labeling strategy is to provide a labeling kit with the basic device. Christopher Goodrich, an industrial designer with Datex–Ohmeda (Madison, WI) says this is how his company solved the problem of labeling components of an anesthesia machine. Datex–Ohmeda delivers a kit with the basic machine that contains plastic insert labels for controls and displays. In the field, one of Datex–Ohmeda's technicians applies the labels to the machine to match the local language. Goodrich says, "Using plastic inserts to label the machine is much more cost effective than stocking several versions of the machine in our inventory."

Tailoring the Software

What can be done to tailor software to local markets? Many products with sufficient computer memory give users a language menu that enables them to change all text from English to German, for example. Eric Smith, formerly a design engineer with Datex Medical Instrumentation (Tewksbury, MA) and now a usability specialist with American Institutes for Research (Concord,

MA), says that Datex's most advanced patient monitor can be configured in six different languages, all stored in memory and selected from an installation menu. Smith says, "We go as far as to differentiate between American English and British English. We have learned that our customers are very sensitive to even small language differences. For example, an American customer may be turned off if our monitor used the British spelling for the words anesthesia (British = anaesthesia) and color (colour). So, we make the distinction so that our customers feel that their monitor is tailored to their needs." Similarly, Datex is careful to display measurements, such as CO2, in units that are familiar to the user. As such, products marketed to Europe display CO_2 in percent, whereas products marketed domestically display CO_2 as a partial pressure (i.e., mmHg).

Products with limited internal memory may require people in the field to install a different version of software prior to product delivery. Obviously, getting the product to speak the local language is an important first step. However, language is just one consideration when adapting a software user interface to a specific user population. More profound changes that relate to how people do their jobs, such as changing the content and order of menus, phrasing messages in a different syntax, or using different icons may be necessary to make a product truly user-friendly. Determining how products should be tailored to local markets takes an investment in user research.

It is easy for manufacturers to develop provincial designs that never consider the needs of foreign markets. In fact, some product developers never get out of their development lab to talk to customers in their own backyard. This is a high-risk approach if you assume that there are critical differences in how products will be used by different user groups. Sequestering oneself in the lab leads to provincial design solutions fraught with usability problems. Therefore, manufacturers serious about user-oriented design need to talk to their potential customers in all major markets.

Such research is bound to show that one design solution will not fit all needs. For example, there are likely to be some tasks that U.S. clinicians perform frequently that Dutch or German clinicians rarely perform, and vice versa. In such cases, a single design solution that attempts to strike a compromise between user group needs may fail to satisfy both groups. Such products are easily overcome in usability comparisons by competing products that not only speak the right language, but also complement the way people think about and perform their jobs.

A future-looking solution to this problem is to design software to accommodate user interface variations. Areas of flexibility may include information presentation format, menu items and ordering, and the amount of online help available to users. Just like plastic insert labels, software variants can be installed in the field, eliminating inventory problems.

Undoubtedly, there are considerable costs to developing, validating, and maintaining several versions of software. However, such an investment may pay off handsomely in terms of increased sales and customer satisfaction. After all, no customer wants to feel they are being stuck with a design solution tailored to someone else's needs. They are likely to gravitate to products that "speak their language" in more ways than one.

Christopher Goodrich points out, "We [Ohmeda] need to think about doing everything we can to tailor designs to users by means of software changes in order to compete globally. Satisfying user needs by means of hardware changes would make us uncompetitive due to the high cost of manufacturing in the U.S. But, we have a lot more freedom to customize the software user interface."

Conclusion

Tailors remain in business because garment manufacturers produce standard-sized clothes that may not perfectly match a particular customer's body. Still, lots of people buy standard-sized garments off-the-rack if they fit reasonably well. Applying this analogy to the medical device industry, mass-marketed medical devices can never achieve a perfect fit with the needs of a particular user or market. Manufacturers must produce variants of their products that afford a reasonable fit (reasonable usability) or else lose sales. This is because there usually is one or more manufacturers who are anxious to address local needs with custom design solutions.

Adjusting hardware to changing needs may be too costly as compared to the usability benefits, leaving manufacturers the option of tailoring the software while maintaining a single, global hardware solution. Translating the user interface into local language is a great start, much like moving down the sportcoat rack from a 38 Short to a 44 Regular. Things get even better for users when designers modify formats, icons, message syntax, and related user-interface elements to match local needs, steps in the tailoring process analogous to adjusting a sportcoat's sleeve length and collar.

Perhaps user interfaces of the future will be smart enough to tailor themselves not only to specific market needs, but also to an individual's needs. Some product features, such as "smart alarms" that adjust their ranges to stable conditions may be a glimpse of what is to come. Then, the challenge will be to avoid personalizing devices to the point that they are unusable by others.

Key Points

- Manufacturers are loath to inventory several variants of a medical device, such as a ventilator or infusion pump, just because its user interface must incorporate local language or special features to meet the needs of a specific market.

- Generic or "global" hardware designs often replace text labels on a control panel with graphical symbols.
- Usability tests of devices that incorporate graphical symbols in place of text often show that such devices are less intuitive to use.
- One way to avoid placing language-dependent text labels on hardware is to shift controls from hardware to software.
- Companies that tailor software user interfaces to reflect local language can run into trouble if they do not anticipate the need for such tailoring in the original design.
- A clever way to retain direct access controls and avoid the need to place text labels on hardware is to use "softkeys" that are common to automatic teller machines (ATMs).
- Designing a good symbol is harder than it may seem, particularly if the symbol will represent an action (verb), as opposed to a recognizable object (noun).
- The American National Standards Institute (ANSI) promulgates a symbol acceptance criteria of 85% correct for symbols incorporated into safety signs.
- If the goal is to succeed in a local market, then maybe address the international market, it may be important to optimize the product for the local market first or "nationalize" the product.
- The considerable costs to developing, validating, and maintaining several versions of software may be offset by increased sales due to immediate customer acceptance and satisfaction.

Reference

1. American National Standard ANSI Z535.3-1991, Criteria for Safety Symbols, National Electrical Manufacturers Association, Washington, D.C., 19–20.

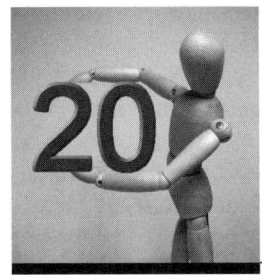

Why Choose Color Displays?

Michael E. Wiklund

There is an entire class of medical devices, such as infusion pumps, blood gas analyzers, and ventilators, that could be considered technological centaurs — part mechanical device and part computer. Intermixing mechanical and computer components has greatly extended the functionality of these devices over the past decade, enabling physicians to develop entirely new therapy regimes. It has also led to a shift in the way people interact with those products. Information display and control actions previously assigned to dedicated-purpose meters, counters, knobs, and switches are now handled via interactions with software. The ubiquitous control panel has been replaced with the increasingly ubiquitous computer display and input devices, such as a trackball, arrowkeys, and touch screen. Turning a knob has been replaced by "highlighting and selecting."

Initially, these centaurlike products incorporated very small displays — typically a 2-line by 16-character liquid crystal display (LCD) or its equivalent. These little displays had considerable value as variable output devices, but also introduced significant usability problems. Comparing interactions with a medical product to a person-to-person conversation, the little displays made conversation overly terse, leading to miscommunication. Because of the lack of screen titles and meaningful prompts, device users found themselves confused about their place in a sequence of tasks, unsure of the meaning of terms abbreviated to fit the available space, and puzzled about the next step of a task.

Fortunately, as soon as prices came down, manufacturers started to incorporate the kind of larger displays found in notebook computers. This step solved many of the usability problems associated with insufficient screen space.

The current trend among medical device manufacturers is to upgrade to color displays. An upgrade to color has considerable allure. Color certainly enriches communications between user and device, boosting a device's usability and desirability. For example, end-users state a strong preference for color-coded warning messages (e.g., white text on a red banner to indicate a dangerous condition), which can be very attention getting and start communicating their message (i.e., there is a problem) upon initial glance. These benefits of color have already been proven in higher-end products, such as integrated patient monitors and advanced imaging devices that are clearly special-purpose computers. But the price difference between monochrome and color displays is still a concern for manufacturers of lower-cost medical devices. Consequently, design decisions regarding the use of a color versus monochrome display often stall and become the subject of endless debate and waffling.

The Advantages of Color

Recognizing that others will champion the cause of low-cost monochrome displays, the balance of this chapter offers arguments in favor of stepping up to color. Some of the arguments may be familiar ones, but others may not. The number of advantages offered by color versus monochrome displays may be surprising.

Image Quality

Image quality varies widely between and within general classes of displays, including cathode ray tubes (CRTs), electroluminescent panels (ELPs), vacuum fluorescent displays, and LCDs. Although there are exceptions to the general rule, image quality increases as display cost increases. For example, a monochrome LCD (twisted nematic/passive matrix) is relatively inexpensive, but has several image quality shortcomings. Such displays are not as bright as others, are prone to viewing-angle limitations, and refresh slowly, blurring dynamic effects such as cursor movement or list scrolling. By comparison, a color LCD (thin-film transistor/active matrix) provides a reasonably bright image that refreshes quickly and affords a wider viewing cone. It is important to note, however, that some monochrome displays such as CRTs and ELPs also provide high-quality images.

Visual Appeal

As common sense would suggest, people generally regard colored screens as more visually appealing than monochrome screens. Anecdotal remarks and quantitative ratings by participants in user studies consistently reinforce this conclusion. For example, if you conduct a focus group or usability test

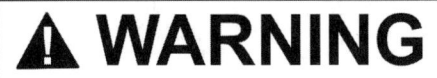

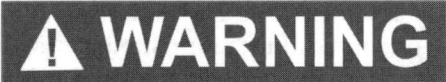

FIGURE 20.1 (See color insert following page 142)
Warning message in black and white versus color.

with prospective customers and show them a version of an information display in color versus monochrome (gray scale), almost all will prefer the color screen. In some sense, this preference is comparable to people's general preference for stereo over monaural sound. Color adds an extra dimension to the visual experience, enabling people to draw upon the full capability of their senses. As such, customers will exhibit a natural attraction to, and preference for, colored displays over monochrome displays, all other things being equal.

Graphic Simplicity

Color monitors afford designers a greater opportunity to produce simple-looking screens. The reason is that adjacent colors of differing hues (spectral wavelength composition) and similar values (lightness versus darkness) create natural borders, whereas adjacent gray tones are incrementally less effective. As a result, colored elements do not always need edge demarcation to assure distinctiveness, for example, where monochrome screens do. In comparison to colored screens, most monochrome displays are burdened with extra on-screen elements, adding to their visual complexity.

Color Coding

Color is a terrific method of coding important information (see Figure 20.1). When color is not available, one must resort to other coding techniques. Alarm messages, for example, can be made larger and bolder than other text, physically segregated from other information, highlighted by means of demarcation lines or an inverse video effect, or be presented using a symbol (e.g., a bell or horn symbol) in place of text. However, color is a most compelling coding technique when it comes to detecting alarm information embedded within other information. In fact, human factors studies have shown that color outperforms other visual codes, such as size, shape, and brightness as a coding technique.[1] It performs particularly well when the task is to search for an item or group of items among many, or to track a moving target.

More Information

Color displays offer the potential to present more information at a time than monochrome displays. As discussed earlier, it is simply a matter of having one dimension for communicating information. Christopher Goodrich is a senior industrial designer with Datex–Ohmeda, Inc. (Madison, WI), a manufacturer of anesthesia delivery systems. He considers a color display essential to the usability of medical devices that present a lot of information in parallel. "Color gives you an effective way to visually separate groups of information so that the information is easier for users to find," he says. "This helps you avoid a trade-off imposed by monochrome screens — putting in less information to avoid visual clutter."

Competitive Advantage

Competing manufacturers often engage in so-called feature wars. In such wars, manufacturers arm their products with extra features (usually software functions that can be enabled or disabled) that appeal to customers initially but rarely get used. As an everyday example, consumers are drawn to CD players that can play songs from several CDs in a preprogrammed sequence, but few use the feature once they own the device. In the medical world, the valued but unused feature might be a special data-analysis feature.

Color displays are different. They provide a continual benefit to users, much the way a good sound system rewards the listener. Color displays also provide a significant competitive advantage, particularly in head-to-head comparisons that take place in clinical environments and trade shows. As many marketing managers can attest, devices equipped with color displays tend to draw more casual interest among people walking the trade show floor. The competitive advantage can be expected to shift toward products incorporating a monochrome display only when minimum cost is the dominant purchase criteria.

Some companies may consider color displays a necessity only when technology matures and manufacturers start to compete on the basis of design quality as opposed to functional capability. As such, companies holding an initial technological advantage may equip their products with monochrome monitors, expecting to sell just as many units and maximize profit. However, this approach offers future competitors an opportunity to break into the market with a me-too product equipped with a color display, meeting a demand for higher user-interface quality. Therefore, an early commitment to color before it becomes a necessity may be an effective way to ward off future competition while also boosting user-interface quality.

Progressive Image

Medical and diagnostic device manufacturers work hard to establish a positive image for their company in the marketplace. Most seek a progressive image, positioning themselves on the leading edge in terms of technology, perceived quality, and actual quality. It is not clear that marketing a product incorporating a monochrome display will erode a progressive image, but it could. For instance, when customers check out products incorporating monochrome displays for the first time, they are prone to label them old-fashioned or cheap. This perception may be a case of transference from people's experience with black-and-white versus color television. In comparison, the same product equipped with a color display might be labeled as progressive and user-friendly.

Meeting Customer Expectations

Today, such consumer electronics as palmcorders, pocketable TVs, cellular phones, and digital cameras incorporate color displays. This has raised the ante for industrial product manufacturers. Customers are becoming accustomed to high-quality color displays in place of monochrome displays. Therefore, some customers may feel neutral at best about using a product incorporating a monochrome display. However, other customers may regard the product as less user-friendly and cheap.

A spokesperson for Aksys, Ltd. (Libertyville, IL), a start-up company developing a system for hemodialysis, agrees that color has a real draw for customers. "Color can raise a customer's perception of product quality and user-friendliness — no question about it. Our customers are certainly used to products in their daily lives, such as televisions and home computers, that use color monitors. Therefore, their in-home experience raises the expectation for color in a medical product intended for use in the home. So, even though competitors might not be forcing us toward color at this time, we have to look seriously at the customer's preference for color."

Goodrich is also convinced that forces outside the medical industry are compelling medical device manufacturers to use color displays. "Customers are starting to expect medical devices to incorporate color displays, largely due to their experience with consumer products. This shift in expectation stands to make monochrome displays obsolete for application to products that require large displays." Speaking for himself and the hundreds of customers he has interviewed, Goodrich adds, "Monochrome displays are just so lacking in overall appeal, you want to avoid them, except in cases where the wide-angle viewing capability of ELPs is essential."

Future Enhancement

In the near future, the struggle of choosing between color and monochrome displays should end. The cost differential will shrink and color displays will be the de facto standard for high-tech devices. Accordingly, the "turn of the century" represents a transition period, posing a shelf-life problem for manufacturers that choose monochrome for their next-generation products. What are manufacturers going to do when the marketplace forces them to upgrade to color? For many, the hardware needed to support a monochrome display will not support an upgrade without major redesign and retooling. Display mounts, power supplies, and display controllers may be incompatible, although some manufacturers have started to engineer commonality into their monochrome and color product lines. Also, a subsequent switch to color may require considerable software changes. So, initial reductions in development and manufacturing costs may be counterbalanced by the costs of design changes or introducing yet another next-generation product to market ahead of the intended schedule.

To hedge their bets, manufacturers can take a hybrid approach: designing for monochrome today, allowing for an easy upgrade to color tomorrow. This approach may result in some overengineering at the outset, but is likely to reduce product development and manufacturing costs in the future. Overengineering may come in the form of a flexible approach to display mounting and higher-capacity display drivers, for example. It may also come in the form of extra software code with setup functions that enable the appropriate code to produce a monochrome versus color image. However, it is possible to develop a single version of the software that works with either a color or monochrome monitor. The effect is akin to starting with a color monitor and adjusting the colors so that everything looks monochromatic. Making this approach work requires care in picking colors of equivalent value (lightness versus darkness) so that the monochromatic image has a consistent appearance.

Customer Choice

Rather than making a display decision, some manufacturers offer both color and monochrome displays and let customers decide between them (see Figure 20.2 and Figure 20.3). The extra costs of engineering and manufacturing both types of units can be recovered by marking up the color units, for example, presuming that some customers will pay the extra amount. Then, as the cost of color displays decreases to meet the cost of monochrome displays (due to economies of scale and competition), the monochrome monitor can be dropped from the inventory. From the beginning, this approach pays off in terms of establishing a high-tech image while also being able to offer a reduced price on an entry-level product. Typically, this approach requires designers to introduce redundant information coding, augmenting a color code with some other coding technique, such as shape coding or size coding. This ensures that a colored screen will still work in monochrome. Redundant coding also benefits people who have impaired color vision (8 to 10% of Caucasian males, about 4% of non-Caucasian males, and about 0.5% of all females).[2]

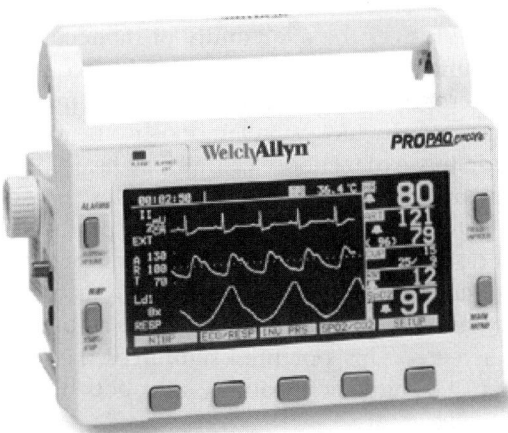

FIGURE 20.2 (See color insert following page 142)
Patient monitor with a monochrome screen. Photo courtesy of Welch Allyn Inc.

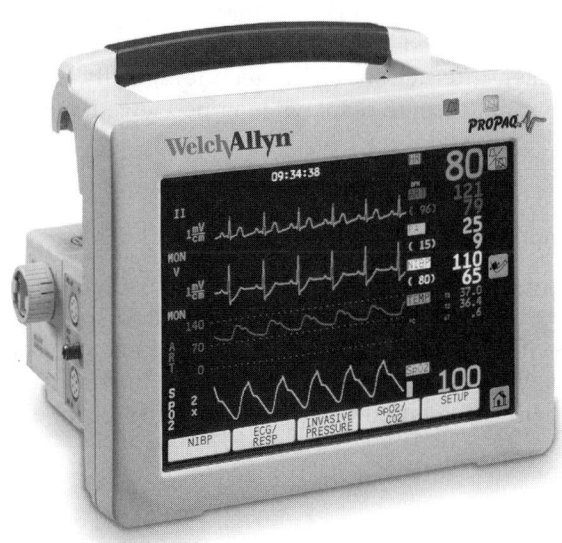

FIGURE 20.3 (See color insert following page 142)
Patient monitor with a color screen. Photo courtesy of Welch Allyn Inc.

Avoiding Supply Problems

Already, there is concern over the availability of monochrome monitors in the future. Many manufacturers wonder if they will face a problem similar to finding low-end microprocessors in a market that has moved on to higher-powered microprocessors. In fact, small monochrome CRTs are virtually obsolescent. However, those that choose color today face a potential problem that stems from volatility in the notebook computer market. Specifically, color display manufacturers are likely to adjust their product lines according to the needs of their dominant buyers — notebook computer manufacturers. In fact, the de facto standard notebook screen size has continued to grow over the past few years to the point that they are as big as conventional desktop computer screens. This potential reinforces the need for medical device manufacturers to engineer flexibility into both their products and manufacturing processes.

Device Integration

Many medical devices are used in conjunction with others. This is particularly true of devices used in the operating room and intensive-care environments. Such environments are not known for high levels of integration between products. However, there is a growing trend toward integration. For example, anesthesia workstations used to be a conglomerate of devices placed on various shelves. Now, companies are working together to produce integrated solutions. If one extrapolates this trend, one can envision entire systems of components that work together, sharing data and control capabilities. Products equipped with color displays fit well with this vision of high-quality user interactions with technology. By contrast, products equipped with monochrome displays may be viewed as impoverished relative to other higher-end devices.

Third-Party Applications

With the advent of medical information highways within hospitals, many products will be sharing information. As a result, displays previously dedicated to a specific function, such as presenting vital signs and waveforms, may also display laboratory results and e-mail. In such cases, the use of a color display will be essential to ensure that third-party applications look correct.

Economies of Scale

Because of the costs involved, equipping certain lower-end products that have limited user-interface requirements with color monitors may be viewed as overkill as well as detrimental to sales. However, companies that also market higher-end products equipped with color displays may discover economies of scale favoring across-the-board use of color displays. The economies may not accrue strictly on cost of goods. Rather, they may accrue from reduced inventory, engineering, servicing, and software development costs.

Using Color to Communicate Better

Information displayed on-screen can be enhanced with the use of color. In many instances, color also allows more information to be presented on-screen. Following are some examples.

- In a breathing circuit diagram, the lungs can be colored pink, making them more recognizable as a body part as well as indicating proper oxygenation.
- Bar graphs associated with anesthesia gas flows can be colored to match standards for the labeling of compressed gases (e.g., green for oxygen in the U.S. market).
- An arterial blood pressure waveform can be colored red to reinforce an association with oxygenated blood.
- On-screen start and stop buttons can be colored green and red, respectively, to reinforce a traffic light metaphor (i.e., green means "go" and red means "stop").
- To indicate high priority, important messages can be printed on a yellow, rectangular square to resemble Post-it notes.
- To help users recognize components, maintenance diagrams can depict the actual appearance of the product using as many colors as necessary or can even show a digitized color photograph.

Conclusion

Applications for monochrome monitors remain. However, for those manufacturers weighing the trade-offs between color and monochrome displays, there are abundant reasons to select color. Presuming a professional application of color in screen design, a color display opens up new dimensions in user-interface design that enhance a product's overall usability and appeal. Still, the added dimension of color may pale in comparison to the benefit of minimizing the cost of a product that must compete in a price-sensitive market. This trade-off is what makes the decision between color and monochrome displays so difficult.

For some product manufacturers, the cost considerations may lead to the continued use of monochrome displays for a few more years while the cost of color displays continues to drop. However, individuals calculating the benefits and costs should take care to consider all of the potential benefits of color that extend beyond the visual appeal of a given product or even the economics of a single product line. Moreover, decision makers should ask themselves the pointed question: Which type of display would I choose if I had to look at it every day for many years? Chances are that the very same individuals use a desktop computer equipped with a color display.

Key Points

- Turning a knob on a medical device has been partly replaced by "highlighting and selecting" on a computer screen.
- Upgrading a medical device display from monochrome to color can enhance communications between user and device, boosting a device's usability and desirability.
- The advantages of a color display include better image quality, increased visual appeal, graphic simplicity, and the ability to use color to assign special meaning to information.
- Color displays offer manufacturers a competitive advantage, give their products a more progressive image, and help them meet the expectations of customers accustomed to color displays found in consumer electronic devices, for example.
- In the future, manufacturers may have difficulty finding a supply of monochrome displays at a reasonable price, while greater economies of scale drop the price of color displays.
- A medical device equipped with a color display will fit in better with other devices found in clinical environments.

References

1. Thorell, L.G. and Smith, W.J., *Using Computer Color Effectively — An Illustrated Reference*, Prentice Hall, Englewood Cliffs, NJ, 7, 1990.
2. Thorell, L.G. and Smith, W.J., *Using Computer Color Effectively — An Illustrated Reference*, Prentice Hall, Englewood Cliffs, NJ, 117, 1990.

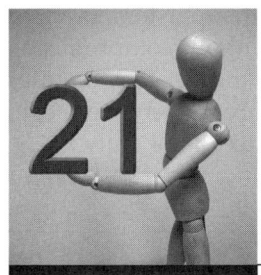

Intuitive Design: Removing Obstacles Also Increases Appeal

Michael E. Wiklund

Imagine that you are an experienced nurse starting a new job at a large teaching hospital. You have been assigned to a cardiac care unit where your first patient is a 65-year-old male with acute hypertension (high blood pressure). The charge nurse asks you to set up an intravenous infusion for the patient using a four-channel pump that you have never operated before.

Fortunately, the comparatively advanced device is intuitive to use. The device's large computer display tells you exactly what to do at every step — from hanging the IV solution bag to inserting the IV tube into the pumping mechanism to programming a flow rate. After the pump checks that you programmed a safe dosage, it directs you to start the infusion by pressing the big green button that dominates the front panel.

Potential delay or compromise to patient care averted! Instead of struggling to understand how to set up and run the unfamiliar pump, the pump helped you draw upon your existing knowledge and skills to operate it correctly the first time. Wouldn't it be nice if all user-device interactions went this smoothly?

Regrettably, many user-device interactions do not proceed this smoothly. Rather, caregivers frequently encounter obstacles while trying to use an unfamiliar device. The device may offer little guidance on its proper operational sequence, leaving the user guessing what to do next. It may require the user to look up and enter a cryptic numerical code to start a function, thereby opening the door to confusion and user error. Or, the device may provide little feedback to judge whether it is working properly.

Caregivers, many of whom consider themselves "can do" individuals, overcome such obstacles by seeking guidance from experienced colleagues or by simply spending precious time figuring things out. Naturally, most caregivers prefer devices that are easy to use from the start, especially considering the large number of devices they use in their work.

The key for medical device developers is to fulfill their customers' need and desire for initial ease of use (i.e., intuitiveness) without compromising operational efficiency (i.e., task speed). It is a balancing act that requires developers to take a holistic view of the user experience, which may begin with in-service training or self-discovery and span a decade of daily use.

Limitations of Training

Developers often cite training, particularly in-servicing, as the cure-all for products that are difficult to learn to use. The average in-service lasts no more than an hour and may include a dozen or more people. Some trainers may wish to provide more training and deliver it one-on-one, but caregivers usually do not have sufficient time to devote to more in-depth training. Typically, a manufacturer's representative teaches the in-service, covering the basic operational concepts and demonstrating the essential tasks. Many hospitals take a "train the trainer" approach that calls for key staff, such as nurse educators, to receive in-service training from the manufacturer's representative, then pass the lessons along to other staff. Caregivers generally much prefer hands-on in-services to reading and following instructions in a user manual.

However, despite the popularity and presumed effectiveness of in-service training, many first encounters between caregivers and medical devices actually occur at the point of care, such as the patient's bedside. A caregiver may have missed the in-service because she or he was busy with a patient or was off duty. In some cases, caregivers "float" from another unit that does not use the particular device and, therefore, did not receive training. Perhaps the caregiver comes from a temporary nurse agency that has supplied RNs to address a staffing shortage. Or, it may be a caregiver's first day on the job, as described earlier, presenting no prior opportunity for training.

Accordingly, it is wrong to assume that all staff will receive formal training before they use a particular medical device, despite the movement to require caregivers to complete training exercises before they are authorized to use a device. Restrictions on device use are simply not the norm at this time. So, the burden remains on manufacturers to design devices that enable users to easily understand a device for themselves — and quickly — before a patient suffers any harm.

Intuitive Design: Caregiver's Perspective

Human factors textbooks offer extensive advice on how to design intuitive user interfaces. However, caregivers are also a good source of guidance. The following recommendations have been distilled from interviews with several

Intuitive Design: Removing Obstacles Also Increases Appeal 205

nurses working in general medical and critical-care environments. Notably, many of the design characteristics that enhance intuitiveness also tend to reduce the potential for use error and increase product appeal.

Provide Extensive Prompts

Nurses want devices to lead them through a clear and consistent series of actions to accomplish a task, almost as if a human guide were leading them. They view prompting (i.e., a series of short, context-sensitive instructions) as the surest way to avoid skipping a critical step. They accept that prompting may increase the time required to complete a task, but feel that extensive prompting speeds up tasks by reducing the need to seek help. They also see prompts as a means for new users to teach themselves to use a device in a fail-safe manner.

One nurse commented that she attended an in-service on how to use an epidural pump, but then did not see it for another few months, leaving her time to forget her training. She felt that step-by-step prompting would have been her savior if she were pressed to use the pump with little notice. She noted that nurses are prone to take any shortcuts that save time, but deep down prefer to follow methodical procedures that prevent errors.

Another nurse commented, "Why keep steps 1, 2, 3, and 4 a secret? Print them right on the product." She was less concerned with making a medical device look too simplistic and more concerned with every person operating the device correctly (see Figure 21.1). So, while literally labeling a product with the numerals 1, 2, 3, and 4 may not always be a viable solution, the underlying intent seems valid: design the user interface to accentuate the proper operational sequence.

One nurse insisted that devices should not only tell users when they do something wrong, but it should also tell them how to correct their mistake. She welcomed the use of voice output as an intuitive means for appropriate devices, such as defibrillators, to communicate with caregivers.

Use Prominent Labels

Nurses applaud the use of prominent labels to conspicuously indicate a device's purpose and proper operation. One nurse offered the example of labeling defibrillator pads with the words *Front* and *Back* in large black letters as a good way to direct users to apply them correctly. She explained that first responders, such as members of a Code team, have little time to figure things out in a crisis. They perform tasks by rote rather than pausing to identify and analyze their options. So, they are better off when a device spells out the operational basics

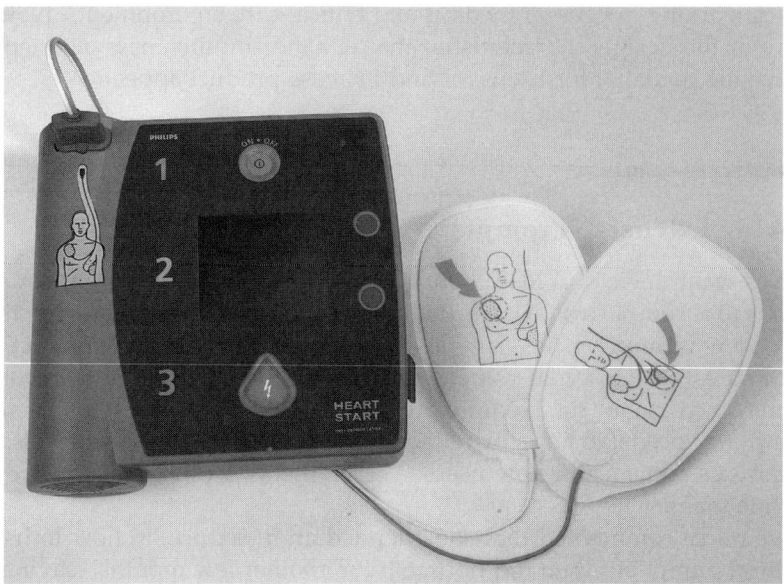

FIGURE 21.1
Heartstart® FR2 SEMI-Automatic External Defibrillator directs the user's attention and actions with bold numbers. Photo courtesy of Philips Medical Systems.

in an almost exaggerated manner. Similarly, it helps nurses perform tasks as seemingly straightforward as applying or releasing the brakes on a hospital bed if the brake includes a prominent label (see Figure 21.2).

Commit to a Single, Optimized Configuration

Contrary to the call for customization, nurses considered device configurability to be a problem. In their view, enabling devices used within the same institution to assume various configurations compromises a nurse's ability to master their operation. Consequently, experienced nurses may encounter new configurations that take time to decipher. Many would sacrifice flexibility for the sake of configuration stability, noting that stability enables the experienced nurse to provide expert support to new users.

Prevent Users from Turning Off Critical Alarms

Nurses recognize that they may give device manufacturers conflicting guidance regarding alarms. They despise nuisance alarms that create more work.

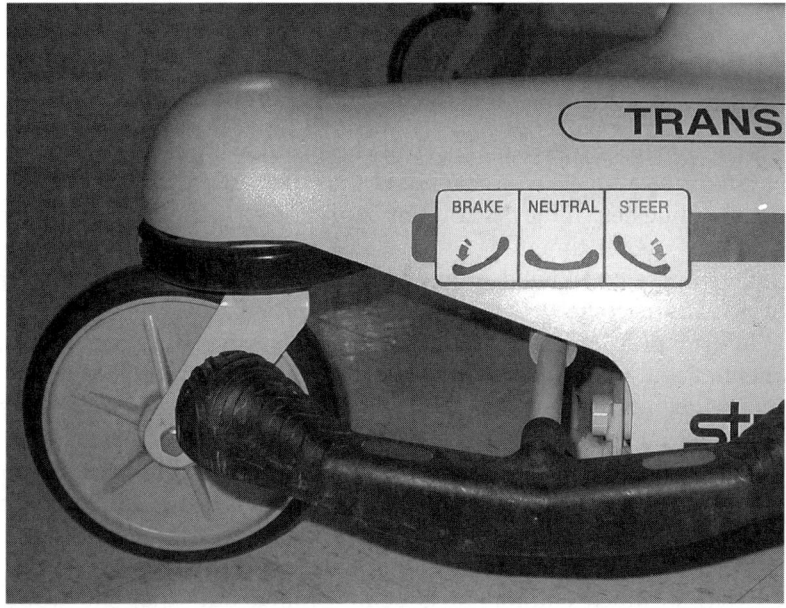

FIGURE 21.2
A hospital bed's brake control is prominently labeled. Photo courtesy of Emerson Hospital (Concord, MA).

However, they recognize the underlying benefit of alarm systems associated with critical therapeutic and monitoring devices. Therefore, they advise manufacturers to prevent users from turning off any critical alarms, presuming that users can silence alarms for an appropriate amount of time.

Provide Large Displays

Large displays have obvious benefits. They provide more space to display larger graphics, text, and numbers, making the information readable from a greater distance. Designers can take advantage of larger displays to emphasize the most important information, which helps both new and experienced users focus on the most important information. Large displays also provide room for prompts.

One nurse lamented that manufacturers seem to design their products for people in their 20s who have better than 20/20 vision and who will view displays in ideal lighting conditions. Noting that the average age of nurses is in the mid-40s, she advised manufacturers to oversize their displays, labels, and other printed materials so they are legible to people who have reduced visual acuity.

Provide Online Help

Nurses like embedded online help systems, as long as the manufacturer invests enough resources to make it truly helpful. One nurse described online help systems as a time saver. She noted that she could direct new nurses to check the online help if they encounter operational problems, thereby reducing demands on her time.

Another nurse considered online help superior to quick reference cards because cards become worn and outdated, whereas online help contains more information and can provide context-sensitive assistance. She also commented that nurses just out of school are quite comfortable with computers and expect a sophisticated device to incorporate online help, just as they expect contemporary software applications to include one.

Another nurse insisted that smart devices, such as those that incorporate an online help system, should tell new users what they need to know about operating the device in three minutes or less. She explained that nurses in her large hospital rarely have time to attend an hour-long in-service. She added that so much equipment is being "rolled out" that she would be attending in-services all the time rather than attending to her patients.

Provide Large Controls

One nurse observed, "I've yet to see a device with buttons that were too big." This comment underscores the view held by several nurses that large controls make a device easier to use and, conversely, that small controls make a device harder to use. The association between large controls (see Figure 21.3) and ease of use may be part perception, but one can understand the preference for controls that provide a good visual target as well as a firm grip. Shape and color coding can make controls even more intuitive. Touch screen-based controls, such as those found on some patient monitors, can also make a device easier to use, presuming that the touch targets are not crowded together and provide effective actuation feedback by means of visual effects and sounds.

Be Consistent

Several nurses recommended that manufacturers standardize their controls and graphical symbols. One nurse noted that people could step into virtually

Intuitive Design: Removing Obstacles Also Increases Appeal

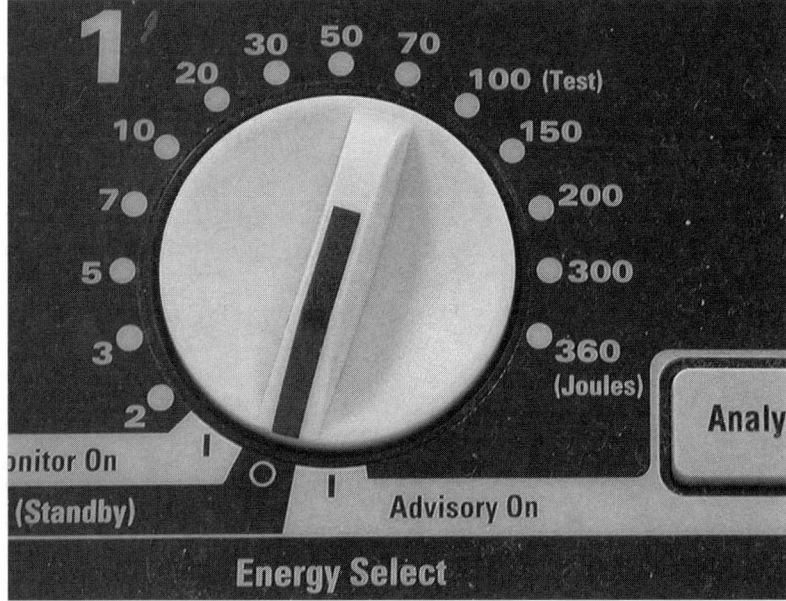

FIGURE 21.3
A defibrillator's energy level control is large, color coded, and shape coded. Photo courtesy of Emerson Hospital (Concord, MA).

any rental car and drive away because the placement and operation of the primary controls is relatively consistent. She challenged medical device manufacturers to achieve a similar degree of design consistency so that caregivers can easily switch from one medical device to another.

One nurse advised manufacturers to make all of the necessary connections obvious, half seriously suggesting that some manufacturers go so far as to hide connection ports from the user. She also recommended using shape and color coding (see Figure 21.4) to the maximum extent possible so that making the proper connections is a simple matter of matching up similar-looking components.

Automate Appropriate Functions

Nurses welcome automation as long as they can remain "in the loop" in terms of understanding a patient's condition so they are prepared to respond effectively to emergencies, including those involving a device failure. For example, nurses feel no strong need to calibrate a device or run a maintenance check if the device can be engineered to perform these functions automatically. Such automation makes devices easier to learn because there is simply less to learn.

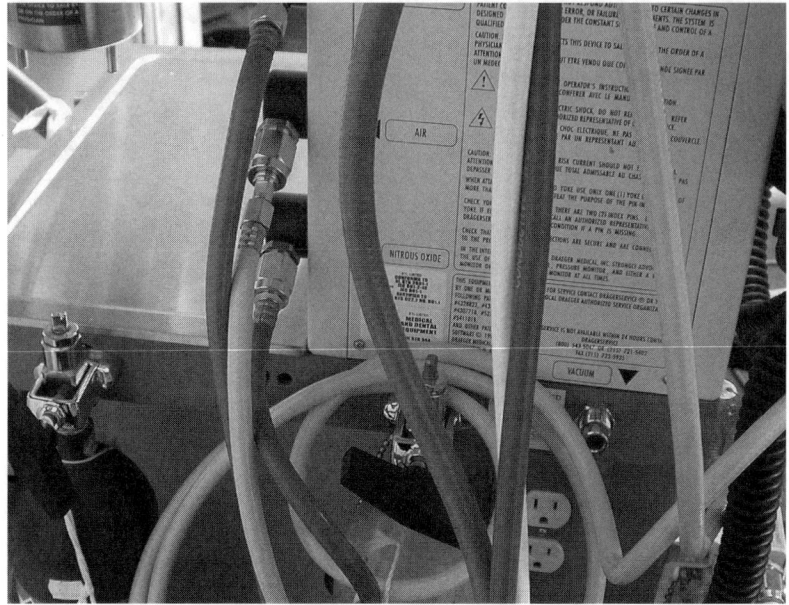

FIGURE 21.4 (See color insert following page 142)
Gas lines running to the back of an anesthesia workstation are color coded. Photo courtesy of Emerson Hospital (Concord, MA).

Avoid Minor Changes

Nurses get frustrated by minor, incremental changes to medical devices that contradict the expectations they develop using earlier-generation products. They recommend that manufacturers stick to one method of operation, rather than a slightly different scheme of operation, until they are ready to launch an entirely new iteration of the device. Minor changes can actually be more confusing than wholesale changes.

Enable Users to Practice Tasks

Nurses welcome medical devices that incorporate a simulation mode and the accessories necessary to practice using them. Such devices enable users to gain proficiency with a device before using it on a patient. However, devices need protections in place to prevent users from confusing simulated performance with actual performance.

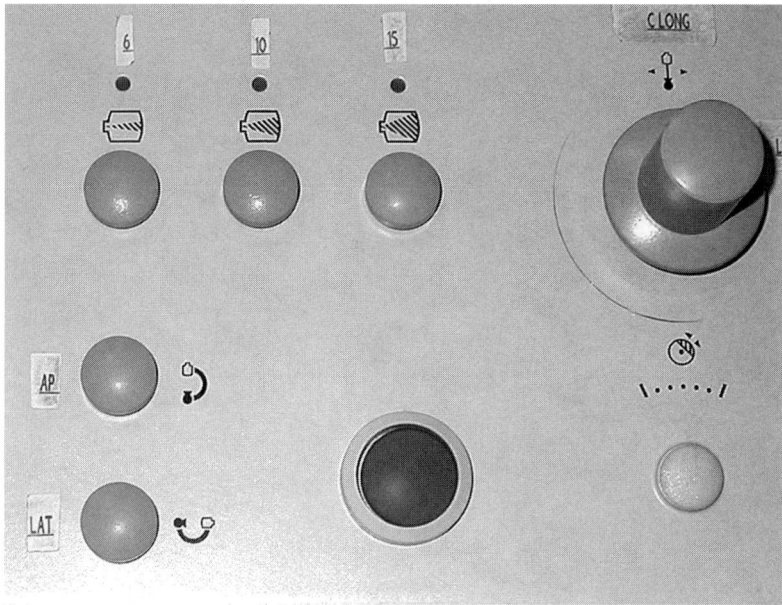

FIGURE 21.5
A red control stands out in a field of light gray controls, although it lacks an informative label. Photo courtesy of Emerson Hospital (Concord, MA).

Perform Checks

Nurses also welcome the increased computing power found in many devices that makes it possible to check user settings, such as a programmed infusion rate. Such power enables them to ensure that the settings fall within the boundaries of normal use established by the manufacturer or health-care institution. That way, if their inputs fall out of the normal range, the device can alert them to the potential hazard, such as a morphine overdose.

Make Important Features and Information Prominent

Nurses recognize that some controls and displays are used more frequently or urgently than others and that some controls and displays perform especially critical functions. They feel that the important controls and displays should grab the user's attention. This may be accomplished by making them larger, segregating them from others, or coding them in a conspicuous manner, such as giving them a special shape or color (see Figure 21.5).

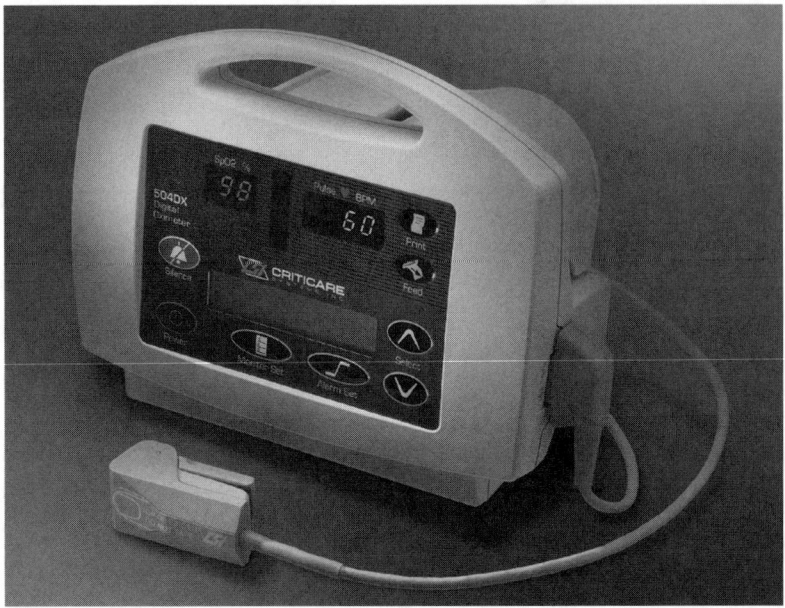

FIGURE 21.6
Criticare Systems' 504DX Portable Pulse Oximeter employs well spaced, large membrane keys. Photo courtesy of Criticare Systems, Inc.

Hold the Extras

Manufacturers feel compelled by market forces to include extra features in their products because procurement processes tend to reward feature-filled products that appear to offer greater value. However, nurses view most extra features as excess baggage that gets in the way of simple operation. One nurse commented, "Our patient monitors have lots of advanced features. I have no idea what they do."

But, is the answer to eliminate the extras altogether? Perhaps, depending on whether the extras are important to a small percentage of potential users or practically nobody. For example, one nurse cited the dose calculators built into some infusion pumps as an extra that is useful to a small percentage — perhaps 20% — of all users. But, other extras may be useful to only a handful of people and not worth keeping. Another solution is to isolate the extra features by placing them behind a panel or in a software menu. However, this solution is antithetical to human factors guidelines, such as creating logical functional groupings and providing easy access to functions. Therefore, the best approach is to scrutinize every feature in terms of its true value and to purge those that increase complexity while adding little benefit (see Figure 21.6).

Conclusion

The medical care environment rivals consumer electronic stores, such as Best Buy and Circuit City, as a technology haven. Within critical-care environments, one finds blood gas analyzers, defibrillators, electrocardiographs, electronic thermometers, infusion pumps, noninvasive blood pressure monitors, patient monitors, patient warmers, diagnostic spirometers, and many other specialized devices. For nurses and other caregivers, these devices present a lot of technology to master, so it is no wonder they gravitate toward intuitive technologies.

In a perfect world, there may be enough time to learn how to use all the features built into all of the medical devices. However, in the real world, most caregivers worry about learning the basics and utilizing the special features only when necessary and, often, only as time permits. This makes intuitiveness a critical design feature and a great opportunity for innovation, even if the innovation is the removal of an extraneous feature.

Key Points

- Caregivers frequently encounter obstacles while trying to use an unfamiliar medical device. Many overcome such obstacles by seeking guidance from experienced colleagues or by simply spending precious time figuring things out.
- Developers often cite training, particularly in-servicing, as the cure-all for products that are difficult to learn. But, it is wrong to assume that all staff will received formal training before they use a particular medical device.
- Many of the product design characteristics that enhance intuitiveness also tend to reduce the potential for use error and increase product appeal.
- Nurses want devices to lead them through a clear and consistent series of actions to accomplish a task.
- Contrary to the call for customization, nurses consider device configurability to be a problem, preferring configuration stability over flexibility.
- Nurses advise manufacturers to design alarm systems that cannot be disabled, use large displays and controls, make important features and information prominent, use prominent labels to conspicuously indicate a device's purpose and proper operation, forego extraneous

features that only get in the way of simple device operation, provide online help, and generally ascribe to industry standards.
- Nurses welcome automation as long as they can remain "in the loop" in terms of understanding a patient's condition.
- Nurses discourage manufacturers from making minor design changes that create inconsistencies between older and newer devices.
- Nurses welcome the means to practice using a medical device before using it on a patient. They also like devices that are smart enough to check if settings fall within the boundaries of normal use.

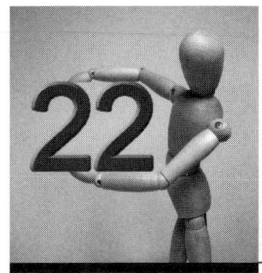

Medical Devices That Talk

Michael E. Wiklund

Talking medical devices can enhance the way users interact with such products. But how can you ensure that your device is actually helpful?

How do you feel about products that talk to you? Do you appreciate automobile navigation systems that direct you to "Turn left ahead?" Or an automated receptionist that invites you to "Listen carefully to the menu options because some have been changed?" And what about talking bottle openers?

If you are like most people, you find some of these things helpful and others annoying. What seems to be the distinction? Whether the voice is a useful aid or just a noisy gimmick? This simple criterion can be applied to talking medical devices as well.

So far, medical device manufacturers seem to have taken a smart, disciplined approach to giving their products a voice. There are some excellent examples of talking devices that enhance the way users interact with them. Voice-enabled medical devices are leading users through some particularly challenging tasks, breaking down barriers to independent use by people with impaired vision, and improving usability as a whole.

Sample Applications

Automated external defibrillators (AEDs) are an impressive example of voice prompts enhancing user interactions with a medical device. An AED is

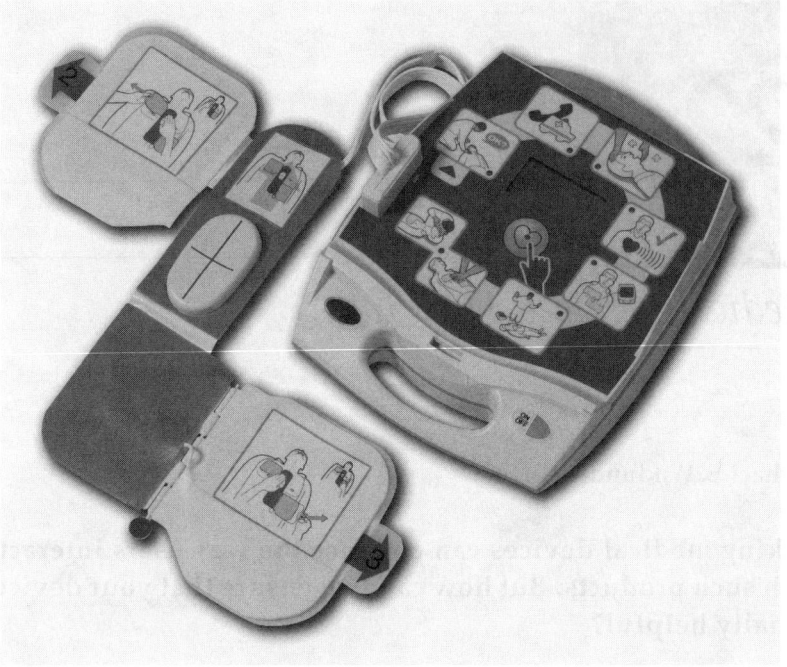

FIGURE 22.1
The ZOLL AED Plus uses voice prompts to guide users through the steps required for a rescue. Photo courtesy of ZOLL Medical Corporation.

designed for use in an emergency when a victim may require resuscitation. The latest-generation AEDs use voice prompts to guide users through the numerous steps required to perform a successful rescue. Spoken instructions, such as stay calm and check breathing, spare the rescuer from having to read textual or graphical instructions, which would be more time-consuming and could create confusion. Clearly, the use of voice prompts in an AED is no gimmick. People who have used devices such as the ZOLL AED Plus (see Figure 22.1) respond well to the voice prompts, finding them both helpful and reassuring during a stressful event.

Talking glucose meters are another exemplary application of speech technology, but focus on a different goal. The value of a talking glucose meter, such as the Roche Diagnostics' ACCU-CHEK® VOICEMATE System (see Figure 22.2), is that diabetics who have vision impairments or total blindness — common outcomes of the disease — can use it independently. A visually impaired person simply needs to follow the device's spoken instructions to "apply blood to a specially designed test strip, insert [the] strip into the device, and listen for the numerical result." This natural means of interaction could also serve the needs of people who have cognitive impairments. Or it might be preferred by people who simply would rather listen to information such as "result is 64 milligrams per deciliter," than to read it on a small

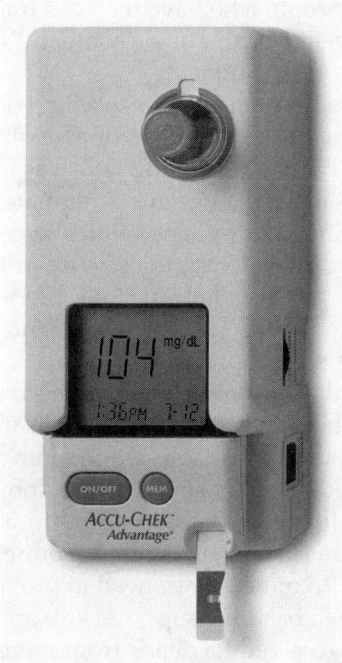

FIGURE 22.2
Roche Diagnostics' ACCU-CHEK® VOICEMATE System can report a blood glucose level aloud. Photo courtesy of Roche Diagnostics Corporation. ACCU-CHEK® and VOICEMATE are trademarks of a Member of the Roche Group.

display. Of course, a user might choose between the two modalities if the device incorporated both a display and voice output.

About the Technology

As in designing other types of user interfaces, there is both an art and a science to producing a well-spoken medical device. Designing a good one is a matter of balancing technical and user-centered needs.

Choosing the right technology is one of the more straightforward design tasks. For medical devices that only talk (i.e., that do not have voice recognition capabilities), developers can choose between digitized and synthesized speech technologies. Digitized speech usually sounds much better because it is based on recording a real person's voice, then playing back the right segment at the right moment. The technology works best with medical devices requiring a relatively small vocabulary. According to Ward Hamilton, vice president of marketing at ZOLL Medical Corporation (Chelmsford, MA), digitized speech is well suited to the firm's defibrillator. The device is intended for use by laypeople who have received training on the fundamentals of resuscitation as well as on use of the company's AED, as recommended by the American Heart Association.

Once ZOLL engineers determined the specific voice segments needed to guide a user through the numerous steps of assessing a victim's status and delivering a shock or CPR, the remaining task was to choose the right voice talent to make the messages. The designers ultimately chose a man with an authoritative-sounding, medium-pitched voice to create the recordings; his résumé included narrating for Nova, the science-oriented public broadcasting program. The software installed in ZOLL Medical Corporation's computer-driven defibrillator holds the voice segments in memory and plays them back according to a rigid protocol.

"We deliberately made the prompts terse based on our general understanding that lots of verbiage is hard to deal with in an emergency," Hamilton says. "People who use our device have stepped into a situation where someone appears to have died. It's very stressful. We don't want to give them too much to remember ... [or they] become numb to it." Developing effective prompts "is a tremendous balancing act that requires lots of customer feedback," Hamilton adds. "In our case, we need to provide enough information so that users recollect their basic life support skills and CPR training." Hamilton estimates that they received feedback from more than 2000 people over several years of development.

Synthesized speech differs sharply from digitized speech in terms of both its sound quality and its application. A synthesized speech segment sounds exactly the way the term suggests: synthetic. A computer, rather than a human, is doing the talking, and you can tell. Often, synthesized speech sounds nasal, emotionless, and strangely accented. Pitch variations, or the absence of them, can also make synthesized speech seem unnatural and hard to decipher.

In the typical application, a software program generates a phrase or sentence to be spoken by the computer. Next, the computer strings together the sounds associated with letter combinations in the words. Over the past decade, voice synthesis technology has improved considerably. Artificially generated speech now sounds more human, and has become more intelligible.

Nancy Lonsinger is vice president of marketing at Roche Diagnostics (Indianapolis). She says that synthesized speech was the best solution for the ACCU-CHEK® VOICEMATE blood glucose meter because of the variability of the device's spoken output. For example, the VOICEMATE speaks the value of the glucose measurement and the identity of insulin vials. It reports back to the user his or her blood glucose level, which can range widely in value, from 10 to 600 mg/dl. Synthesized speech clearly makes sense in this case. It would be impractical to record all of the possible combinations of words and values, some of which would be unknown at the time of device production.

"Before the VOICEMATE, visually impaired patients would have to wait for assistance from a family member or other helper to test their blood," Lonsinger

Medical Devices That Talk

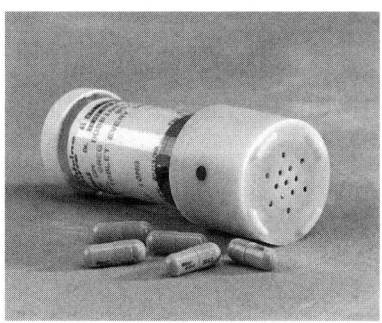

FIGURE 22.3
The Talking RX Prescription Reader employs a recording and playback device.

says. "Now, they can perform the task by themselves." She describes the VOICEMATE as an important addition to the company's line of blood glucose testing devices, addressing the needs of a special market segment.

The device is priced in the range of $400 to $500, making it 5 to 10 times more expensive than standard blood glucose meters aimed at the general consumer market. The product's high price is reportedly due to its high development cost and relatively low sales volume. "VOICEMATE has been wildly successful within its relatively small market," Lonsinger notes, "but it hasn't generated substantial financial rewards for the company." Still, she says, "VOICEMATE has generated considerable goodwill toward the company. It also gives our employees a deep sense of satisfaction because we are helping people take care of themselves."

A hybrid technical approach to producing medical devices that talk involves building whole sentences from individually digitized words. In such applications, the sentence "Your temperature is ninety eight point six degrees Fahrenheit" is produced by stringing together the words *your, temperature, is, ninety, eight, point, six, degrees,* and *Fahrenheit*. One can add inflection to specific words to make the final sentence sound more natural. Accordingly, a device's vocabulary may include multiple versions of the same word, each one spoken with a different inflection to sound, for example, inquisitive vs. directive.

Another speech technology of note, albeit a rudimentary one, is just another version of digitized speech. It is the voice recording and playback technology found in stuffed animals, greeting cards, and picture frames. Millennium Compliance Corp. (Southington, CT) is a small company started by John Dobbins, a pharmacist originally from the University of Connecticut (Storrs, CT). The company has put a relatively inexpensive recording and playback device into its Talking RX Prescription Reader (see Figure 22.3).

The cuplike device, which attaches snugly to the bottom of a medium-sized medication container, enables the pharmacist to record essential information about the contents (normally found on a pill bottle's paper label).

The device, which is sold over the counter, is targeted toward visually impaired consumers, who may have previously relied on others to read the information on their pill bottles. Millennium's product can record a 60-second segment. However, Dobbins says, "the 60-second capacity is usually far more than pharmacists need to record the vital information."

What about Two-Way Communication?

The applications previously discussed in this article are examples of one-way communication: devices that talk to users but cannot respond to voice commands. What about two-way communication? An example of this is the automated telephone prompts that airlines use to get callers to speak their origin and destination cities. The technology involves both digital or synthesized speech and speech recognition. It has great promise and is already emerging within the consumer electronics marketplace in products such as cellular phones. However, achieving a reliable level of recognition of commands — close to 100% — continues to be a challenge. Even a recognition rate as high as 95% can cause significant operability problems and user frustration. Getting the systems to work well can seem like a magic act that involves fine-tuning how the system samples, compresses, and buffers the sound data even before they are fed into the recognition software.

To increase reliability, systems may either limit the number of recognized words to a relatively small vocabulary or require users to train the system. Training is accomplished by repeatedly speaking the words to be recognized so that the computer can create a database of spoken words in preparation for determining a match. Despite these limitations, two-way communication technology seems an inevitable next step beyond medical devices that simply talk. One can imagine a wide range of voice-activated medical devices, particularly for people who need their hands for other purposes than pressing buttons and people who have physical disabilities. In fact, some such devices already exist.

The da Vinci Surgical System from Intuitive Surgical (Sunnyvale, CA) is used to perform minimally invasive bypass surgery on a beating heart. It uses voice activation to activate robots that harvest the arteries used for the bypass. The Socrates Telecollaborative System, also made by Intuitive Surgical, uses voice input to control cameras, lighting, and operating table functions.

Voice activation is also being used to control the movement of an artificial arm developed by students at Johns Hopkins University (Baltimore). The arm responds to the commands *raise, down, open, close,* and *stop*. Such applications seem only the beginning in terms of meeting the needs of people with physical impairments.

Design Guidelines

There are some general guidelines on the design of effective voice prompts that can help ensure simpler, one-way applications of speech technology.

Learn about the User

User-centered design philosophy involves device users throughout the user-interface design process. Designing the voice-based user elements of a medical device is no exception. Developing effective voice prompts calls for substantial input from the intended users. For starters, users can provide valuable feedback on the concept of using speech at all. They can then make suggestions about wording and provide feedback on prototype designs.

Ensure Proper Task and Information Flow

It is helpful to chart the flow of the voice prompts and associated device and user-related actions. This way, you can be sure that the process is logical and intuitive, thereby helping to avoid confusion and use errors. In addition, device makers should identify the likely use errors and ways to recover from them.

Prompt Users at a Suitable Pace

Prompts should not outpace users' ability to listen, understand, and follow instructions. Conversely, the pace should not be so sluggish that users lose their concentration, become annoyed, or are unnecessarily delayed from performing urgent actions. Dobbins's advice to people recording a talking prescription is to speak slowly and deliberately, particularly if the patient has diminished mental capacity.

Synchronize Prompts with Actions

It is easy for prompts to get out of sync with user actions, particularly if the user does not perform tasks in the anticipated order. Thus, designers need to consider the full range of possible user behaviors to determine the best way to maintain synchronization. Ultimately, it may be necessary for users to press a button to indicate that they are ready to progress to the next step.

Make Prompts Sufficiently Loud

Some medical devices are used in quiet environments, such as a bedroom or office, while others may be used in louder environments, such as a factory floor. Designers should consider incorporating a volume control. Setting a device to emit prompts at the maximum required volume may make them too loud. However, in cases such as an AED, it may be better to keep the device's user interface simple by excluding a volume control and presetting the sound level so that prompts are intelligible against typical or worst-case background noise. Further, ensure that the sound-production hardware has enough power to achieve the required sound levels.

Use Plain Wording

Even a sophisticated user is better served by plainly worded prompts. Simple wording usually gets the point across faster and avoids confusion, particularly in cases where users must divide their attention between performing tasks (e.g., checking for breathing) and listening for the next instruction. Plain wording also promotes better understanding among people who have limited vocabularies and nonnative speakers. One strategy for developing plainly worded prompts is to analyze people giving instructions to each other, or "natural dialogues." The assumption is that natural-sounding prompts will be easier to understand and follow.

Be Consistent

When designing voice prompts, it is important to employ consistent terminology and syntax. Avoid inconsistencies such as those reflected in the following examples:

- "To start the test, press the red button."
- "Push the green key to stop the test."

Note the arbitrary use of the terms "button" versus "key" and the different sentence structures, which may complicate matters for some users.

Keep Prompts Short

People are better at following short prompts than long ones that may cause them to forget details. Assume that users have a short attention span. However, take care not to make prompts so terse that they fail to communicate their point.

Provide Clear Direction

When trying to move a task along efficiently, there is no room for extraneous detail. Unnecessary detail can obscure the primary message. For example, aircraft warning systems emphatically state "Pull up!" if a plane is going to crash into the ground. This prompt is clearly superior to "The plane is descending toward the ground at a dangerously high rate of 100 feet per second." The more detailed prompt never actually tells the pilot what to do in the face of an imminent hazard. So, particularly in the case of emergency treatment devices, get to the point quickly. Thus ZOLL's AED Plus states, "Don't touch the patient" instead of "Do not touch the patient because an ECG analysis is in progress or about to begin."

Ensure a Suitable Tone

An emphatic-sounding prompt may be appropriate when guiding a task that must be performed quickly and correctly, such as attaching an AED's electrodes to a specific spot on a victim's chest. However, the same tone might not be appropriate for a blood glucose meter intended for daily use.

Designers also need to consider the ramifications of recording speech passages using a particular tone of voice, including variables such as pitch and inflection. Tone is easier to manipulate when dealing with digitized speech, as compared with synthesized speech. In most cases, a polite, non-judgmental-sounding voice is warranted.

The speaker's gender is a key variable. In some cases, designers may want to give users the choice of a male-sounding vs. female-sounding voice. Some evidence suggests that a female voice is more attention getting, but either a female or male voice can do the job.

Ultimately, developers should probably choose a voice with a tone that a majority of the users can relate to. Avoid an especially high-pitched female voice or a low-pitched male voice, which may be off-putting to some users and may be clipped by the recording and reproduction technology, which is likely to deliver low-fidelity sound.

Ensure Proper Translation into Other Languages

Avoid translating prompts word for word because syntax and common word usage vary widely among languages. It is better to take a more holistic approach to translations, ensuring that the final prompts sound natural to native language speakers. Accordingly, it may be best to engage native speakers to perform the translations into their first language.

Provide Alternative Prompts

For medical devices that may be designated for exclusive use by either laypersons or medical professionals, it may make sense to offer alternative sets of voice prompts. Each set can be tailored to speak the language of the target user population. The set intended for use by medical professionals would employ common medical jargon, while the set intended for use by laypersons would not. In certain cases, developers may want to leave open the possibility of tailoring prompts to a particular customer's needs or demands.

Validate the Prompts through User Testing

A set of prompts may look good and logical on paper, but they may not work when presented in context. Therefore, plan to conduct a usability test of the prompts at several stages of development. Keep refining the prompts until they promote the desired user behavior and, in appropriate cases, the users like them.

Conclusion

Medical devices that talk sound like progress. However, as with most enabling technologies, there are perils to avoid. Voice prompts should be reserved for cases where they truly enhance user interactions. Guiding users through an emergency procedure during which attention is split between device interactions and direct patient care seems to be a good application. Enabling people with visual impairments to use medical devices without assistance is another. Voice prompts may be universally beneficial to all users because they can use their eyes and hands for other tasks. But medical device developers should guard against overusing the technology. The world does not need a bunch of chatty medical devices that speak out for no compelling reason.

Key Points

- Voice-enabled medical devices are leading users through some particularly challenging tasks, breaking down barriers to independent use by people with impaired vision, and improving usability as a whole.
- For medical devices that only talk (i.e., that do not have voice recognition capabilities), developers can choose between digitized and synthesized speech technologies.
- Digitized speech usually sounds much better because it is based on recording a real person's voice, then playing back the right segment at the right moment.

- A hybrid technical approach to producing medical devices that talk involves building whole sentences from individually digitized words.
- Two-way communication technology that combines speech output as well as human voice recognition seems an inevitable next step beyond medical devices that simply talk.
- Voice prompt designers should learn about the user and seek their input during the course of prompt design; ensure proper task and information flow; prompt users at a suitable pace; synchronize prompts with actions; make prompts sufficiently loud; use plain wording; provide clear direction; ensure a suitable tone; and ensure proper translation into other languages.

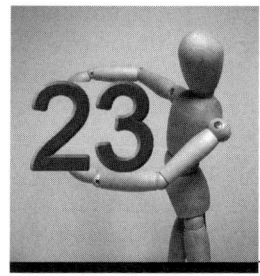

Home Healthcare: Applying Inclusive Design Principles to Medical Devices

Stephen B. Wilcox

As more and more complex medical devices are being operated at home, manufacturers need to develop them with disabled users in mind.

As the trend toward minimizing patient time in the hospital continues, one notable consequence has been the migration of medical devices from medical facilities to patients' homes. This phenomenon means that, increasingly, the patient, rather than the medical professional, is the device user. The effect of this change on the design of many medical products is substantial.

Patients and generally healthy medical professionals can be quite different. Medical professionals are less likely than the general population to suffer from various disabilities and more likely to be above average in the capabilities required to operate medical devices. In contrast, users of home-healthcare devices may suffer from chronic diseases, or experience dexterity or mobility problems, or visual, auditory, or other perceptual deficits, or even cognitive disabilities. Indeed, it is obvious to say that the very conditions that a medical device is designed to address are often associated with various disabilities.

From the device designer's point of view, the trend toward home healthcare changes the nature of the task. Smart, highly trained users are good at overcoming device limitations, as anyone can testify who has spent time in the operating room or any other area of a hospital. Thus, in effect, the physicians, nurses, and technicians who use medical equipment allow the medical device designer to be a bit sloppy, because the users are smart enough, strong enough, and healthy enough to forgive a multitude of sins. They readily develop "work-arounds" to overcome the device problems they face. That is how they achieve their reputations as "can-do" people.

Because patients are, by comparison, much less able to overcome device limitations, there is greater pressure on the designer of a home-healthcare device to reduce those limitations. The designer must assume that the user may have physical, perceptual, or cognitive disabilities. At the same time, no one, the user of a medical device included, wants to be treated as "special" in the sense of "special education." This logic is the impetus for applying "universal" or "inclusive" design principles to home-healthcare products.

Inclusive Design

The idea of *inclusive* design, also sometimes referred to as "universal design," is to provide products that are easy for everyone to use, including those with various disabilities. The key is to make a product usable by a person with a dexterity problem or a visual or cognitive deficit, but not to "telegraph" the fact that the product has been designed for the disabled. Because people do not like to be stigmatized or reminded that they are disabled, they often simply refuse to use an assistive device. As Laura Gitlin puts it, "[A] reason for device abandonment is ... that devices symbolize a change in competencies that is associated with negative social judgments."[1]

Inclusive design is a strategy with two parts:

1. To make home-healthcare products appear as normal as possible
2. To accommodate those with disabilities, who will inevitably be over-represented in the population of users

The first part is largely a matter of the designer's approach; it does not necessarily require special knowledge. Larger text for labels and lower-force control mechanisms, for example, are better for people with various disabilities, but they are also easier for everyone to use (see Figures 23.1, 23.3, and 23.4). The device designer just has to think in these terms, and the incentive structure of the organization has to incorporate the consideration of inclusive design.

The second part is trickier, because there is a natural tendency for product designers to use themselves as their benchmark users. Thus, when the user is significantly different from the designer, there is a need for the designer to obtain additional information.

What follows, then, is a summary of some of the disabilities from which people suffer and some techniques that device developers can use to help them better understand the needs of disabled users.

Home Healthcare: Applying Inclusive Design Principles to Medical Devices

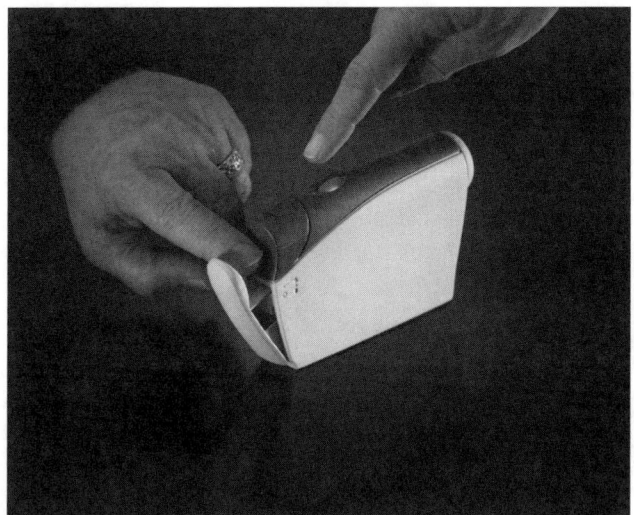

FIGURE 23.1 (See color insert following page 142)
The Personal Lasette from Cell Robotics (Albuquerque) is designed for easy use by people with or without disabilities. Image courtesy of Cell Robotics International, Inc.

Disabilities

According to the U.S. Census Bureau, more than 20% of the general population suffers from some form of disability.[2] The distribution of these disabilities is shown in Figure 23.2. Fortunately, there are effective design strategies for the various conditions.

Mobility/Dexterity

An estimated 1.8 million Americans are in wheelchairs; 13.6 million have limited use of their hands. Difficulty with fine control of the fingers, which is often caused by arthritis, is one of the most common problems. Another common problem is loss of limb control as a result of spinal damage, cerebral palsy, multiple sclerosis, muscular dystrophy, or overuse injuries such as carpal tunnel syndrome.

Some design strategies include:[3]

- Making buttons large and widely spaced so that fine motor control is less necessary and errors are less likely
- The use of spoken commands for device activation to eliminate the need for physical manipulation of controls

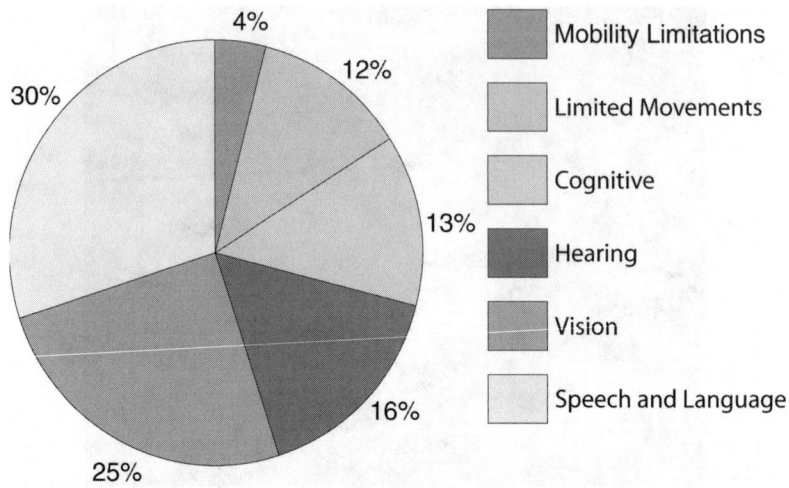

FIGURE 23.2
Limitations involving vision, speech, and language make up more than half of all disabilities in the United States.

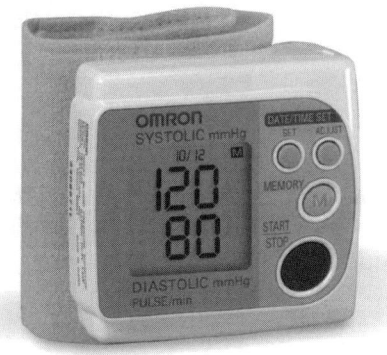

FIGURE 23.3
The Omron HEM 712C blood pressure monitor has large text, simple operation, automatic inflation, and just slips over the wrist. Image courtesy of Omron Corp.

- Minimization of the need for simultaneous actions (so the user will not have to perform two things at once)
- Minimization of the need for sustained pressure on controls (to accommodate people with poor finger or hand strength)

Cognitive

Between 6.2 and 7.7 million people in the U.S. suffer from mental retardation. Another 5 to 10% of the population suffers from learning disabilities. Other

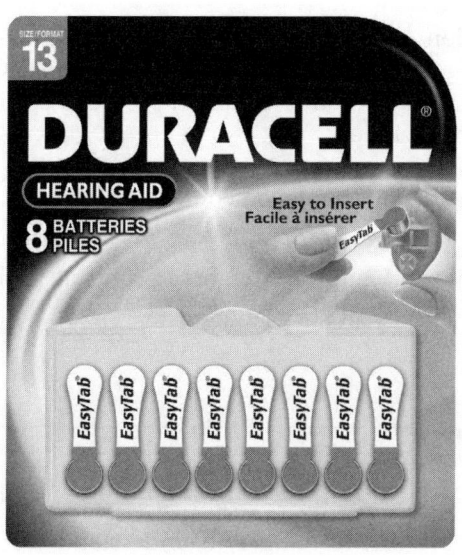

FIGURE 23.4 (See color insert following page 142)
Duracell's EasyTab hearing-aid batteries make loading the battery much easier for a person with dexterity problems. Image courtesy of The Gillette Company.

cognitive deficits include the mental confusion associated with psychosis, various language problems, and the difficulty of concentrating, known as *attention deficit disorder*.

Design strategies for accommodating such users include:[4]

- Incorporating automatic rather than user-activated adjustments
- The use of simple, unambiguous language
- Placement of advanced features under a separate menu
- Making all actions reversible
- Avoiding time constraints

Auditory

Auditory deficits affect 10% of the U.S. population. They vary from total deafness to various levels of partial deafness. The elderly tend to lose higher pitches first.

Design strategies include:[5]

- Providing redundant visual or tactile cues for operating information
- Volume adjustability
- Wireless coupling to hearing aids

Visual

Close to nine million Americans suffer from visual deficits severe enough to make it difficult for them to read an ordinary newspaper. Over half a million people are legally blind. Another common problem is color blindness.

Design strategies include:

- Providing tactile landmarks on control surfaces
- Providing a voice mode redundant to visual information
- Adding tactile and auditory detents to controls for blind users
- Allowing speech as an input mode

Understanding Disabled Users' Needs

One way for the product developer to understand the needs of disabled users is to obtain technical information about the various deficits[6] — what frequencies of sound are the most problematical, how arthritis affects the hand, etc. There is a great deal of literature available on these subjects.[3] Some other strategies are described below.

Including People with Disabilities in the Design Process

A company developing a particular device will probably have access to patients who are likely to use it. However, the problem is to identify the "worst cases," so to speak, who may not be contained in a small sample of patients. Thus, it can be useful to recruit people who have particular disabilities. Some methods for doing so include:[7]

- Contacting organizations, such as the American Foundation for the Blind or the Arthritis Foundation
- Placing ads at retail stores that sell assistive devices
- Contacting the occupational or physical therapy departments of local universities

Such people can play a number of roles. They can critique designs, participate in brainstorming sessions, or participate in usability testing.

Including Experts in the Design Process

Local universities or organizations can also be used to identify experts in particular disabilities. They can be a rich source of advice.

Creating Heuristic Design Criteria

Accommodating the needs of disabled users can be translated into various objective criteria. Experts can be helpful in developing these criteria, which then can be used as a "filter" to evaluate alternative design approaches.

Simulating Disabilities

A way to give device designers an intuitive sense of what the problems are for disabled users is to simulate disabilities by, for example:

- Wearing blindfolds or translucent glasses
- Wearing earplugs
- Wearing gloves
- Wearing an "empathy belly," used to simulate pregnancy
- Working from a wheelchair

Such techniques should be used with caution. Having a disability is never the same as experiencing a simulated disability. However, simulating disabilities can provide some insight and can provide quick tests for alternative prototypes

Conclusion

As more medical devices migrate into patients' homes, an inclusive design strategy becomes more important for making products usable. Successful inclusive design for these products requires a different approach than the one many medical device companies now use. However, it is an approach that has been widespread for years in the consumer products world, and one that any product development group should be able to learn.

Key Points

- Home-healthcare products require a different approach to product development than products that are designed to be used by medical professionals.
- Taking an inclusive design approach is a way of meeting the needs of home-healthcare product users.

- Disabilities to be accommodated, in order of frequency, include mobility and dexterity limitations, cognitive deficits, auditory problems, and visual problems.
- Inclusive design involves designing products to be used by all users, including those with disabilities, without making it obvious that disabilities have been accommodated.
- Strategies for meeting the needs of disabled users include gathering technical information about the capabilities, limitations, and tendencies of disabled users; including people with disabilities; in the design process; consulting with experts on the various disabilities; creating design criteria that address the needs of people with disabilities; and simulating disabilities.

References

1. Gitlin, J., Why older people accept or reject assistive technology, *Generations, Journal of the American Society on Aging,* 29, 41–46, 1995.
2. McNeil, L., *Americans with Disabilities: 1994-95, Data from the Survey of Income and Program Participation,* Bureau of the Census Current Population Reports, U.S. Department of Commerce, Washington, D.C., 1995.
3. Kanis, H., Operation of controls on consumer products by physically impaired users, *Human Factors,* 35, 305–328, 1993.
4. Robertson, G. and Hix, D., User interface design guidelines for computer accessibility for mentally retarded adults, *Proceedings of the Human Factors and Ergonomics Society,* Human Factors and Ergonomics Society, Santa Monica, CA, 300–304, 1994.
5. Dugan, *Keys to Living with Hearing Loss,* Barron's Educational Series, Hauppauge, NY, 1997.
6. Pirkl, J., *Transgenerational Design: Products for an Aging Population,* Von Nostrand Reinhold, New York, 1994.
7. Petrie, H., User-centered design and evaluation of adaptive and assistive technology for disabled and elderly users, *Informationstechnik and Techniche Informatik,* 39, 7–12, 1997.

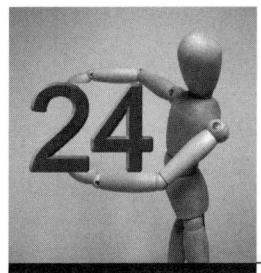

Designing Usable Auditory Signals

Stephen B. Wilcox

Designing an alarm or other auditory signal that will be clear, distinctive, and not annoying can be a challenge, particularly when it has to go into the complex auditory environment presented by a hospital.

The purpose of an auditory signal is to inform users of the state of a device, which, in turn often relates directly to the state of a patient. In the case of alarms, the purpose is to alert the user that something is wrong. A good auditory signal is one that can be clearly heard and that is distinctive enough to unambiguously indicate what it means. Another requirement for any signal is that it avoid annoying the user. Annoying signals increase the user's stress level and provide an incentive to disable them.

An alarm has the additional burden of getting the user's immediate attention.

A key fact about auditory signals for medical devices is that they cannot be designed in a vacuum. They will typically be used in a complex auditory environment that will include alarms and other sounds emitted by various devices (e.g., the regular beeps of pulse oximeters, blaring music, particularly in the OR, white noise from a number of sources, etc.) (see Figure 24.1). Thus, an alarm that seems perfectly appropriate by itself may not make sense in the real environment of use.

Furthermore, auditory signals, particularly alarms, should conform to relevant standards, the identification and interpretation of which can be far from trivial. It follows, then, that the design of an auditory signal requires careful consideration of the user, of the auditory environment, and of the standards and other technical requirements that apply. In what follows, we propose a multistep procedure for designing alarms and other auditory signals that addresses these and other issues.

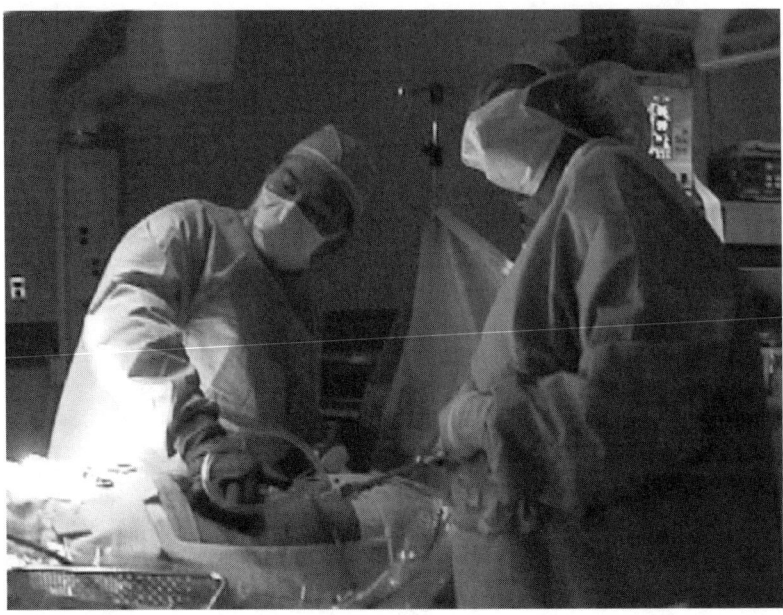

FIGURE 24.1
The sound environment of the OR can be very different from that of the product developers' offices.

Step 1. Determine What the Signals Will Indicate

It would seem obvious that the designer of auditory signals for a given system must begin with a clear idea of the array of conditions that will be indicated by the auditory signals. Unfortunately, this is not always the case. How many different conditions will be indicated? Will a given signal indicate a "yes-or-no" condition or the level of some variable? What is the hierarchy of importance of the various conditions? Should the user be made consciously aware of a particular condition or simply be given background information? How many separate conditions will be indicated by a given signal? These sorts of questions have to be answered carefully.

A good starting point is to make a list of all of the system states that will be indicated and to classify these states on relevant dimensions (e.g., in terms of their implications for the patient and in terms of their overall importance), then to determine which of these system states require auditory signals. Auditory (vs. visual) signals are particularly useful when it is important for the user to be informed of a condition regardless of where he or she is looking.

Step 2. Gather Information

Two basic categories of information are standards and general human factors guidelines for the design of an auditory signal. Examples of standards include IEC 60601-1-8,[1] and ANSI/AAMI HE49-1993.[2] The latter will eventually be superceded by ANSI/AAMI HE75, which is currently under development and will have sections on auditory displays and alarms.

Examples of guidelines include those contained in monographs such as Stanton's *Human Factors in Auditory Warnings*[3] and Stanton and Edworthy's *Human Factors in Alarm Design*.[4] There are also a variety of articles and other documents that can be useful for a given type of signal (e.g., "The design of auditory signals for ICU and OR environments",[5] "Managing the monitors: an analysis of alarm silencing activities during an anesthetic procedure"[6]).

Standards and guidelines provide constraints that signals should conform to — constraints regarding parameters such as sound frequency, loudness, and temporal pattern.

Step 3. Record and Analyze Sound from the Expected Environment of Use

It is crucial to understand the auditory environment of a new signal. The best way to do this is to obtain high-quality recordings from the types of environments where the product will be used. This requires a good nondirectional microphone and a good recorder. The microphone should have a frequency range of at least 20 to 20,000 Hz. The recorder should have a frequency range of at least 20 to 40,000 Hz (to assure good frequency response up to 20,000 Hz), and both should have flat frequency response curves. Of course, it is important to obtain a good representative sample of use environments and for the use environments to be realistic, in the sense they include the sounds that will typically accompany the new device — e.g., music, people talking on the phone, etc.

Once these recordings are obtained, they should be analyzed with a spectrum analyzer to determine what frequencies are represented (see Figure 24.2). A key goal will be to design auditory signals that do not share frequencies with existing sounds. Everything else being equal, a given sound can be heard better to the extent that it is not "masked" by other sounds with similar frequencies.

238 Designing Usability into Medical Products

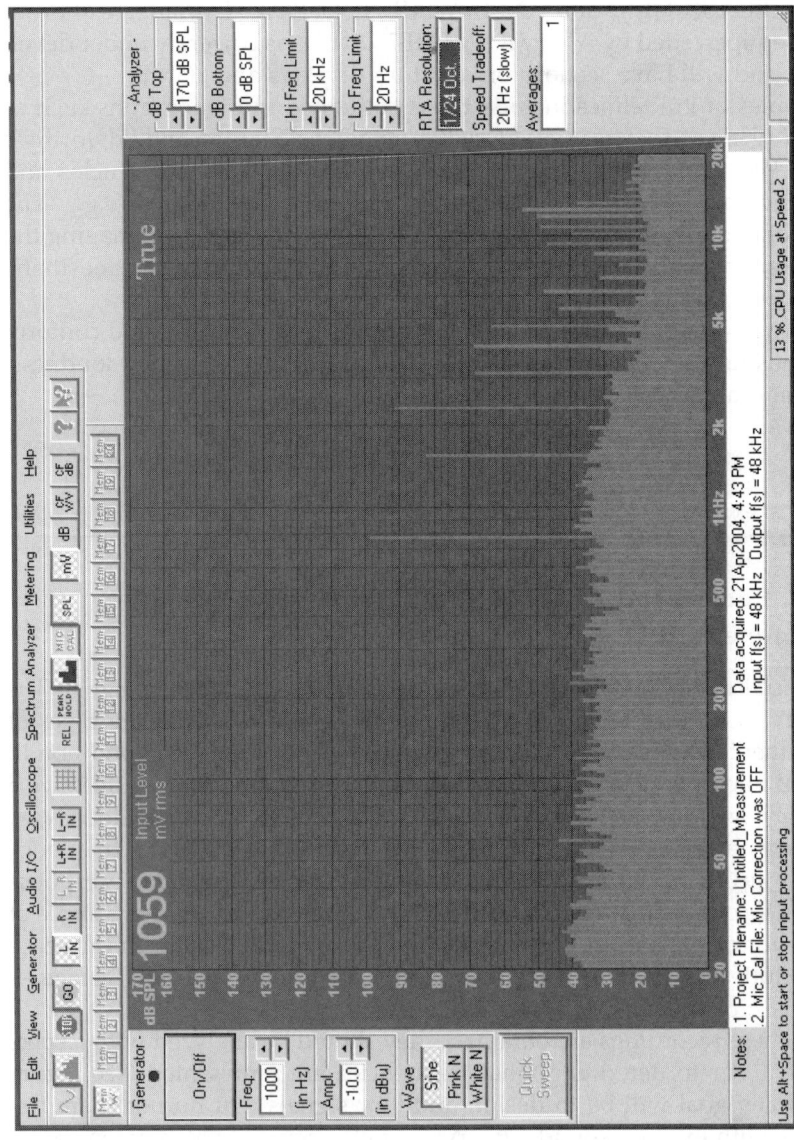

FIGURE 24.2
Output of a spectrum analyzer.

Step 4. Recreate the Ambient Sound

In addition to formally analyzing the ambient sound, it is important to recreate the sound environment so new signals can be tested realistically. As with sound recording, this requires good equipment. Again, it is important to have an amplification and speaker system that supports a 20 to 20,000 Hz range with a flat frequency response. Remember that sound degradation is cumulative. Suppose, for example, that each of your components (microphone, recorder, amplifier, and speakers) degrades the sound by 10%. The end result will be a 34% degradation.

The other part of the equation is to play the sound back in a room as similar as possible to the room where it was recorded, particularly with regard to its size.

Step 5. Choose the Sound Frequencies

Once you have a recreation of the ambient sound with which to work, you need good sound-generation software to create the auditory signals (see Figure 24.3). As mentioned above, it is useful to find sound frequencies that are as different as possible from the ambient sound. You should create sounds (i.e., chords) with at least four frequencies, then add additional harmonics to create a sound that is distinctive and that sounds appropriate for what it indicates (see Figure 24.4). Of course, relevant standards and guidelines should be consulted here. These sources will inform you, for example, to avoid sounds at the extremes of the spectrum because that is where hearing loss tends to begin.

We also advocate working directly with sine waves so that you know what you have. Sound generators have alternative wave forms, such as "square waves" or "triangular waves," but these other wave forms are made up of complex combinations of sine waves.

Sounds that are "semi-musical" seem to work best, that is, chords that are somewhat musical but that are not commonly used in music. A sound that is too musical can be confused with music and may not attract attention, particularly if it is used in an environment, such as an OR, where music is played. On the other hand, if the sound is too "nonmusical," or dissonant, it can be grating. Sources of such semi-musical chords are early twentieth-century composers, such as Stravinsky or Bartok. One idea is to find possible chords in the sheet music of one of these composers, then to recreate candidate chords in sine waves (i.e., not containing the additional harmonics of the notes as they would be played on a musical instrument). Next, you will have to adjust the key and the octave to make sure the frequencies that you choose are as different as possible from the ambient sound.

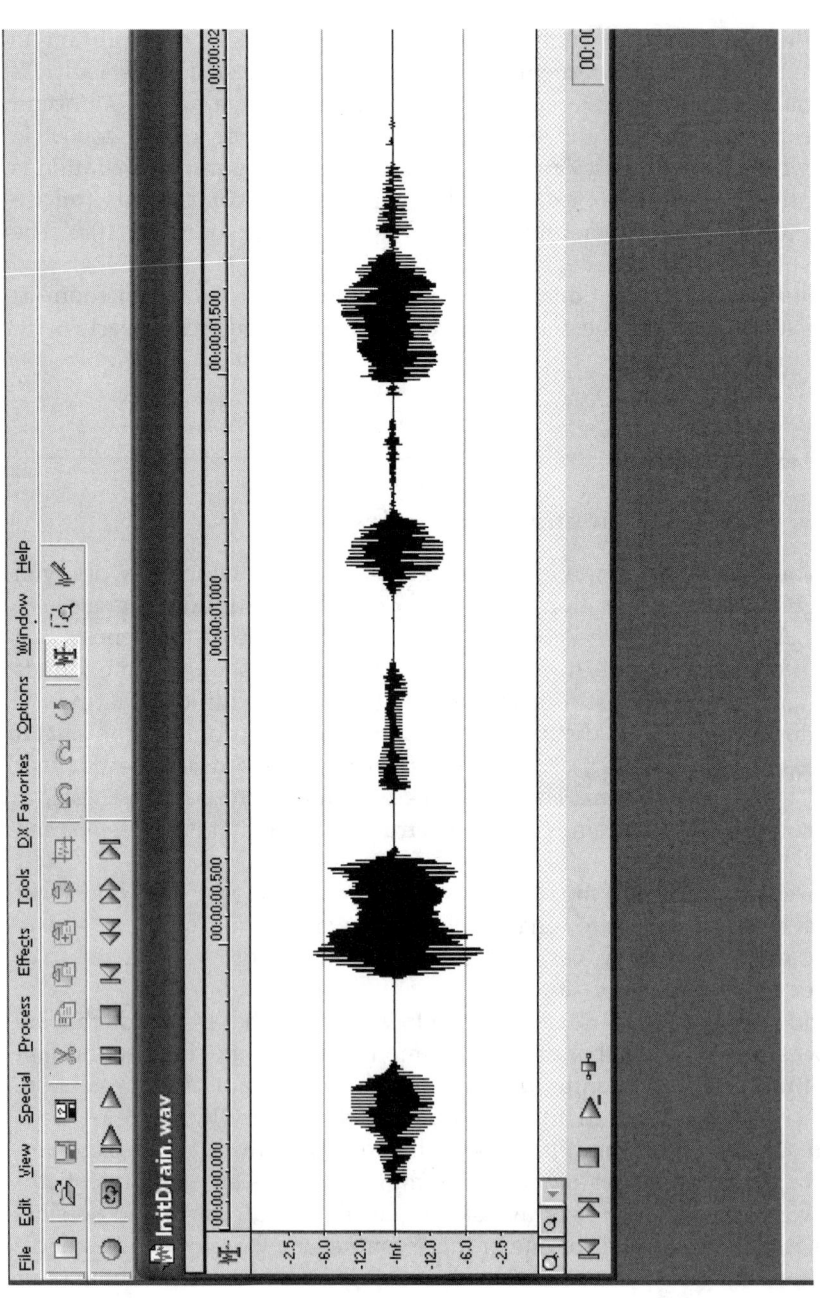

FIGURE 24.3
Sound editing software showing a temporal sound pattern.

Designing Usable Auditory Signals

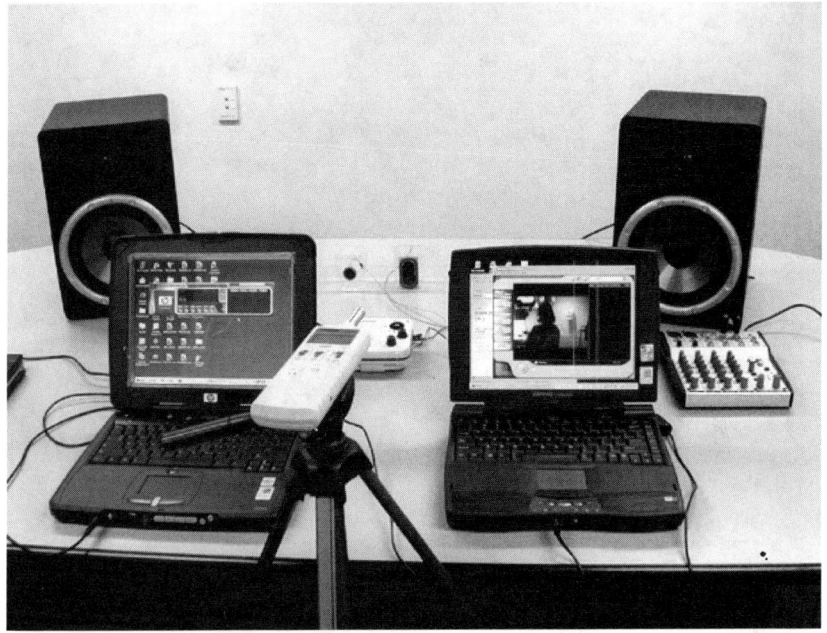

FIGURE 24.4
Setup for reproducing sound — sound editing software, sound meter, mixer, and sound meter.

At this stage, it is good to generate various candidate signals and to listen to them in the recreated ambient sound environment until you have a "short list" of signals that are appropriately conspicuous, distinctive, and reasonably pleasant to listen to. It is even better if you can find sounds that have an intuitive relationship to what they indicate, but this can be difficult to achieve. As with the ambient sound, the generated signals should be as realistic as possible, ideally, generated by the actual system (speakers and amplifier) that will be incorporated into the ultimate device (see Figure 24.5).

As should be clear from the foregoing discussion, it helps to have a person on the design team for an auditory signal who is familiar with the basics of music and musical notation.

Step 6. Choose the Sound Pattern

As with the choice of frequency, the choice of the temporal pattern of a signal will be constrained by various standards and guidelines. However, within the constraints imposed by standards and guidelines, there is still room for a great deal of variation. As with the choice of chords, composers such as Stravinsky and Bartok can be a fruitful source of sound patterns, i.e., partial melodies, that are somewhat musical but not too musical. Again, you should

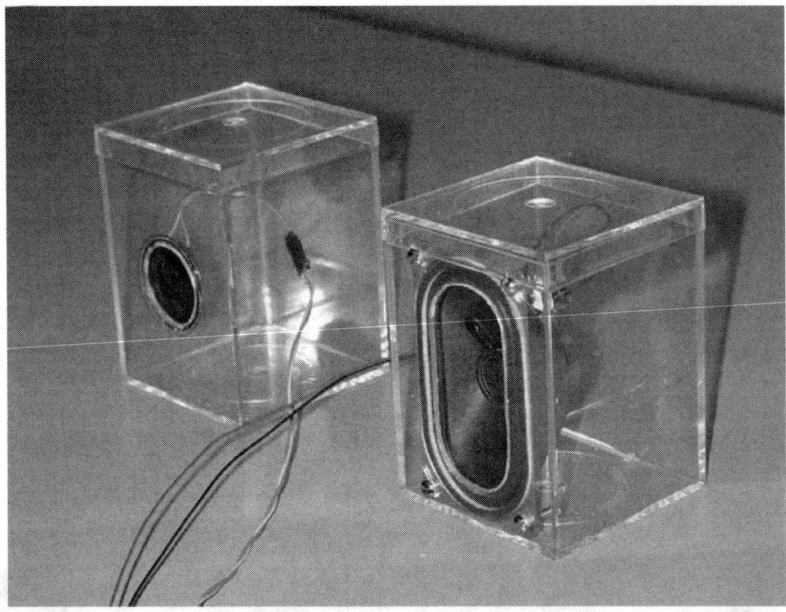

FIGURE 24.5
Speakers to be used in a medical product rigged for testing.

experiment with various sound patterns (incorporating the chords created in Step 5) until you have signals that appear to meet the various criteria just discussed.

Step 7. Test the Candidate Signals with Users

As we have advocated throughout this book, usability testing is crucial to assure that a device works like it is supposed to work with users. The same is true of auditory signals. They should be tested either with recreated ambient sounds, as discussed earlier or, even better, in the real environment of use.

Often, auditory signals can be tested along with other prototyped aspects of a new design so that you do not need separate testing sessions for the former.

For usability testing of auditory signals, the criteria for success include:

- Conspicuity
- Distinctiveness
- Freedom from annoyance
- An intuitive relationship to what is indicated

The latter cannot always be achieved, but it is a bonus if it can be. Within limits, the more alternative candidates for the signals that can be included, the higher the chances of creating a superior one.

Conclusion

The creation of good auditory alarms and other signals requires a systematic, multistep process that includes consideration of the functions of the signals, the auditory environments they will be emitted in, and the characteristics of the intended users. Even then, creating a superior auditory signal involves a certain amount of art as well as science. One source for the art is early twentieth-century music.

Key Points

- Designing good auditory signals begins with the understanding of the functions to be indicated by the signals.
- Given the importance of the auditory environment for a given signal, it is useful to record representative ambient sound and to test candidate signals in the context of that ambient sound.
- It is also important to gather and review relevant standards and guidelines.
- A useful source for sound patterns for ambient signals is early twentieth-century music.
- As part of the design process, auditory signals should be subjected to usability testing, as with any design element that has an impact on users.

References

1. Medical electrical equipment — Part 1–8: General requirements for safety — Collateral standard: Alarm systems — in medical electrical equipment and medical electrical systems, IEC 60606-1-2-8, International Electrotechnical Commission, Geneva, Switzerland, 2003.
2. Human factors engineering guidelines and preferred practices for the design of medical devices, ANSI/AAMI HE48-1993, Association for the Advancement of Medical Instrumentation, Arlington, VA, 1993.

3. Stanton, N., Ed., *Human Factors in Alarm Design*, Taylor & Francis, London, 1994.
4. Stanton, N. and Edworthy, J., Eds., *Human Factors in Auditory Warnings*, Ashgate Publishing, Aldershot, U.K., 1999.
5. Haas, E., The design of auditory signals for ICU and OR environments, *Journal of Clinical Engineering*, 23, 33–36, 1998.
6. Xiao, Y., Mackenzie, C., Seagull, J., and Jaberi, M., Managing monitors: an analysis of alarm silencing activities during an anesthetic procedure, *Proceedings of the IEA/HFES 2000 Congress*, 4-250–4-253, 2000.

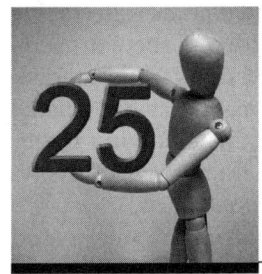

Medical Device User Manuals: Shifting toward Computerization

Michael E. Wiklund

Will manufacturers digitize their medical device user manuals as readily as they have digitized other aspects of their operations?

Consider the challenges facing technical communicators (i.e., technical writers) who design and produce medical device user manuals: First, their work must address the needs of an especially diverse audience, starting with caregivers and extending to trainers, biomedical engineers, sales personnel, government regulators, and many others. Because of its broad potential audience, the typical medical device user manual must be several documents in one. Second, technical communicators often have only limited resources and time to produce high-quality manuals as their companies speed products to market. Third, a user manual's primary audience — arguably the nurses, physicians, and technicians who deliver direct care to patients — tend to prefer engaging in hands-on training over reading user manuals. The popularity of the hands-on approach creates a perception of user manuals as perfunctory — a perception that could take the wind out of any technical writer's sails.

As computer technology grows ever more ubiquitous, a popular trend toward computerizing learning tools is cause for new excitement among technical communicators and allied professionals alike. As more caregivers gain computer access, the practicality of their viewing instructions on a medical device's computer display, on the Web, or on an interactive CD-ROM, for example, will increase. Such technological progress will enable content developers to think beyond the printed page and embrace alternative delivery mechanisms that may be more compatible with a particular user's learning style. In addition to the benefits it might afford users, computerization will assist manufacturers in updating content as readily as they install new versions of software into devices. As a result of this emerging multimedia approach, the hard-copy medical device user manual is swiftly evolving toward a system of both print and electronic components.

Since some institutions and individuals will embrace computer-based learning more readily than others, device manufacturers will be challenged to make their transition to a systems approach easy and comfortable. Manufacturers will also have to prove to the FDA and other certifying bodies that a multimodal approach to documentation will help ensure the proper and safe use of devices. It appears certain, however, that dynamic, interactive user manuals viewed on computer displays will be a desirable adjunct to paper-based documents, and the cost savings associated with computerization are likely to make it imperative.

Current Practice

As mentioned earlier, caregivers usually prefer to determine how devices work through hands-on experimentation or by being tutored by another person. Spending hours reading a user manual hardly suits their need to get things done under the pressure of a critical-care environment. Most device end-users would rather sit through a 30-minute in-service session to learn a device's essential functions and then rely on intuition or the experts from biomedical engineering to solve any technical problems that arise (see Figure 25.1). End-users' preference for interactive, person-to-person instruction makes them a challenging audience for the people who develop conventional user manuals that lack an interactive element.

Nevertheless, the FDA requires device manufacturers to supplement their products with printed manuals. The applicable law (21 CFR 801 and 809) considers user manuals to be an extension of a device's labeling that clarifies its proper and safe use.

As a result, some manufacturers view user manual writing as a regulatory mandate rather than a facet of product design excellence. They reason: why invest so much time and money into producing high-quality user manuals when we know that few people read them? In fact, medical device salespeople frequently encounter customers — the chair of a hospital's device selection committee, for example — who insist on judging a product based on how easy it is to use *without* any training, assistance, or referrals to the user manual.

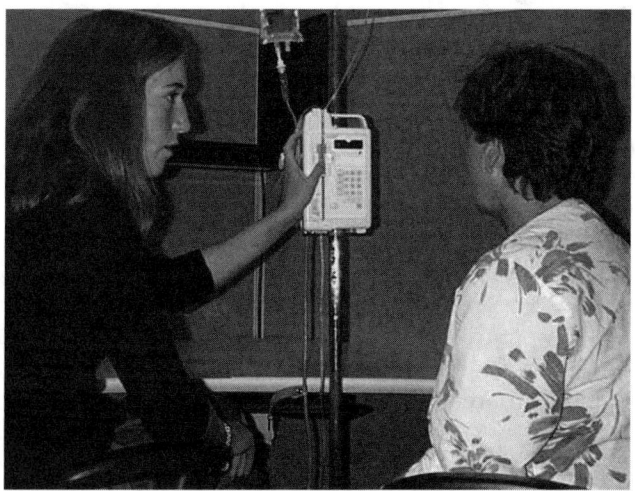

FIGURE 25.1
Nurse receiving hands-on training on the operation of an IV infusion pump. Photo courtesy of American Institutes for Research.

The Negative Reinforcement Loop

Unfortunately, when a manufacturer views the user manual as merely an obligatory measure to meet regulations in the U.S. and other countries, this "peg-in-the-hole" mentality establishes a negative reinforcement loop. These manufacturers are less inclined to invest heavily in product documentation because, presumably, nobody is reading the manuals. Caregivers who then try to solve a problem by checking one of these manuals discover that the manuals are not particularly helpful and not worth consulting again, thus reinforcing the manufacturer's perception that no one reads the manuals. This unfortunate cycle causes considerable waste of user-manual development effort, and it renders manual production, distribution, storage, and final disposal incrementally less efficient.

Meanwhile, companies that choose to invest substantially in producing excellent user manuals should be commended. Ultimately, there will always be caregivers who prefer to read a manual; as a courtesy to those individuals, manufacturers should produce good ones. Europeans, in fact, are generally regarded as avid manual readers in contrast to their American counterparts. Moreover, user manuals have confirmed value to biomedical engineers and staff educators who often use manufacturers' manuals as a starting point for developing their own in-house training materials. So, good user manuals are helpful to some, even if the primary beneficiary is not an end-user.

Unfortunately, most people would be unable to cite a company known to produce extraordinary user manuals. Because excellent documentation is not generally perceived as a competitive advantage, good user manuals do not receive special recognition. More likely, companies that produce high-quality user manuals are better known for producing products that are customer oriented and that feature good user interface designs, and for offering outstanding customer service.

On the other hand, the shift toward computerization may garner a new visibility for user manuals and the people who produce them. Recognizing the downstream cost savings and the potential to use high-quality learning tools to their competitive advantage, companies may be driven to make greater up-front investments in educational resources than they do now.

According to Brian French, a nurse who serves as the professional development coordinator at Massachusetts General Hospital (Boston), his institution expects computer-based learning to play a significant role in nurse education within the next three to five years. The new technology will augment current in-service training programs. "An institution likes ours," French says, "needs to address staff training needs on a 24/7/365 basis. Computer-based learning tools will be particularly important to us because we can make them continuously available. Printed materials will serve as a backup to the computer." French represents a large teaching hospital with more than 800 beds and a staff of about 15,000 employees, including more than 2,500 registered nurses. Surprisingly, his institution faces the same challenges many smaller hospitals do in terms of providing staff with access to computers and the Internet. "Current technology and space are designed to meet the clinical needs of patients, our first priority. The new challenge is to increase the number of computers and the amount of design space to meet the learning needs of staff at the bedside, while maintaining our ability to meet patient-care needs. But computerization is coming and we will have no choice but to adapt our facilities accordingly."

Paper Manuals versus Electronic Versions

In light of the computerization trend, will paper-based user manuals become as archaic as the typewriter? It is starting to look that way, despite paper documents' portability and their survival through power outages and operating system crashes. It is likely that they will always have a permanent quick-reference and backup role (see Figure 25.2). And because of different learning styles, there will always be individuals who prefer to read a user manual over taking other learning approaches.

Still, little evidence exists to suggest that the majority of caregivers will dedicate more time to reading manuals, the quality of the documents notwithstanding. Busy caregivers have little time or inclination to search for

Medical Device User Manuals: Shifting toward Computerization 249

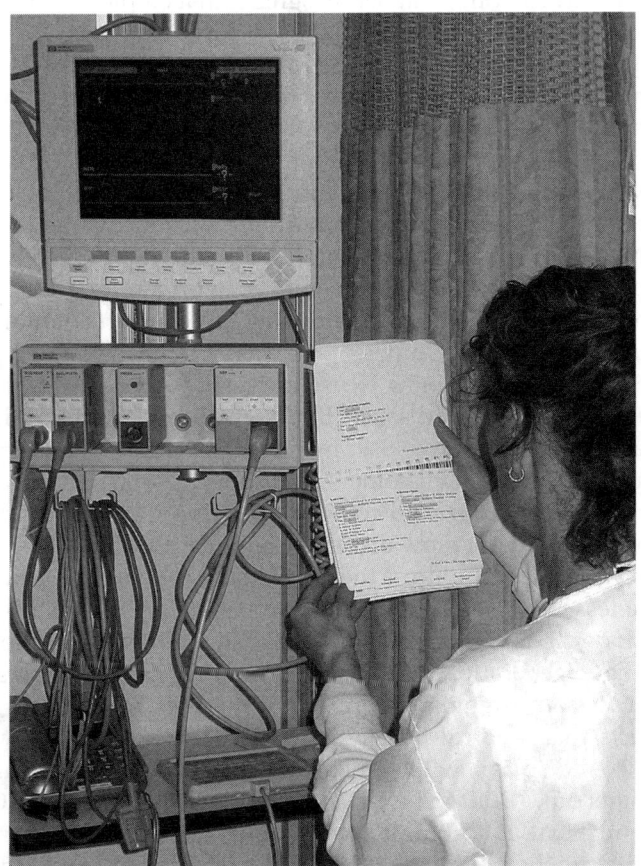

FIGURE 25.2
Nurse checks the operators guide to a patient monitor.

guidebooks; in their parlance, they need solutions "stat" and at the point of care. User manuals are rarely within easy reach during a crisis.

Debra Wagner, a technical writer with GE Medical Systems Information Technologies (Milwaukee) shares the view that while computerization is inevitable, traditional paper manuals will always have a role in instruction. Wagner's company, which produces a range of high-technology devices, including cardiographs and patient monitors, expects computers to revolutionize the way medical device manufacturers support customer training efforts. "We pay close attention to the voice of the customer," she says. "Right now, our customers are seeking customized resources they can use to build their own training programs. Every institution has its own way of doing things, so a flexible approach is best. At GE, we are looking toward delivering content through many electronic means, including over the Web. In doing so, we will move toward a new paradigm involving the establishment of a generic-content warehouse that can be used by people responsible for training, marketing, and sales." Still, Wagner recognizes that employees have different learning styles and that some prefer hard copy to pixels. Therefore, GE Medical Systems expects to continue making content available in many formats, including traditional hard copy. She points out that hospitals are "loaded with lots of high-tech equipment. But there is currently a relatively low percentage of people who are comfortable with accessing information over the Web. Of course, this is changing quickly."

Peg Rickard, manager of information design and human factors at Datex–Ohmeda (Madison, WI), a manufacturer of anesthesia delivery systems and monitoring products, also sees the need for a hybrid approach to producing learning tools. She reports that her company has conducted studies on how people learn to use Datex–Ohmeda products. "As you would expect, most people prefer being shown how to use the devices by one of our people or the people we train," Rickard says. "But there are still a substantial number of individuals who do read the user manual." She adds, "Our surveys show that as many as 50% of our customers read some portion of the user manual, though not necessarily cover to cover. These people tend to be the over-40 crowd: those who did not grow up using computers and who may find them intimidating. We need to address their preference for hard copy, even though it would be less expensive to put the materials on a CD-ROM."

Rickard adds, "Looking ahead, we have to be prepared to serve the needs of the younger generation, which has grown up on computers and will expect to access our training materials by computer."

She expects that medical devices, such as patient monitors with laptop computer-sized displays, will be their own conduit for educational content. But, she points out, "Built-in help systems have their limitations. Obviously, online resources are not going to help you troubleshoot a patient monitor that has a malfunctioning display. You will always need to include with the product some sort of quick reference card or troubleshooting guide."

The Hybrid Strategy

Plotting the future of her information design efforts, Rickard envisions a hybrid strategy: taking a systems approach to address the variety of customer learning styles and infrastructural constraints. She says, "To address the needs of one group of customers at the sake of another would be a missed opportunity." For now, her company plans to produce educational materials in various formats. Datex–Ohmeda will continue to deliver paper-based user manuals along with CD-ROMs containing the same basic document in electronic form. Looking ahead, the company envisions delivering content over the Internet and opening the door to new methods of content organization.

GE's Wagner has similar expectations for her company over the next few years. She says, "The kinds of Web-based content delivery systems that we are pilot testing today should be mainstream within the next five years. However, we are likely to continue to provide critical product information, as well as the content necessary to fulfill regulatory requirements, in hard-copy form."

As the nature of product documentation changes, so will the nature of the teams developing the material. Today, GE Medical Systems Information Technologies maintains a group of five writers to support its clinical systems development work. However, in the near future the company expects the work to involve additional people with database management and Web development expertise, while the writers continue to focus on producing high-quality content.

Massachusetts General Hospital's French anticipates that the movement of manufacturers to computerize their education materials may outpace customers' demand and their ability to accommodate the change. He expects the cost savings realized with Web-based delivery, as opposed to those of printing and shipping documents, will be the driving factor that leads manufacturers to computerize. For this reason, he advocates that manufacturers adopt a hybrid approach during the transition and let the market dictate the pace of change.

The Benefits of Computerization

The medical device industry's movement toward computerization of user manuals parallels similar movements in the medical industry as a whole. Paper is disappearing all over the hospital with the advent of information networks and the related software applications. Caregivers have already been participating in distance-learning sessions associated with building their clinical and reporting skills.

Fortunately, many vendors are prepared to help those medical device developers who lack the expertise or time to develop their own online resources. These vendors claim that computer-based learning tools offer the following benefits over the more traditional forms of printed manuals and in-service training sessions:

- Greater knowledge retention on the part of the learner
- Reduced learning time
- Fewer disruptions to normal hospital operations
- Ease of documenting participation
- Around-the-clock access to quality education
- Reduced costs
- Simplified updating of content

Despite the alleged benefits of computerization, getting busy caregivers to actually sit down in front of computers and realize these benefits might still pose a challenge, especially because in-service sessions often include social interaction, which computer-based training activities do not necessarily provide. That is a challenge for administrators to address with infrastructural improvements and other motivational efforts. The ultimate payoff should reflect a greater ability of staff to operate devices safely and effectively.

The Regulatory Perspective

Patricia A. Kingsley, deputy director of CDRH's Division of Postmarket Surveillance and coauthor of *Write It Right: Recommendations for Developing User Instruction Manuals for Medical Devices Used in Home Health Care*, acknowledges that "written documents are not the professional caregiver's preferred source of guidance." As a registered nurse with more than two decades of clinical experience, she has observed that nurses strongly prefer being shown how to use a medical device rather than reading about it. And CDRH research supports this observation. Nonetheless, one of her major initiatives at the FDA following her move to the agency was to improve the quality of instruction manuals written for professional caregivers and laypersons buying a medical device over the counter.

About the professional users she says, "They tend to read the user manual if a device has reported problems or when they have an unusual patient who may require the caregiver to use a device's more complicated features." Kingsley also mentions the legal role that manuals fill. "The manual serves as a legal document that offers manufacturers liability protection by informing users of the risks and benefits associated with a device, and by describing its proper uses," she says.

Kingsley also cites the anecdotal evidence that nurses, who are the primary users of most medical devices, are looking for more convenient forms of guidance than paper documents provide. In fact, Kingsley says, she is "very excited" about the potential of computer-based learning. "I think it is suitable for sophisticated users as well as laypersons who are unable to read English." She adds, "The agency has been discussing, both internally and with industry, the topic of computer-based learning and other electronic means of educating users." Many within the FDA anticipate a future in which end-users learn how to operate a device by means of computer-based learning tools in addition to other resources.

So how can device manufacturers pursue innovative solutions to user training while the FDA continues to uphold the existing paradigm of requiring printed manuals that demonstrate the safe and effective operation of devices? Kingsley advises manufacturers to work with the FDA in a partnership to "explore innovative options." More specifically, she says that manufacturers "should work with the FDA's policy people to discuss new conceptual approaches. If a manufacturer has a specific solution in mind, then it should work directly with the appropriate division of the Office of Device Evaluation [ODE]. Tell the office what you have in mind. See what options ODE will consider. The agency is moving cautiously because it needs more data on the effect of these new labeling approaches on users' ability to operate the devices safely and effectively. Have research available to support your idea so FDA can be assured that the proposed learning tools will ensure the safe and effective operation of the given device."

Kingsley's remarks suggest an open door to nontraditional approaches to user-oriented documentation at the FDA. But she expects the agency to assume a reactive posture, and she notes that "industry groups such as AdvaMed need to suggest the agenda. The FDA could go in many directions but would prefer to let industry tell us where it wants to go with labeling requirements. This type of industry-led brainstorming is how we originally got involved in looking at standard symbols for use on medical devices."

Conclusion

Hospitals taking a paperless approach to patient medical histories, patient billing, vital-signs recording, and laboratory test reporting seem to represent the future of medical information management. But does the future leave room for the paper-based user manuals that have traditionally been shipped along with medical devices? Will hard copy remain a regulatory requirement? The emerging computerization trend in nearly all industries will leave little room for paper. Even professional airline pilots are turning away from paper documents and toward electronic forms of critical checklists, operating manuals, and maps. Still, the concept of the electronic book has been slow to catch on with consumers who have already embraced personal organizers, such as the ubiquitous PalmPilot. So one cannot be sure about the pace or completeness of the shift away from paper user manuals to electronic formats.

While computerization is already happening to a meaningful degree (industry insiders expect the shift to occur within the next three to five years), some expect that critical information about the operation of a medical device will still be provided in printed form for years to come. To accommodate both possibilities, medical device manufacturers will undoubtedly benefit from producing a core set of content that can assume either print or electronic form to match a customer's preference. Meanwhile, manufacturers should continue to explore innovative solutions and work closely with regulators to determine the viability of their potential solutions.

Key Points

- The FDA requires device manufacturers to supplement their products with printed manuals. The applicable law (21 CFR 801 and 809) considers user manuals to be an extension of a device's labeling that clarifies its proper and safe use.
- Some manufacturers view user manual writing as a regulatory mandate rather than a facet of product design excellence.
- Because excellent documentation is not generally perceived as a competitive advantage, good user manuals do not receive special recognition.
- As more caregivers gain computer access, the practicality of their viewing instructions on a medical device's computer display, on the Web, or on an interactive CD-ROM, for example, will increase.
- Paper is disappearing all over the hospital with the advent of information networks and the related software applications.
- Recognizing the downstream cost savings and the potential to use high-quality learning tools to their competitive advantage, companies may be driven to make greater up-front investments in educational resources than they do now.
- The potential benefits of computer-based training, as compared to reading a user manual in print, include: greater knowledge retention on the part of the learner; reduced learning time; fewer disruptions to normal hospital operations; ease of documenting participation; around-the-clock access to quality education; reduced costs; and simplified updating of content.
- Medical device manufacturers will undoubtedly benefit from producing a core set of content that can assume either print or electronic form to match a customer's preference.

For additional information, visit the following Web sites:

1. C. Bac Kinger and P. Kingsley, August 1993, U.S. Dept. of HHS, Public Health Services, FDA, CDRH, www.fda.gov/cdrh/humfac/hufacpbc.html "Write It Right — Recommendations for Developing User Instruction Manuals for Medical Devices Used in Home Helath Care."
2. Blue Book Guidance on Labeling, www.fda.gov/cdrh/g91-1.html
3. 1997 Draft Labeling Guidance, www.fda.gov/cdrh/ode/labeling.html
4. Patient Labeling Guidance, www.fda.gov/cdrh/ohip/guidance/1128.html

Corporate Human Factors Programs

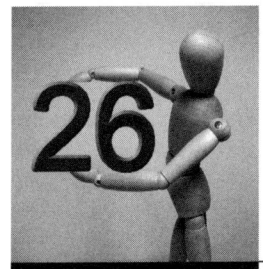

User-Centered Design at Abbott Laboratories

Edmond W. Israelski and William H. Muto

Abbott Laboratories is a diversified health-care company that discovers, develops, manufactures, and markets innovative products and services that span the continuum of care — from prevention and diagnosis to treatment and cure, including pharmaceuticals, medical devices, and nutritional products. The case study authors — Edmond W. Israelski and William H. Muto — collaborate on the implementation of good human factors practices across the large company by teaching workshops, providing expert consultation on product development projects, and helping development groups establish contracts for services from qualified human factors consultants.

Introduction

Abbott Laboratories is a broad-based health-care company that develops medical devices such as in vitro diagnostic devices (IVDs), vascular devices, spinal implants, and feeding equipment, as well as pharmaceuticals and nutritional products. The company operates in 130 countries, has more than 55,000 employees, and generates annual revenues in excess of $18 billion. Abbott's therapeutic technologies address the needs of patients with diabetes, respiratory infections, and HIV/AIDS. The company's technologies enhance the health of adults, children, and even animals.

Goals

Abbott's human factors program was created to establish design processes that lead to safe medical products with best-in-class usability. Specific program goals include:

- Meeting all U.S. and international regulations and guidance pertaining to the human factors engineering of medical technology
- Creating tools and training to enable development teams to implement a user-centered design process
- Assisting and guiding the execution of human factors research and development activities, where possible

Process

Abbott follows a rigorous set of design controls in the course of developing new products. A central corporate organization writes policies that direct the technical work that takes place in various divisions, including those that develop and market medical products. In turn, each division writes their own policies and procedures to best fit their specific market needs. The central organization has a human factors program manager who oversees the related work occurring in the various divisions and who develops corporate policy and helps deliver human factors engineering process training. The corporate person also leads a cross-division, multidisciplined team that provides guidance and review of practical implementation issues relevant to the development process, as well as maintains an intranet Web site that provides human factors information, tools, templates, and other resource materials.

Abbott also employs a "broker model" to facilitate the use of human factors consultants in the user-interface design and evaluation process. The human factors program manager and an additional division-level specialist provide teams with guidance on screening and selecting human factors consultants (i.e., vendors). After the consultants are selected, Abbott's human factors professionals work with the teams to ensure that the chosen company follows the company's policies and best practices.

An internally trained staff performs some human factors activities, such as simple usability tests, under the direction of Abbott's human factors professionals. Whenever possible, the human factors professionals on staff play an active role in various projects involving design, evaluation, and risk assessment.

Methods

Human factors is fully integrated with all of Abbott's relevant development functions, including:

- Engineering
- Marketing
- Medical affairs (former and practicing clinicians who are strong user advocates)
- Regulatory affairs
- Labeling and training development
- Quality assurance

Abbott's product design process (see Figure 26.1) stretches from concept development and design inputs to design outputs, verification, and validation. Listed below each major development phase are the associated user-centered design methods.

Abbott's two human factors specialists have trained more than 400 other staff members on the basics of human factors, including usability testing. To date, trained staff members have conducted numerous usability studies and contextual inquiries as part of product development. However, on most projects, they have left key user-interface design decisions to the formally trained human factors staff as well as to outside consultants.

Abbott conducts most of its usability tests off-site at market research facilities, independent laboratories, simulated hospital facilities, and healthcare facilities. To facilitate usability testing, the corporate headquarters group makes portable usability testing equipment available to teams that need it. The portable lab has seen extensive use in hospital and diagnostic laboratory settings and has been used by medical affairs persons as well as engineering quality personnel. Figure 26.2 shows the portable usability testing equipment including video cameras, computer screen capture, and video taping console.

Project 1: Developing the Architect™ ci8200, i2000, and c8000 Laboratory Diagnostic Systems

For more than two decades, "special chemistry" blood tests have been conducted in hospital and commercial diagnostic laboratories using two categories of analyzers: immunoassay and clinical chemistry instruments.

In an effort to increase laboratory efficiency and reduce the chance of use errors in processing and reporting results, Abbott conceived a system called

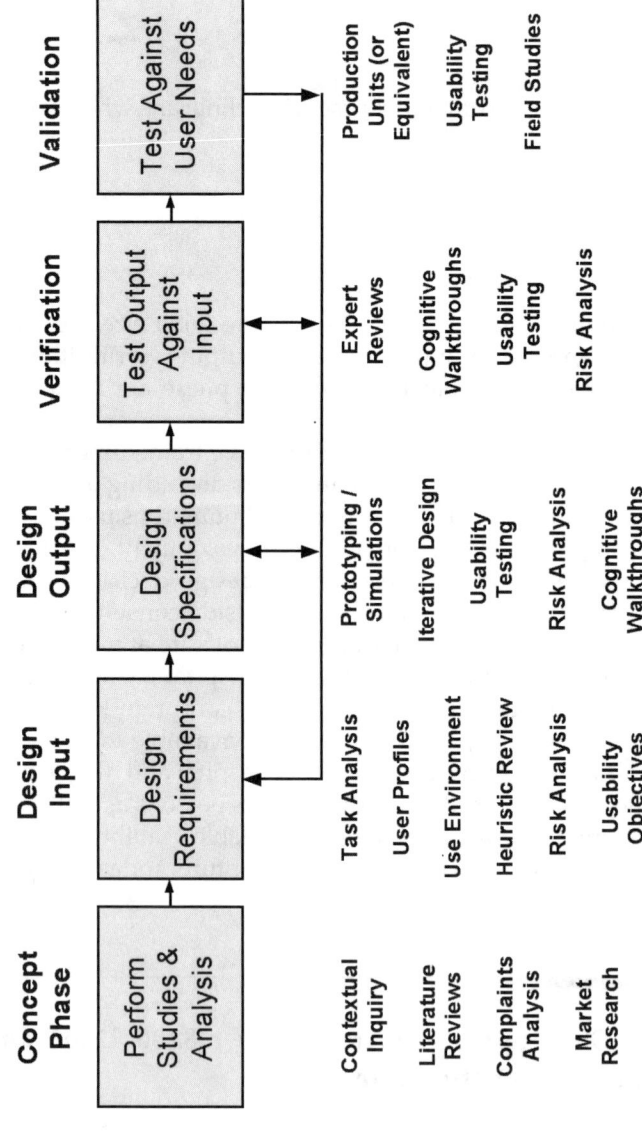

FIGURE 26.1
Diagram of the Human Factors in the Design Process Resources.

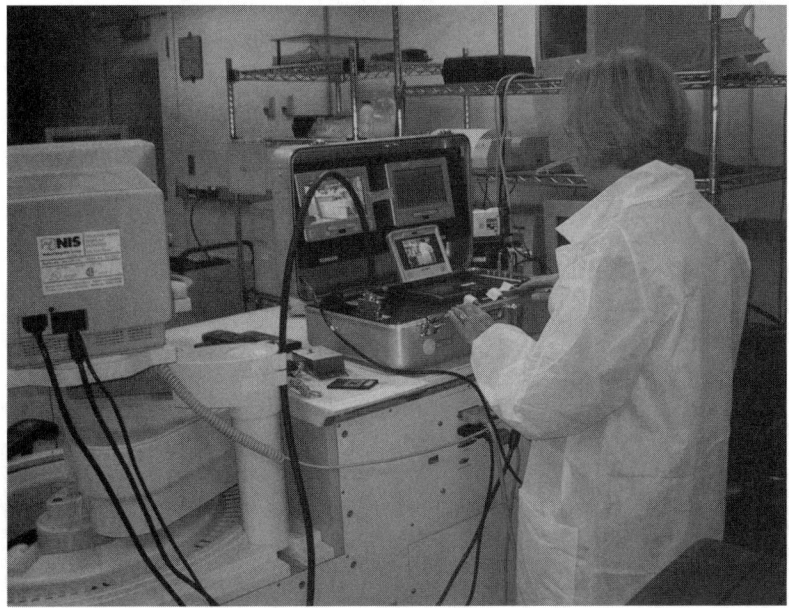

FIGURE 26.2
Illustration showing the portable usability testing equipment suite and its control console.

ARCHITECT™ to integrate the two technologies into a single integrated system — the ci8200 (see Figure 26.3). Human factors played a vital role in defining and assessing the system's essential design elements.

Over the multiyear development effort, internal and external human factors specialists performed:

- Workflow and workload studies
- Function/task analyses
- User requirements definitions
- Graphical user-interface design and prototyping
- Software prototype usability testing and redesign
- Hardware prototype usability testing and redesign
- Final usability testing

The result was a modular family of products that allow the use of separate (stand-alone) systems, as well as integrated systems. In all configurations, intuitiveness and consistency of the user interface were of utmost importance. Some of the design features resulting from the human factors involvement and iterative usability testing included:

- Touch screen-activated graphical user interface (see Figure 26.4)
- Graphical representation of system elements and supplies

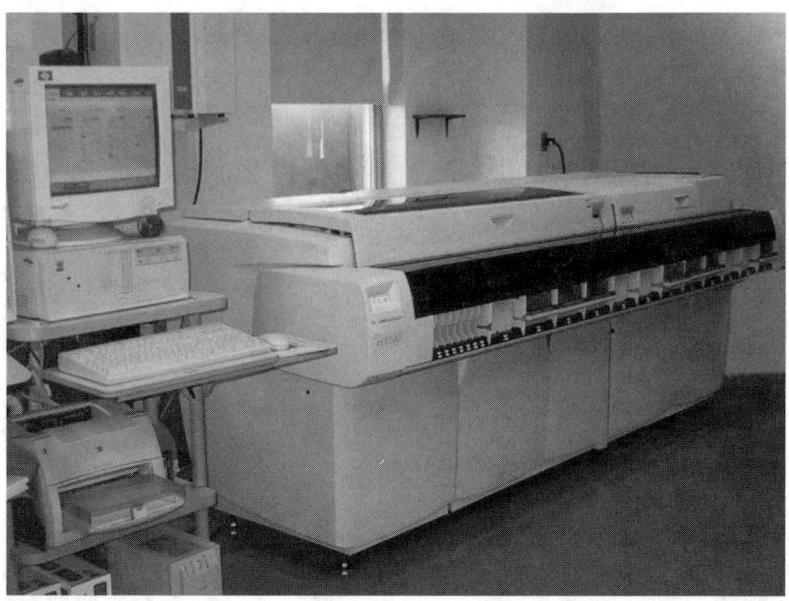

FIGURE 26.3
ARCHITECT™ Integrated System ci8200 is comprised of the c8000 (near end), a chemistry analyzer and i2000 (far end), an immunoassay analyzer. Users load samples into the front through a sample handler that employs a robotic arm to transport samples to the appropriate locations within the instrument and returns them when completed.

- Intuitive menu structures
- Extensive online help
- Automated maintenance procedures
- Automatic patient data collation
- Intuitive quality control system
- Color-coded supplies
- Intuitive, flexible sample handling

Project 2: Developing the Q2+™ Cardiac Output Monitor

The Q2+™ Cardiac Output Monitor measures continuous cardiac output and blood oxygen saturation through the use of a specialized patient catheter. Abbott initiated the Q2+ project due to complaints from users of Abbott's earlier generation product that, despite its advanced functionality, was difficult to learn and use. The main goal of the Q2+ project was to improve the user interface through hardware and software design modifications without changing the underlying sensing technologies or overall packaging.

User-Centered Design at Abbott Laboratories

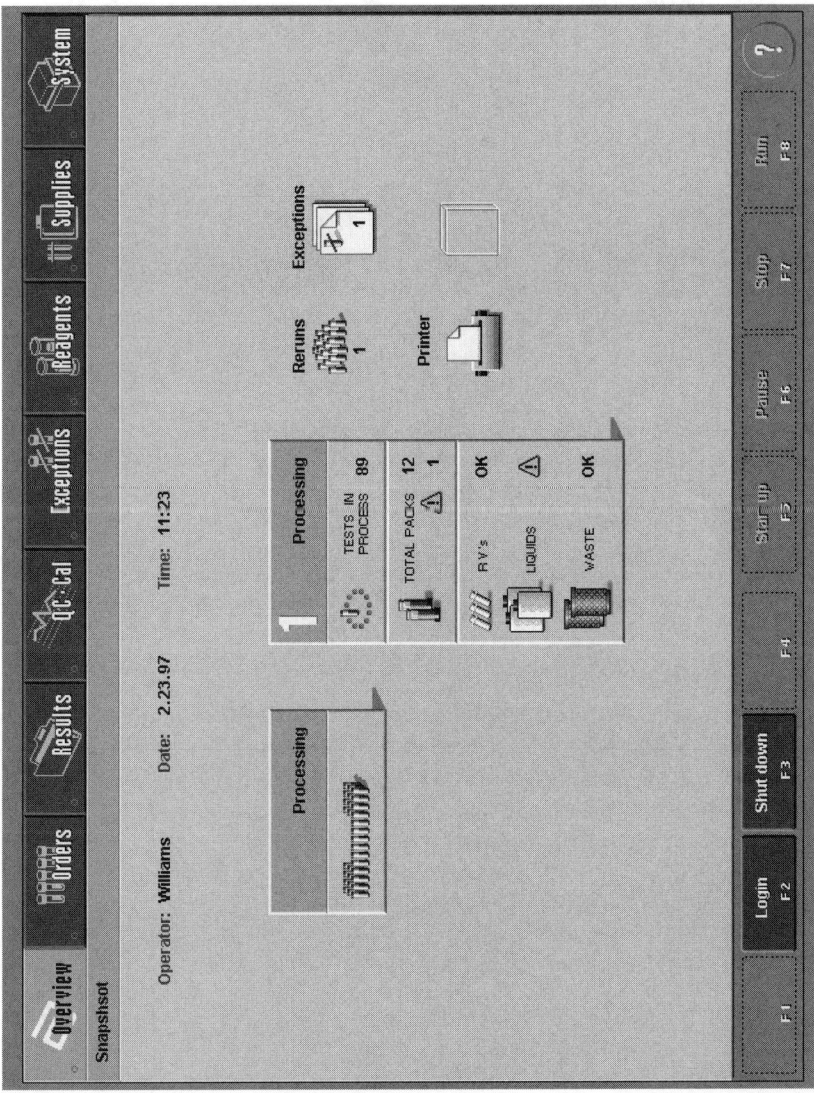

FIGURE 26.4 (See color insert following page 142)
Sample touch-activated screens from Abbott's ARCHITECT[TA] analyzer.

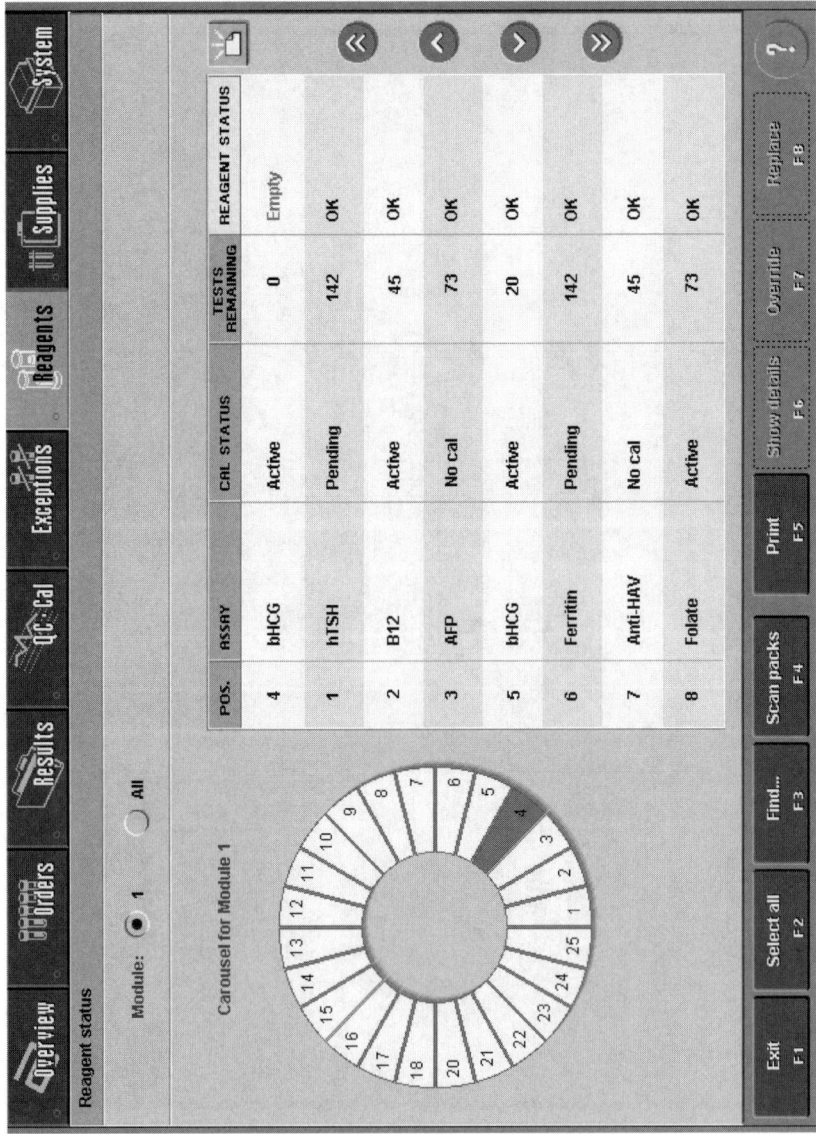

FIGURE 26.4 (continued)

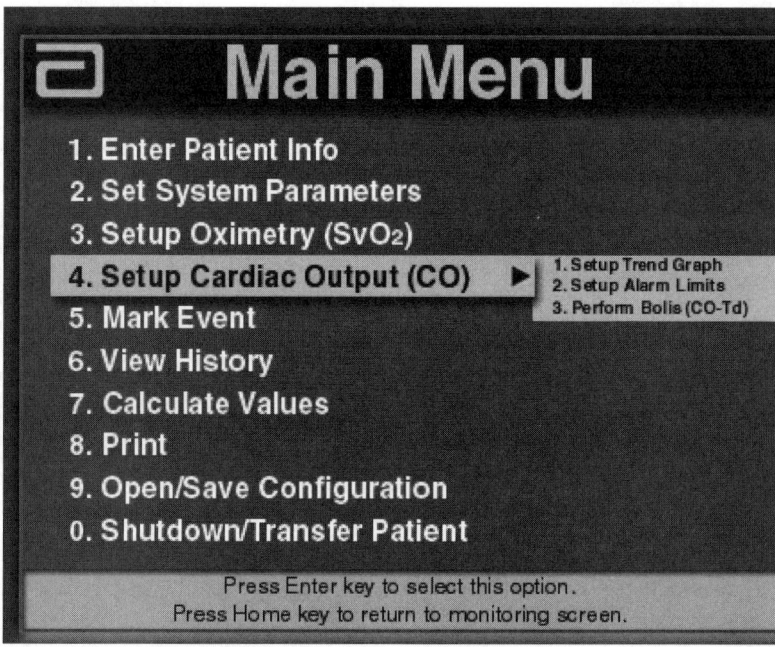

FIGURE 26.5
Q2+™ computer prototype depicting early proposed front control panel layout and main menu with cascading submenu.

Internal and external human factors specialists performed the following tasks:

- Observation-based task analyses
- Observation of nurses and doctors as they set up and used the earlier generation instruments. This activity identified basic functional requirements and identified opportunities for improvement
- Definition of user-interface requirements
- Definition of flat panel screen requirements
- Definition of user requirements for software user-interface redesign
- User interface design and prototyping
- Multiple rounds of usability testing and redesign
- Usability testing of preproduction prototypes

The new product's most significant attributes include (see Figure 26.5 and Figure 26.6):

- Simplified control panel functions and layout
- Flat panel color LCD display screen, replacing monochrome CRT
- Redesigned software user interface

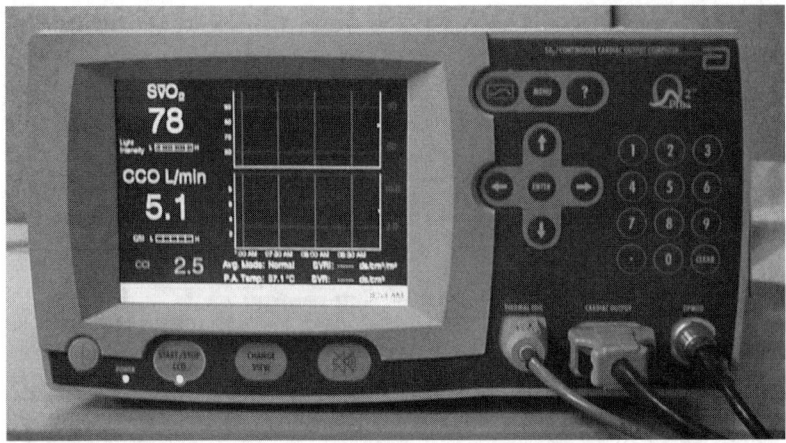

FIGURE 26.6
Actual Q2+™ front control panel with color LCD showing patient monitoring screen.

- New software user interface that employs a hierarchical menu-based approach
- Redesigned monitoring screens with color-coded elements

Usability test participants (doctors, nurses, and anesthesiology technicians) who participated in several rounds of comparative usability tests exhibited significantly improved task performance (execution time and errors) using the new Q2+ over the previous system. The test participants could perform most tasks on the new device with no instructions or training. In short, participants greatly favored the Q2+ user interface over that of the previous system.

Pitfalls

- Convincing company statisticians that formative usability studies can be done with as few as six to eight subjects, and that summative usability tests can also be done with relatively small sample sizes
- Convincing development teams that marketing research methods, such as focus groups or preference surveys, are not substitutes for user-centered design methods, such as usability testing and contextual inquiry
- Making development engineers aware that they are not appropriate surrogates for the product's users and to avoid "self-referential" designs

Lessons Learned

Abbott Laboratories has learned that the biggest obstacle to getting development teams to embrace user-centered design is lack of education and communication. Once staff members have taken even a one-day overview of human factors, they clearly see the discipline's value. For example, many previously uninformed development teams had the false notion that human factors (usability) testing requires large sample sizes. These teams have compared usability tests to medical clinical trials with hundreds and sometimes thousands of test subjects and therefore expected human factors methods to be costly and time-consuming.

Some development staff members had their eyes opened to the importance of human factors after witnessing nurses, physicians, and laboratory technicians struggle with usability problems that typically were easy to remedy. As such, usability testing converted many disbelievers into people who became evangelists for a user-centered design within Abbott, rapidly spreading the "faith" to other project teams.

The old adage is true that success breeds more success. A successful human factors program leads to many more. It also helps that Abbott has now codified user-centered design methods in corporate policies and design control procedures.

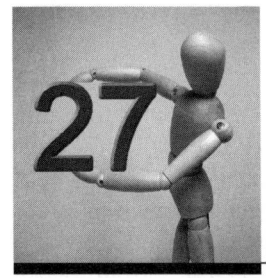
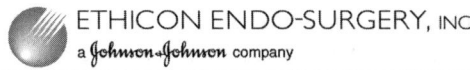

User-Centered Design at Ethicon Endo-Surgery

Larry Spreckelmeier

Ethicon Endo-Surgery, Inc. (EES) is a Johnson & Johnson company that develops and markets a broad portfolio of advanced innovative, procedure-enabling devices for less invasive and traditional general and thoracic surgery, breast disease, gynecology, oncology, and urology. Larry Spreckelmeier heads the human factors efforts at EES. Trained as an industrial designer, Larry addresses human factors with the help of a number of in-house resources and outside consultants.

Introduction

Ethicon Endo-Surgery, Inc. was founded in 1992 as an offshoot of Ethicon, Inc., another Johnson & Johnson company. Since 1995, the EES core market has been disposable minimally invasive surgical instruments. Achieving excellence in human factors has been an important component of the company's strategy for success. Its product line includes surgical linear cutter/staplers, clip appliers, and trocars for open and endoscopic surgery, as well as the Indigo© Laser Sytem, Harmonic Scalpel© UltraCision© line of ultrasonic energy devices, and the Mammotome© line of breast biopsy devices.

Goals

The key goal of the EES human factors program is to assure that the company's products are safe, comfortable, and easy to use. The company must also assure conformity to relevant requirements, particularly the FDA requirements of 21 CFR 820.30. EES optimizes the degree to which its products generally appeal to the medical professionals who will use them. A general attitude at EES is that physicians take it for granted that an instrument will work well. Thus, ease of use is often the differentiator between alternative instruments.

The human factors program, closely associated with Industrial Design, addresses these goals by providing support to the various internal teams that develop EES products. As described in the next section, this support takes the form of:

- Information provided to development teams on an ongoing basis and the maintenance of a body of information on human factors
- Liaison with outside human factors consultants who support specific programs
- Ongoing educational efforts to improve the ability of EES designers and engineers to address human factors issues
- The creation of specific design procedural guidelines to assure that human factors issues are successfully addressed in the product development process

Process

For many years, the company has had a systematic approach to product development that involves interdisciplinary teams working through a series of steps to develop products that fit the intended needs for those products. In the spirit of continuous improvement, a more formal approach evolved in 2002. The *Design Excellence Process* includes a series of steps designated, respectively, *define, measure, analyze, design*, and *verify/validate* (DMADVV). It is the primary responsibility of the human factors and industrial design group to incorporate a user-centered focus into this process.

The HF/ID staff are directly integrated into team activities utilizing Design Excellence DMADVV. A user-focused "discovery" methodology incorporating early field research is also in place to explore and evaluate iterative concepts that appropriately fit user needs, but are not necessarily engineered solutions.

This concept effort feeds into multi-generational product planning which helps define the New Product Pipeline.

For a given project, a team is formed that includes someone from the Industrial Design group. That person then handles the human factors issues associated with the project — alone if the issues are relatively straightforward or, as is typically the case, with the help of outside human factors consultants. Thus, in those cases (which is the majority of projects) when dedicated human factors professionals work as part of the team, Industrial Design acts as the liaison between them and the rest of the team.

Methods and Tools

The company addresses the usability of its products primarily through three basic families of methods: reliance upon technical documents, observational and interview research, and usability testing. These methods are used with the help of outside consultants, and their use is communicated by seminars to sensitize product development professionals of various types to the issues involved.

Technical Documents

When the EES product line began to expand dramatically into laparoscopy in the early 1990s, the company recognized a need for better information about human factors. With a rather small line of products that had been on the market for some time, and were similar in many ways to other surgical instruments, the problem of developing usable products was not terribly intimidating. However, the company faced the prospect of creating products that could no longer be directly visually monitored and that were no longer manipulated in a conventional 3-D space. Laparoscopic instruments are visually monitored by a video image, and they are manipulated via a pivot point formed where the trocar penetrates the patient's tissue wall. Thus, for example, to move an instrument's end-effector to the left, the hand has to be moved to the right.

In order to meet this need for a better human factors information base, the company commissioned an outside human factors consultant to create a reference document to which the designers could refer as they worked on a given design problem. The document contains technical human factors information that is relevant to each major step of the industrial design process, which, for EES includes:

1. Determination of an overall product geometry
2. Specification of control mechanisms and information displays for each function, based upon desired functioning of the device

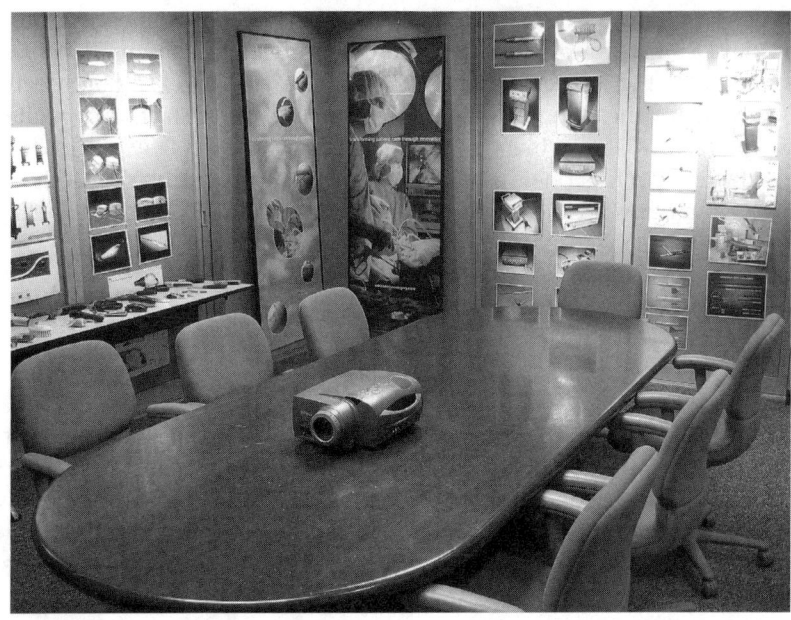

FIGURE 27.1
The industrial design meeting room showing various product concepts.

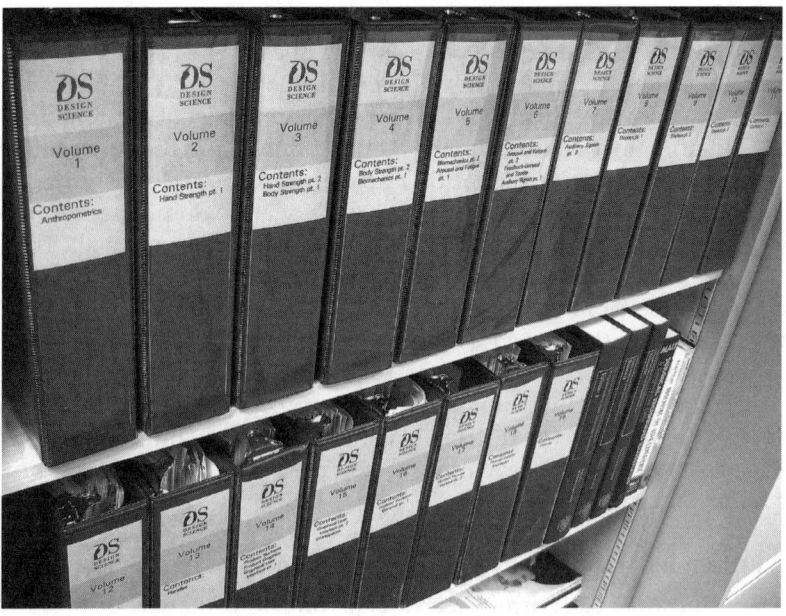

FIGURE 27.2
Human factors reference documents.

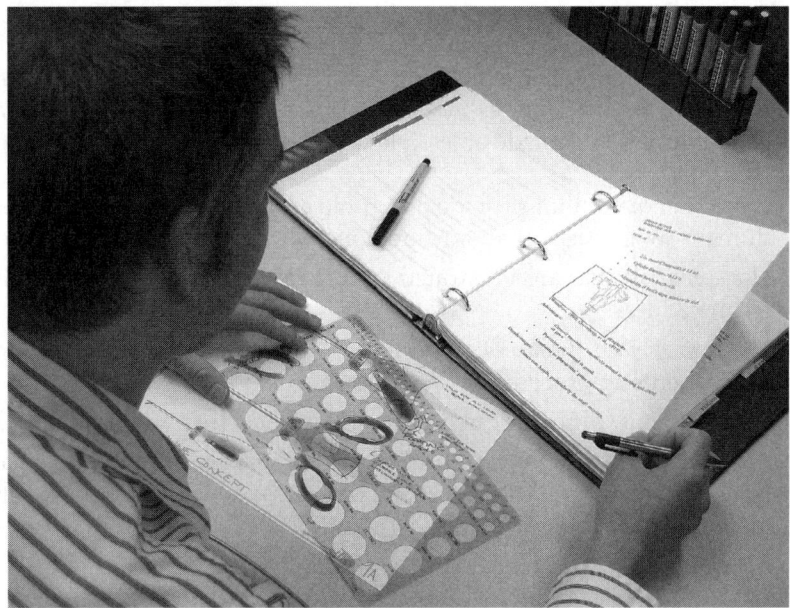

FIGURE 27.3
Using a human factors reference document.

3. Determination of detailed parameters for each of the control mechanisms and information displays, with a particular emphasis on making the product as intuitive and easy to use as possible

So, the EES human factors reference document contains recommendations for various types of grip architectures, the characteristics of different controls and displays, and basic information about potential users, such as force limits for different types of hand movements, range of motion of the joints, size and shape of the hand, and so on. As an adjunct to this document, EES began a human factors library containing technical human factors information.

Over the years, these materials have been added to and amended, and they still serve as an important source of information during the design process. They allow the designers to address "everyday" human factors issues, and the library provides the sort of technical support for decisions that satisfy the engineering members of teams.

Observational and Interview Research

EES uses a number of methods to understand user needs for new products. An important step is to determine the surgical procedures that a given new instrument will be used to perform and to study those procedures. This is done by observing and video-recording procedures, then analyzing them in depth. The team generates a list of design-related questions to be addressed, and a research protocol is created for addressing these questions. Typically, the protocol includes both observation and interviews with the relevant medical professionals. This sort of observational research, supplemented by interviews, then serves as a key resource as the design process unfolds. Some of the ways that such information is made accessible to the team include the following:

- *Procedural maps*, that provide a graphic and text overview of procedures — who does what, for how long, with what instruments, etc.
- *Use scenarios*, that are illustrated summaries of specific components of procedures
- *Searchable video resources*, that allow the team to observe desired components of procedures on demand
- Environment/procedure room diagrams and illustrations
- *Personas*, which are hypothetical users that serve to summarize what is learned about the characteristics of users, particularly from interviews

Usability Testing

As soon as the team begins to create product concepts, these concepts are tested iteratively in as realistic a setting as possible. At the early stages, this may mean testing with nonworking visual models or very crude working models in a setting that, at most, includes training devices or other forms of simulated surgery. Toward the end of the process, testing will usually include animal labs with looks-like/works-like prototypes or even early production parts. At each stage, the EES goal is to create a testing environment that will yield behavioral data as well as attitudes and opinions of potential users. Thus, the testing normally involves realistic tasks with minimal instruction, and the testing is nearly always videotaped. Then, alternative designs are chosen based upon the testing, and concepts are altered to reflect the results of each round of testing.

When conducting usability testing, EES attempts to conduct it in an environment representing reality as closely as possible, to test real users, and to evaluate devices that are as real as possible, in both function and appearance, for that stage of development. Also, when evaluating prototypes, it is often important to assign tasks that mask the actual purpose of the testing in order to obtain objective information.

Documentation

EES has created a formal system for creating a design history file that includes attention to human factors. The system emphasizes what is done

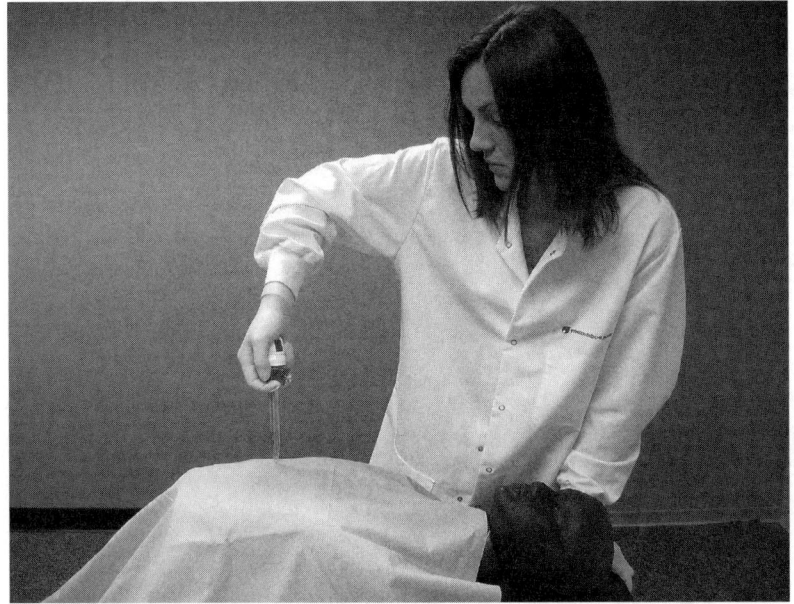

FIGURE 27.4
Early stage usability testing with a simulated patient.

at each stage, the conclusions that are drawn, and what impact it has on the design of the product.

Lessons Learned

EES has learned quite a bit over the years about how to develop usable products. Some key lessons include the following:

- User-centered design requires strong support from the top.

    There are always competing product goals besides usability — time to market, ease of manufacture, cost, etc. Unless there is a strong commitment to usability on the part of upper management, usability can be at risk of being crowded out by this competition.

- It is important for industrial design and human factors people to engage in discussion and observation with medical professionals as early as possible in the process and to begin evaluation of device concepts via usability testing at an early stage.

    Without early input from users, error mitigation is much more difficult and potentially costly to achieve.

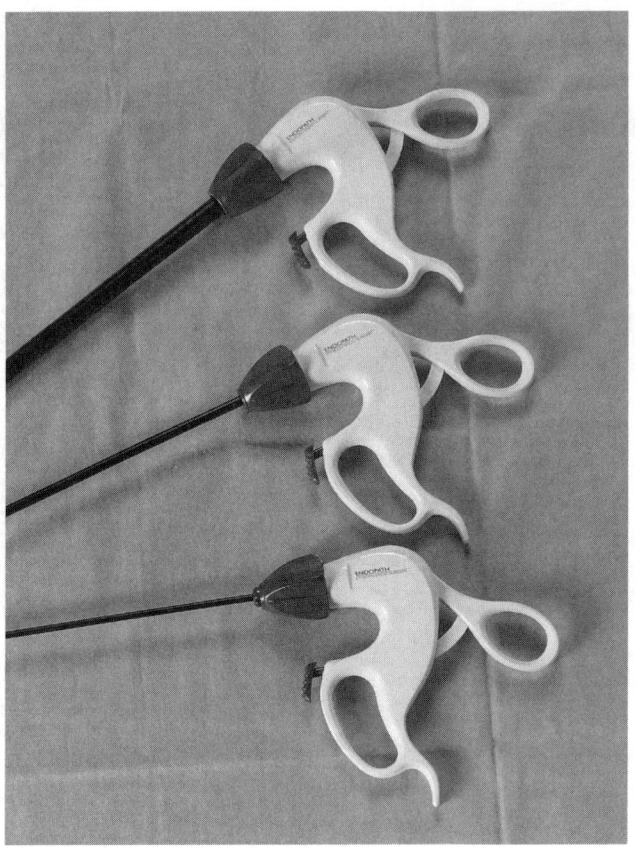

FIGURE 27.5
Laparoscopic instrument handles.

- The formal design systems, such as QFD and Six-Sigma, need to be considerably modified to achieve true user-centered design.

  Such systems usually emphasize the "voice of the customer," but not necessarily the "behavior of the user" as a key focus, and the latter is more important than the former for creating a truly usable and safe product. Also, the inherently iterative nature of user-centered design can be somewhat at odds with the seemingly "mechanical" approach to product development of the formal systems.

- Adopting a user-centered approach to design has far-reaching implications for personnel and corporate structure.

  As the EES product development system changed, some company functions were inadvertently duplicated, others became obsolete, and new functions had to be added.

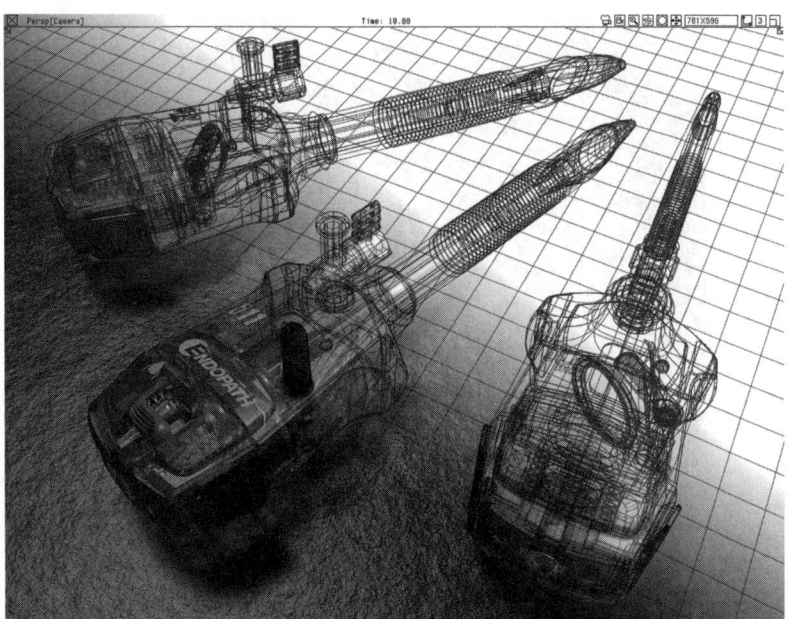

FIGURE 27.6
Trocars.

- Human factors has to be sold.

    It cannot be taken for granted that product development personnel will instantly accept a user-centered approach to design. Thus, it is crucial for those responsible for human factors to be "salespeople" as well as human factors professionals. Surprisingly, most people do not immediately understand the principles behind human factors.

    Voice of the customer is the proxy for capturing and articulating user needs. Human factors success is best achieved when fully addressed through discussion, behavioral observation, usability studies and user verification of the final design concept. It is this iterative process that evolves the concept into the final product. This is best characterized by architect Sir Denys Lasdun:

    > "Our job is to give the client,
    > On time and on cost,
    > Not what he wants,
    > But what he never dreamed he wanted,
    > And when he gets it,
    > He recognizes it as something
    > He wanted all the time."

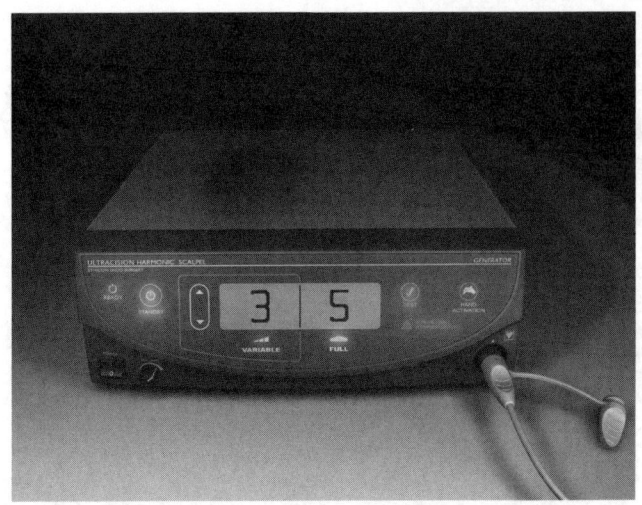

FIGURE 27.7
Generator for EES's Ultracision harmonic scalpel.

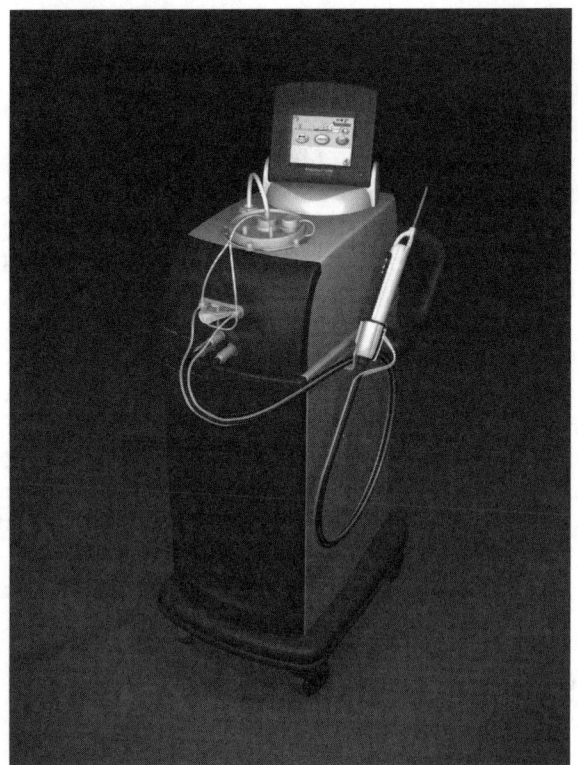

FIGURE 27.8
Mammotome breast biopsy system.

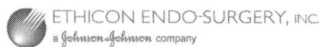

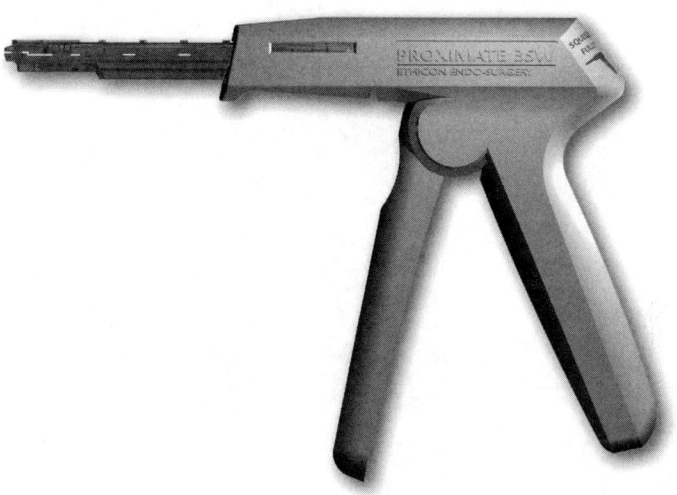

FIGURE 27.9
Surgical stapler.

- Industrial design is a good home for human factors.

    While industrial designers certainly need help from dedicated human factors professionals to do the complete job, there is a lot of merit in fully integrating human factors with industrial design. The designer is the one who actually applies the input from human factors, so it eliminates a great deal of translation to make sure that designers are sophisticated with regard to human factors. Making the designers the liaison between human factors professionals and the rest of the team is one good way to assure that the two disciplines are integrated and that designers continue their human factors education.

Product Design Case Studies

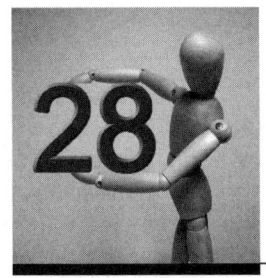 

Home feels better.

Case Study: Personal Hemodialysis System

This case study illustrates how a venture capital-funded company's investment in human factors helped them to (1) simplify user interactions with a fundamentally complex hemodialysis machine, (2) ensure the machine's safety and usability, and (3) secure FDA approval for their groundbreaking technology.

Background

The Company

Chicago-based Aksys, Ltd. was established to develop hemodialysis products and services for patients coping with renal failure (i.e., kidney failure). Specifically, the company sought to develop an automated personal hemodialysis system that would enable patients to receive therapy on a daily basis in alternative care settings, particularly their own homes. Aksys planned for the system to enable more frequent but substantially shorter treatments than are typically delivered in hemodialysis clinics. They also expected the system to improve the quality of life enjoyed by hemodialysis patients by improving their health and freeing them from having to visit treatment clinics several times a week. Aksys also hoped to reduce the total cost of treating patients with end stage renal disease (ESRD), a desirable outcome from the perspective of health-care payors.

The Product Need

End stage renal disease (ESRD) results in a slow, progressive loss of kidney function. The disease often becomes life threatening. Most patients with ESRD can only be treated by means of dialysis. It is estimated that more than a quarter of a million people in the U.S. alone require dialysis, and the number is growing rapidly. By 2010, the number of patients receiving dialysis treatment may approach half a million in the U.S., with at least that many more people on dialysis worldwide. It is estimated that Medicare and Medicaid reimbursements for dialysis treatments in the U.S. will be in the range of $5 billion and growing rapidly.

Traditional Dialysis Treatments

Traditionally, dialysis patients receive hemodialysis treatments three times a week at a clinic or have daily peritoneal dialysis treatments at home. Hemodialysis involves passing a patient's blood through an "extracorporeal circuit" that includes an artificial kidney (dialyzer) and a tubing set. The process normally calls for the patient to sit beside a clinic's hemodialysis machine for several hours while blood cleansing takes place. Peritoneal dialysis involves infusing a patient's peritoneal cavity with fluids that absorb body toxins that would otherwise be removed from the body by the kidneys, then removing the fluid. Both treatments have limitations in terms of their medical effectiveness, comfort and convenience to the patient, and total cost.

The Product

In March 2002, Aksys received the Food and Drug Administration's approval to market the PHD® Personal HemoDialysis System that permits daily hemodialysis in alternate care settings (see Figure 28.1). The company believes the product has the potential to revolutionize dialysis treatment, and thereby the quality of life, for many current and future patients with ESRD. The company claims: "[The] PHD System (1) is designed for operation through a computerized, user-friendly interface, (2) is automated, requiring minimal operator involvement, (3) includes an integrated automatic disinfection system which is designed to enable safe and effective reuse of several key components, (4) requires fewer consumables and (5) is relatively compact."[1]

Many of the first PHD users had positive impressions of the new technology, as captured in the following testimonials*. A particularly pleased patient attests: "I've been on dialysis for 26 years, and for 26 years I haven't felt

---
* Aksys MC-0005-03A PHD Brochure 2004

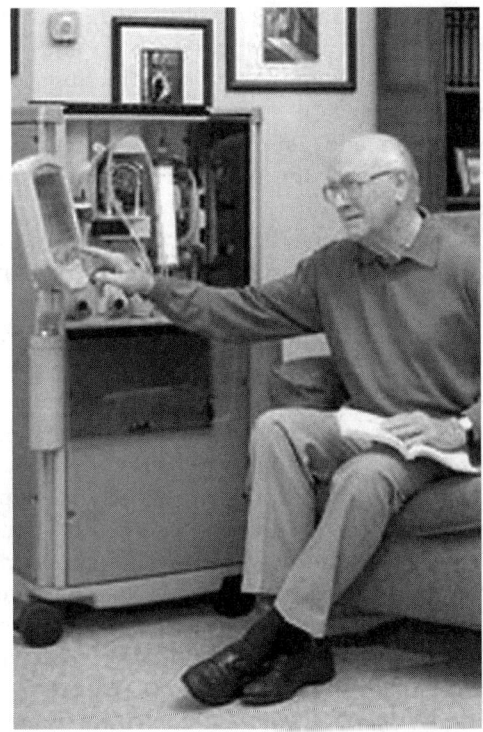

FIGURE 28.1
Aksys, Ltd's Personal HemoDialysis System enables patients to perform hemodialysis at home.

good. But now my friends and family are seeing a real change in me because I'm excited; I'm feeling better. PHD makes it easy for me, and others like me who want to be active members of their families. With PHD, I'm able to live a life that's more normal." Another satisfied patient states, "One of the benefits of the PHD system is that you can stay at home, which allows you the freedom to set your dialysis times at your convenience. The multiple safety features of PHD provide an added sense of security. Also, I no longer experience the large energy swings and the night cramps as I did with in-clinic dialysis. Overall, treatments with the PHD have allowed me to maintain a more normal lifestyle."

User-Interface Development

Early in the development process, Aksys recognized that the PHD's usability and safety were critical to the product's success. Accordingly, they engaged human factors experts to help ensure that end-users — patients and their personal assistants — would be able to use the machine safely and effectively and with satisfaction. They did not want to make medical efficacy and the core dialysis technology the prime focus only to end up with an overly complex device. They also recognized that conducting a robust human factors program was an important step toward meeting the FDA's human factors-related regulations and gaining the regulatory agency's confidence that laypersons could operate the machine with appropriate amounts of training.

Aksys's investment in human factors consulting support cost about $250,000. There were additional costs associated with the internal staff, who worked closely with the consultants. Rather than running a "turnkey" program in which a consultant would develop a user-interface design in isolation, Aksys and its consultant worked collaboratively throughout the development process. This ensured good communication between Aksys's engineers and programmers and the consultant. It also helped Aksys increase its understanding of good human factors methods so they would be better prepared to conduct the work in-house when the next opportunity arose.

The user-interface development process began with a period of user needs research and analysis, proceeded with the design, modeling, and testing of user-interface design concepts, and continues today with incremental refinements resulting from field experience. Feedback from professional caregivers who used the PHD during clinical trials and laypersons who use it at home suggest that it is quite user friendly and empowering — a positive return on the company's investment in good human factors practice.

User Needs Research and Anaylsis

Much of the early user needs research and analysis took place in hemodialysis clinics in the metropolitan Chicago area. In one clinic after another, researchers observed and spoke to professional caregivers administering hemodialysis as well as to the patients hooked up to dialysis machines. Some of the most compelling insights leading to user-interface design goals and requirements came from the patients. They spoke frankly about the pain and inconvenience of hemodialysis and how it interfered with their enjoyment of life. However, they also expressed their appreciation for the lifesaving therapy. Most were enthused at the prospect of performing hemodialysis at home, despite their varying levels of anxiety about taking control of their therapy, as opposed to relying so much on others. It became clear that some patients would be ideal candidates for home treatment, while others would not.

The research suggested the development of a user interface with the following features:

- Touch screen to avoid the need to use a less-natural pointing device than one's finger
- Clear, step-by-step instructions written in a conversational tone using nontechnical terms

Case Study: Personal Hemodialysis System

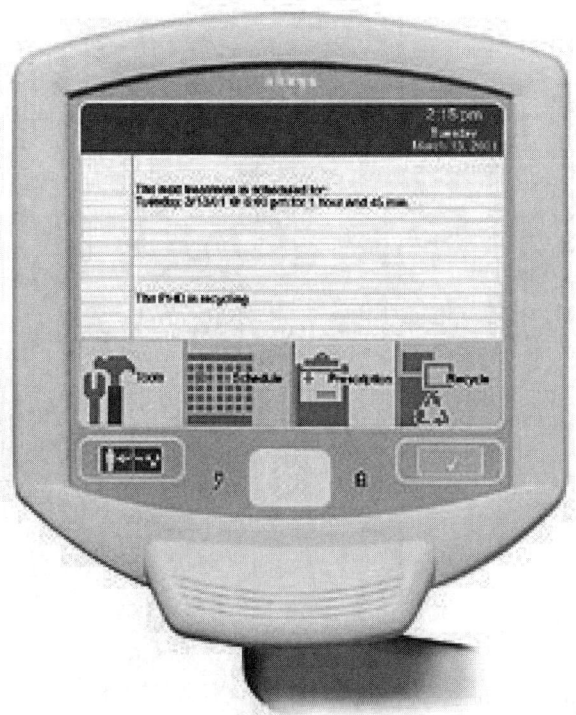

FIGURE 28.2
The PHD's components include a touch screen control panel (left) and a base unit (right) that contains the extracorporeal circuit that cleanses the user's blood.

- Pleasing graphics to imbue the user interface with a more pleasant and less computer-like appearance
- A limited set of top-level choices so users do not feel overwhelmed
- The option to request more detailed information about the therapy in progress to satisfy more technologically oriented users' needs to understand the machine's functions
- Controls that would enable the user to stop therapy immediately if need be
- A user interface (touch screen display) that the users could adjust to suit their physical characteristics, sitting position, and preferences

User Interface Design

Human factors specialists developed a range of conceptual design options before converging on one (see Figure 28.2) that presented information and control options through a top-level screen and a menu consisting of four options: tools, schedule, prescription, and recycle. The top-level screen

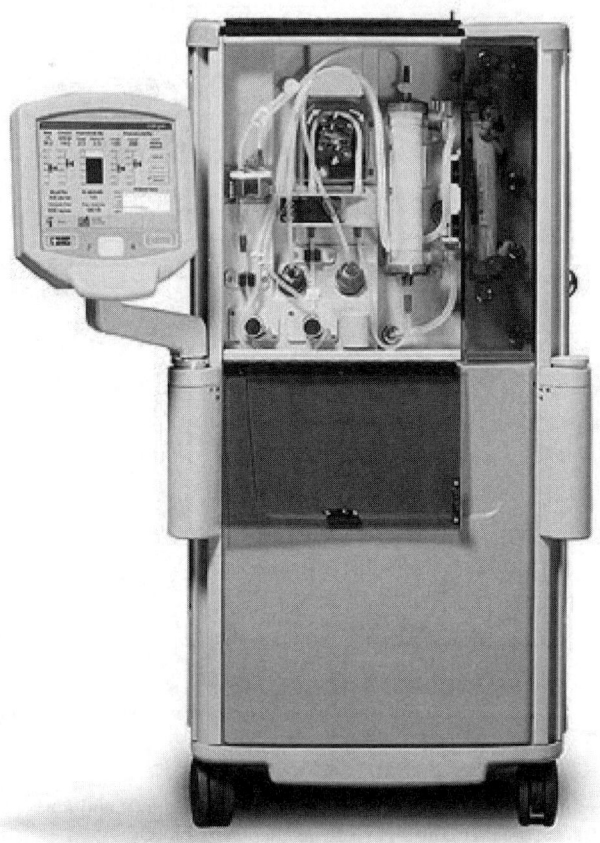

FIGURE 28.2 (continued)

assumed the appearance of a sheet of lined paper that included a greeting and instructions for interacting with the machine. The menu options were placed at the bottom of the screen to minimize the need to raise one's arm to make a choice and to avoid blocking on-screen information with one's hand. The actual menu keys included both text and graphics to ensure that users understood each key's function, as well as to give the user interface a more friendly appearance. To optimize the screen's legibility for individuals with vision impairments, all of the on-screen text is larger than normally found in conventional software applications.

The user interface leads users through a series of phases and steps to complete the hemodialysis process (see Figure 28.3). It also provides continuous feedback regarding the dialysis process and the patient's physiological status (see Figure 28.4). The human factors specialists established several therapeutic stages to create a clear mental model of the machine's functions and to reduce the perception of hemodialysis as an interminable number of steps.

User-interface prototypes that enabled users to perform tasks but did not actually control a hemodialysis machine enabled the developers to perform

Case Study: Personal Hemodialysis System   289

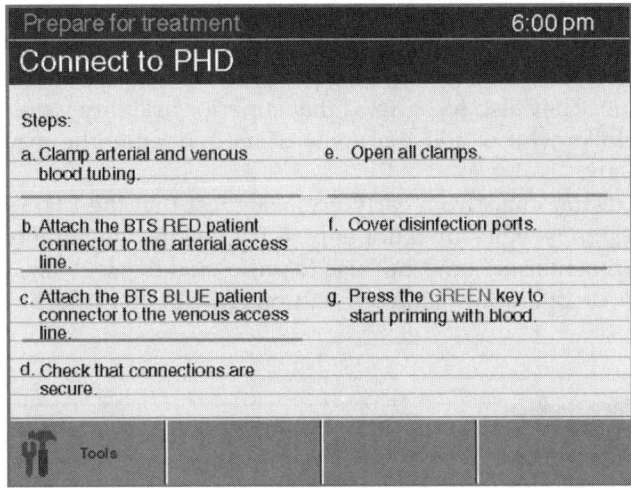

FIGURE 28.3
The PHD's user interface leads users through the setup and treatment process in a step-by-step manner.

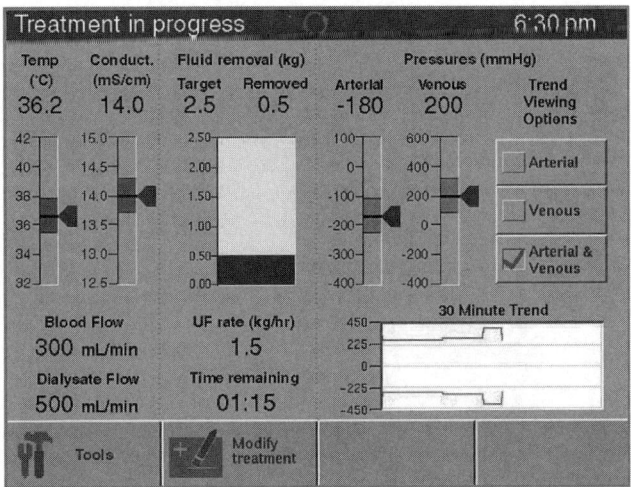

FIGURE 28.4
The PHD's user interface provides feedback on the progression of the dialysis process and the patient's physiological status.

early usability tests of the user-interface design. Such testing showed that the user interface was generally well suited to the needs of the intended users, but did indicate opportunities for further refinements. The user-interface design also evolved in reaction to technological constraints and feedback on the design during clinical trials.

By the end of the user-interface design process, Aksys executives switched from being concerned about the PHD's usability, to viewing it as one of the machine's greatest assets and selling points, nicely complementing its therapeutic value. They also recognized that superior usability would be important to the folks who would train new users to operate the machine safely and effectively.

Personal testimonials from early users suggest that the PHD's final user-interface design is well suited not only to laypersons who will be trained to operate the machine at home, but also to professional caregivers, people who are capable of operating complex equipment but like the PHD's simple operation.

References

1. Aksys, Ltd Web site, www.aksys.com/corp/company.asp, current as of January 2004.
2. Aksys, Ltd Web site, www.aksys.com/phd/testimonials.asp, current as of January 2004.

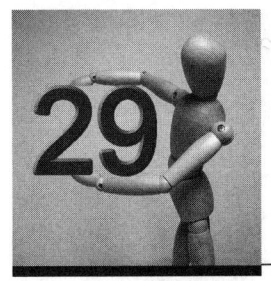 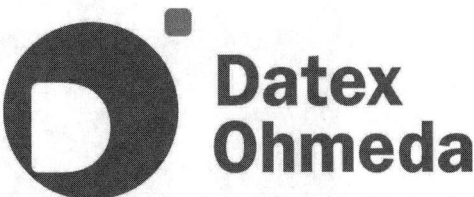

Case Study: Patient Monitor

This case study reveals how a company's investment in human factors influenced its entire product line and continues to pay off a decade later.

Background

The Company

In the mid-1990s, Datex was enjoying considerable success marketing patient monitoring products in Europe. In fact, they had captured considerable market share by selling an integrated monitoring product called *Cardiocap* and a subsequent version called *Cardiocap II* (see Figure 29.1), which was capable of monitoring several hemodynamic as well as respiratory parameters including expired CO_2. But, the Finnish company still was not very well known in the large U.S. marketplace. That changed when the company introduced the AS/3 — a modular patient monitor incorporating a color display and designed specifically for use in the operating room by anesthesiologists and nurse anesthetists (see Figure 29.2).

The AS/3 was extremely successful both in terms of sales and establishing Datex's reputation within the U.S. market as a high-quality, high-value equipment provider. Since the AS/3's introduction, Datex merged with Ohmeda, a leader in the anesthesia delivery equipment field, to form Datex–Ohmeda. Subsequently, GE Medical Systems bought Datex–Ohmeda, cementing its position as one of the three major players in the medical equipment manufacturing industry.

291

292   *Designing Usability into Medical Products*

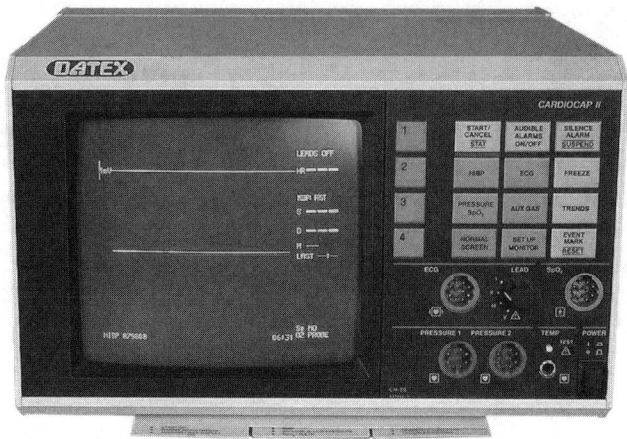

FIGURE 29.1
Datex's *Cardiocap II* integrated patient monitor. Photo courtesy of Datex–Ohmeda Division, Instrumentarium Corp.

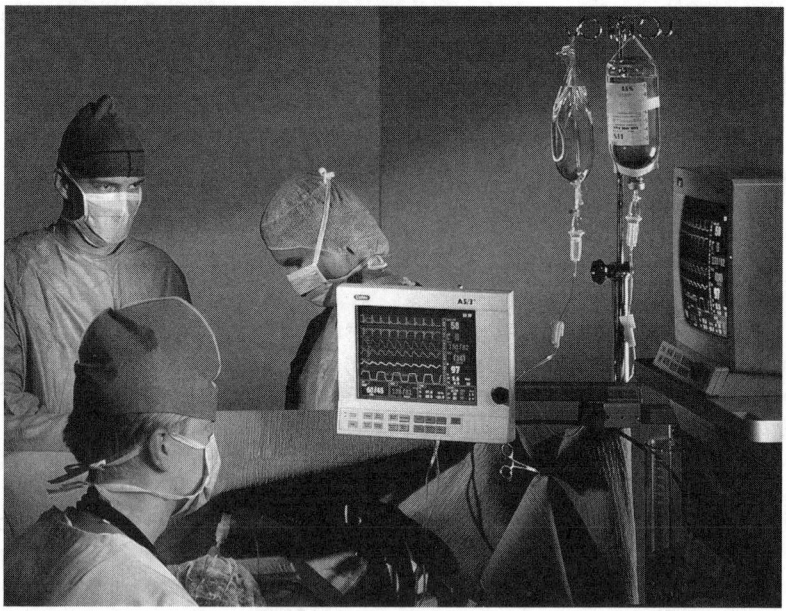

FIGURE 29.2
Datex's AS/3 patient monitor. Photo courtesy of Datex–Ohmeda Division, Instrumentarium Corp.

By 2001, the AS/3 had evolved into the S/5 (see Figure 29.3), available in a stand-alone form and as an anesthesia workstation built-in. It also grew more capable through the addition of new parameters, such as the measurement of *entropy*, an indication of a patient's state of consciousness. It has also

Case Study: Patient Monitor

been engineered to share information over a hospital's network. Still, the S/5 retains the AS/3's overall functional organization, means of menu navigation, and simple outward appearance. Moreover, the AS/3's general interaction style became Datex's model for related products, such as their anesthesia recordkeeper.

The Product Need

Datex developed the AS/3 in response to market demand for integrated (i.e., all-in-one) and modular patient monitors, such as the Component Monitoring System already introduced by Hewlett-Packard (now Philips Medical Systems). Datex recognized the advantage of one monitor over separate monitors. For starters, a single monitor enabled users to focus their attention on one location to acquire interrelated information about the patient's condition (i.e., vital signs). Second, integrated monitors stood to be less expensive in some cases than several stand-alone devices requiring their own cabinets and power supplies. Third, an integrated monitor offered the potential to organize information and present alarms, for example, in a more consistent, usable form. Fourth, an integrated monitor opened the door for an investment in better hardware, leading to the use of a large, color CRT display (since replaced by a color LCD). At the time of its development, a color CRT was almost considered a luxury feature. Today, color displays are critical to presenting information in a readable fashion that relies heavily on color coding.

The Product

The original AS/3 was a medium-size (15" diagonal) color monitor sitting on top of a slim base unit equipped with 20 or so membrane keys and a rotary control that Datex now calls their *ComWheel*. Datex was not the first to employ the rotary control that users rotated to highlight menu options and press to select an option. It was also one of the first to utilize less expensive, mass-produced components originally designed for personal computers. Several medical and consumer electronic devices were already sporting a knob that performed comparable functions. But, Datex used the rotary knob to great effect. Its intuitive operation (turn and press) pleased new users and it emerged as one of Datex's signature features. Similar to Hewlett Packard's patient monitor, the AS/3 received data from modules that received and preprocessed signals from sensors attached to the patient. Today, the evolved monitor is available in several forms that incorporate different size CRTs and LCDs.

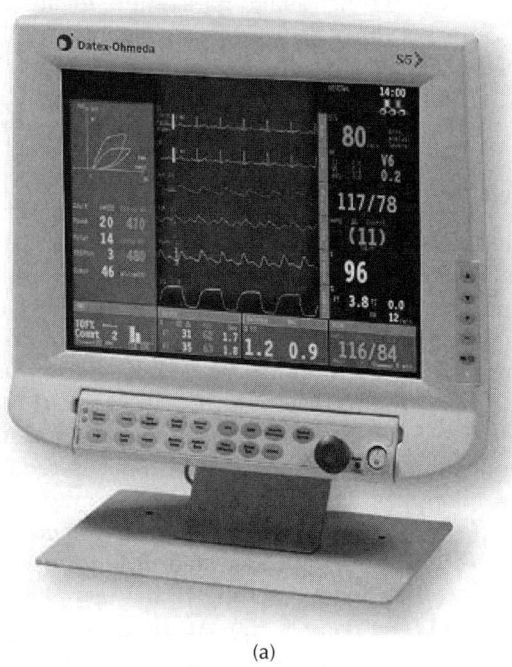

(a)

FIGURE 29.3
Datex's S/5 critical care monitor (a) shares basic features with the original AS/3 patient monitor. Datex's S/5 Anesthesia Delivery Unit (b) is equipped with a comparable monitor. Photo courtesy of Datex–Ohmeda Division, Instrumentarium Corp.

User-Interface Development

User-Needs Research and Analysis

Datex assembled a team of in-house engineers and human factors consultants to develop the AS/3. The company's goal was to develop the detailed user-interface design mostly on their own, but to use the human factors consultants at various stages to accelerate and enhance their in-house efforts.

The team started by visiting several hospitals to observe patient monitors in use during several surgical procedures, including hernia repairs and coronary artery bypass grafts — cases that varied widely in terms of procedure length and patient acuity. During their observations, team members documented tasks performed by the anesthesiologist (or nurse anesthetist) in conjunction with the stages of anesthesia (i.e., preparation for surgery, induction, surgery, emergence, and recovery). This data helped the team form a better sense for the pace of work and how the clinicians used their patient monitors. Follow-up interviews with the clinicians served to clarify user needs and expectations.

Case Study: Patient Monitor 295

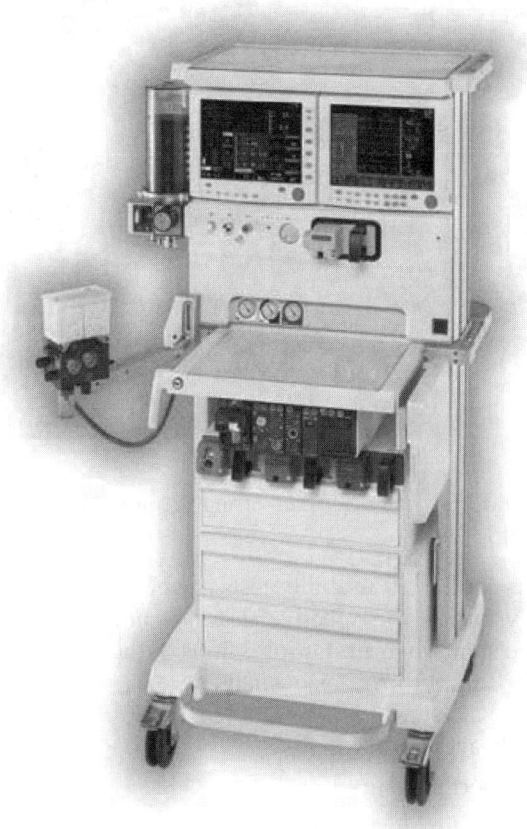

(b)

FIGURE 29.3 (continued)

After completing the field research, the human factors specialists performed a detailed task analysis of the anesthesia practices observed in the hospitals to define urgent and frequent tasks. They also wrote usability goals for Datex's next generation patient monitor, focusing on the time required to perform specific tasks and the desired level of clinician satisfaction with the design in terms of its intuitiveness, perceived speed of use, and the perceived ability to recover from a use error.

User-Interface Design

The development team's next step was to design the hardware and software user interfaces in parallel, recognizing that the hardware requirements would depend heavily on the software's functionality and navigation requirements. Once sample screens and a hardware mock-up became available, the human

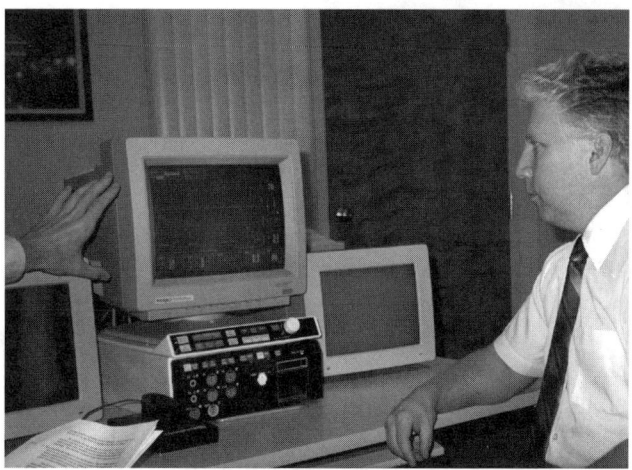

FIGURE 29.4
Anesthesiologist participates in a usability test of an AS/3 prototype. Photo courtesy of American Institutes for Research.

factors specialists conducted usability tests to obtain feedback on the designs. Specifically, they invited prospective users — anesthesiologists and nurse anesthetists — to share their first impressions of the designs (see Figure 29.4) as well as attempt to perform tasks such as:

- Adjust the heart rate alarm
- Display a blood pressure trend
- Set up the monitor for a new patient
- Perform a cardiac output measurement

The development team revised the user-interface designs according to the usability test findings as well as evolving technical requirements. Once Datex produced a working AS/3 prototype, it conducted additional usability tests to refine and validate the design.

Conclusion

When Datex launched the AS/3 development program, it was only a minor player in an American market dominated by companies such as Hewlett-Packard, Spacelabs, Marquette, and Siemens. However, Datex made the strategic choice to tailor the AS/3 specifically to the needs of anesthesia providers, rather than produce a more generic design to serve the purposes of critical-care units as well. Anesthesia providers immediately recognized the benefits of a monitor designed for them and AS/3 sales grew. Within a few years, Datex had established itself as a major player in the U.S. market — one of the company's major goals. New customers perceived and extolled the monitor as the most usable on the market.

As previously mentioned, the AS/3 evolved into the S/5 while sticking to the same basic style of user interaction made possible by the *ComWheel*. Almost 10 years later, the company's investment in human factors continues to pay off in strong product sales and a sustained reputation within the marketplace for producing user-friendly products.

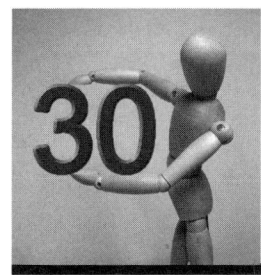

Case Study: Development of a Contrast Medium Injector System for CT Scanning

This case study illustrates how a relatively mature product line can be immensely improved (and can increase market share) by incorporating a user focus into the design process from the beginning. It also shows that making a more effective product involves numerous incremental changes that, taken together, add up to a better product.

Background

The Company

Medrad, Inc., located in Indianola, PA, outside of Pittsburgh, was founded by Dr. Stephen Heilman, a physician, in 1964. The initial purpose was to develop Dr. Heilman's new invention, the first angiographic injector. The company has gone on to develop a viable market share in contrast medium injection systems, providing systems for magnetic resonance (MR), computed tomography (CT), and ultrasound, as well as various other products to enhance imaging. Beyond receiving numerous local, state, and national awards, Medrad is the recipient of the 2003 Malcom Baldrige National Quality Award in the manufacturing sector.

299

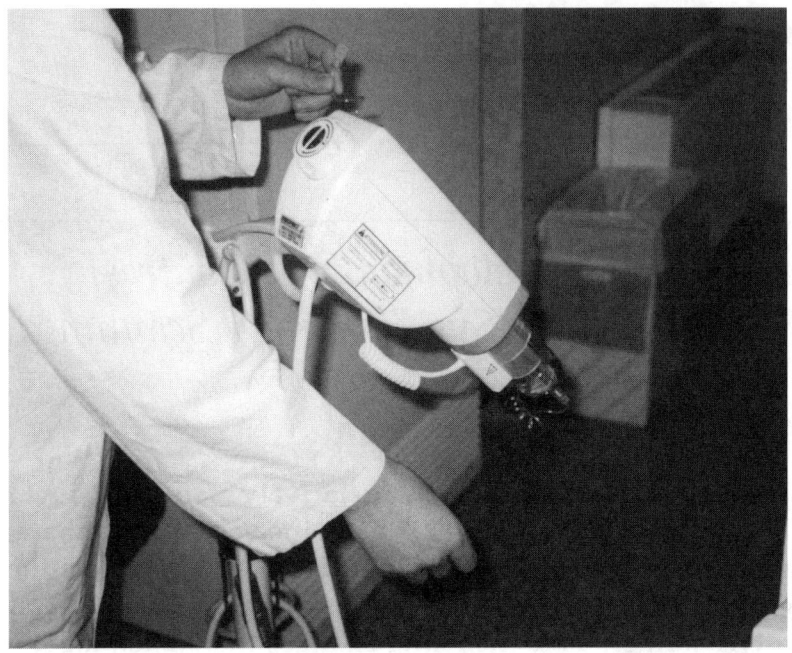

FIGURE 30.1
The predecessor injector in the field, with the syringe mounted at the end.

The Product Need

Medrad began the development of a new contrast medium injector system for CT scanning in 1999. At that time, Medrad's existing CT product was over five years old (see Figure 30.1). In the five years since its introduction, the technology had changed, competitors had progressed, and Medrad believed that there were opportunities for providing new features and developing a better user interface (see Figure 30.2). Also, Medrad had already begun the development of a different product, a new MR injection system, and had created a new graphic user interface for it. The development of a new CT injector provided the opportunity for applying a common operator interface to the new CT products, as well as MR products, in order to amortize the investment over multiple products, and to maintain a consistent "look and feel" and style of interaction across Medrad's product lines.

One challenge for the program was to improve on a successful system, which had already rendered a substantial market share for Medrad with its largest product line, the CT injector system.

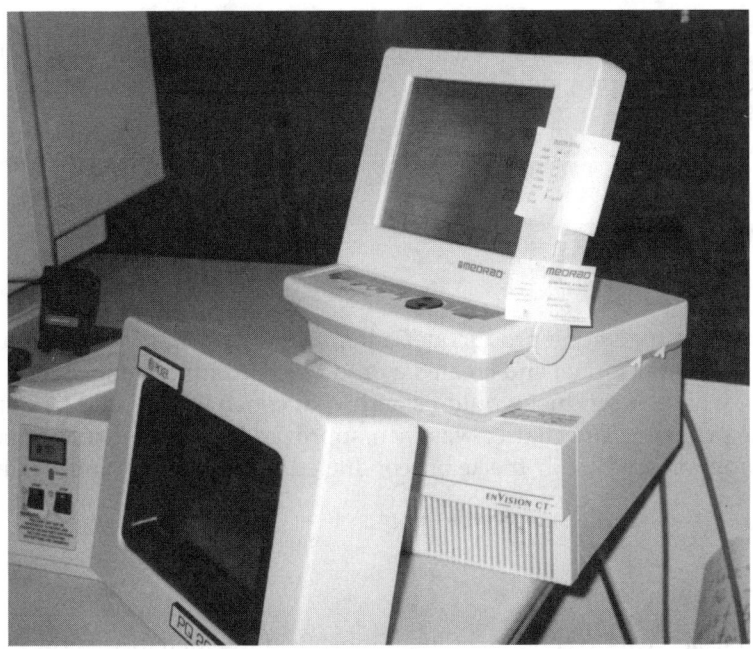

FIGURE 30.2
The touch screen unit of the predecessor in the field, showing posted notes.

The Product

A typical contrast medium injector system consists of three components:

1. A disposable syringe, which contains and injects the contrast medium fluid, through tubing, into the patient as the plunger of the syringe is advanced
2. The injector head, which contains basic controls and displays as well as the mechanical drive mechanism which engages the plunger of the syringe
3. A separate graphic user interface, which allows the user to set the various parameters of the injection — e.g., timing and volume — and to initiate an injection

Because the product was designed specifically to support CT imaging, it had to be compatible with existing CT scanners. The goal of a CT injector is to deliver the right amount of contrast medium into the right blood vessels with the right timing, so that the resultant CT images are as diagnostic as possible.

At the outset, Medrad was determined to do what it could with each part of the system to provide additional functionality and make it as easy to use as possible.

The Process

Medrad put together a product definition team consisting of marketing and engineering personnel and created a product charter that defined, in general terms, what the product would be and what constraints would be imposed on the program. The charter was then approved by senior management. As the program unfolded, the team conducted ethnographic and evaluation research.

Ethnographic Research

The first step was to conduct ethnographic field research to see how existing Medrad, as well as other CT injectors, were currently used in the field. The goals of the research were to develop a solid understanding of users, their patterns of use, and the use environment, and to identify opportunities for improving any part of the system or process.

The team went to various hospitals, spending a full day at each site, watching procedures, taking measurements, and asking questions. This research provided background information about existing user procedures and use environments, and it yielded a list of opportunities for product improvements. It captured ways that the procedures could be streamlined, that annoyances could be eliminated, and where patient safety could be improved. The results of this research were then shared with the entire product development team so they had first-hand information on the problems the customers were facing.

Some key findings from this research included the following:

- Existing injectors had some features that were seldom used and/or were poorly understood.
- Loading the syringe onto injectors was unnecessarily difficult.
- Excessive manual movements of the syringe by the operator took time that slowed throughput.
- The information provided on the graphic user interface was not as clear or as well laid out as it could be.

- Improving the safety of the system was a very high priority of the users.
- There were opportunities to decrease the waste of contrast medium.
- The use of saline for priming and flushing fluid lines could provide benefit, but the existing equipment would not easily accommodate the injection of saline.

Evaluation Research

As soon as possible, the team began to generate prototypes of the hardware components of the system and of the software interface and to test these prototypes. As the program unfolded, the prototypes went through stages from low to high fidelity. The software interface was prototyped using VisualBasic and, until relatively late in the program, was developed on a separate track from the hardware development. Hardware was tested iteratively (3–4 rounds of testing), as it evolved. The software interface was also finalized iteratively (10–12 rounds). As the graphic user interface evolved, the team developed, in parallel, a user interface description that the software engineers used to write the final code. The team retained as much of the common-platform interface (mentioned above) as possible, but altered it as needed to support CT injections.

The New Product

Once the team was satisfied that the product was where it needed to be, the design was frozen, and, to prevent potential chaos, the product definition team was not allowed to interfere with the implementation team as the working prototype and the user interface description were turned into actual code. In fact, the disciplined process adopted by Medrad resulted in a need for only one minor operational change to the very complicated interface once it was coded. The process illustrates the value of using "throw-away" coding for prototyping and testing, prior to actual coding. Using such prototyping tools (VisualBasic, in this case) dramatically reduces the time it takes to create prototypes and the time it takes to alter those prototypes, resulting in an overall savings in time due to fewer coding revisions at the end of the cycle (the quickest path to the end is to do it right the first time). It also yields a better product because there is less reluctance to make changes at the end of the process, based upon evaluation research with users.

The resulting product is shown in Figure 30.3 — the new Stellant® CT Injection System. Some key features include the following:

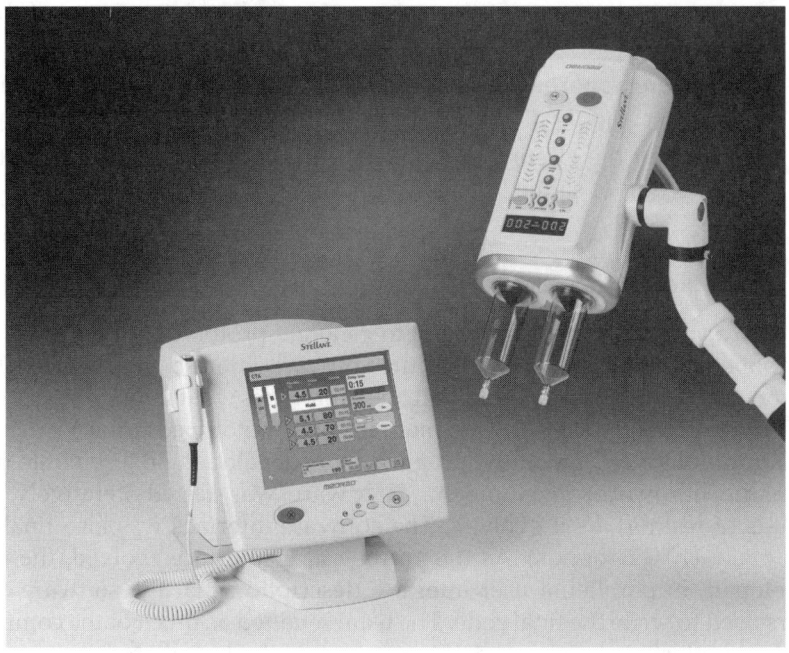

FIGURE 30.3 (See color insert following page 142)
The Stellant CT Injection System — the injector to the right showing the disposable syringes at the bottom; the touch screen interface unit to the left.

- Two rather than one syringe can be loaded at a time to improve efficiency of use and better support complicated injection protocols and easier use of saline for flushing lines
- Accommodation of saline for pre- and post-injecting and for flushing lines
- One-step priming
- A real-time pressure monitor graph that provides additional information to the user about the status of the injection as it progresses
- One-step syringe installation and removal
- Automatic plunger advance and retraction to save time and steps
- Automatic syringe filling to the precise required volume, eliminating waste
- The addition of a mini-reservoir to reduce contrast spillage
- Clearer and more logical real-time presentation of information on the color touch screen
- Presentation of the information required by users on the touch screen — e.g., flow profiles and timing information

Introduced in 2003, the system has been very well received by users and has exceeded all sales forecasts.

One of the Major Keys to Success of the Total Project

When the marketing representative of the project was asked about the biggest key to success for the program, he responded as follows:

> We performed research at the beginning of the project to understand what users were going to need in the future to accomplish their job. Through rapid prototyping and continually reviewing working models internally, we locked into the design early in the process and didn't change it during development. You can have the best new product development organization in the world, but you can't improve business results if you quickly develop the wrong product.

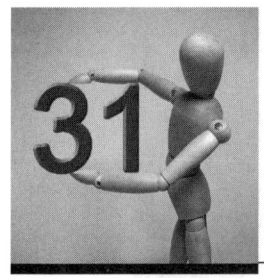

GUIDANT
Case Study: Remotely Controlled Defibrillator

This case study details how a large medical company drew upon human factors resources at several stages of product development and verification to ensure the usability of a defibrillator used primarily by older individuals.

Background

The Company

Guidant is a relatively young company (incorporated in 1994) that has since grown to $3.4 billion in revenue and more than than 11,000 employees. Many of the company's products are designed to help patients with heart disease maintain or return to active, productive, and satisfying lives.

The Indianapolis-based company strives to develop leading-edge products, including defibrillators, pacemakers, catheters, and stents, that enable physicians to deliver quality care. Its development process treats user needs and preferences as a priority.

Many of Guidant's products are designed for use by cardiac surgeons, electrophysiologists, interventional cardiologists, nurses, and cardiac-care technicians in the course of relatively complex medical procedures. However, this case study focuses on a defibrillator that is actually controlled by the patient.

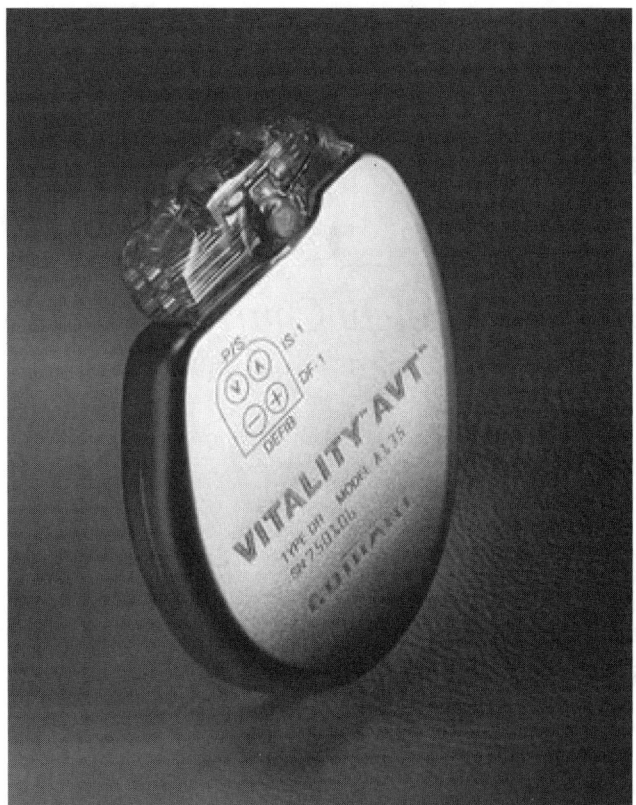

FIGURE 31.1 (See color insert following page 142)
Guidant's PARTNER Rhythm Assistant and VITALITY™ AVT® Defibrillator (Implantable).

The Product Need

Guidant determined the need for a device that would enable patients afflicted with chronic atrial fibrillation (AF) to normalize their heart rhythms without assistance from a caregiver. Notably, AF afflicts about two million Americans and millions more worldwide. Therefore, a device intended for operation by the patients stood to revolutionize AF treatment and fulfill a large market need.

A heart in AF is a temporarily weakened blood pump. Instead of beating 60 to 80 times per minute, a fibrillating heart beats 300 to 600 times per minute, but each beat is more of a flutter that moves less blood from the atria into the adjacent ventricles. As a result of not filling completely with blood prior to contraction, the ventricles have to work much harder to pump the same amount of blood throughout the body. There is a tendency for blood to pool in the atria and for the level of oxygen in the blood to drop.

AF is not necessarily life threatening, principally because the ventricles continue to do their job, even if to a diminished degree. Also, a heart in AF

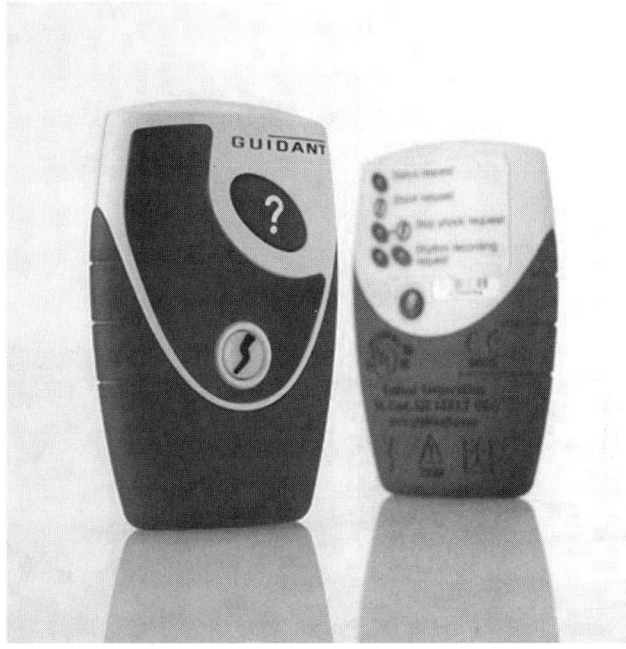

FIGURE 31.1 (continued)

naturally returns to a normal rhythm at some point. However, frequent and protracted episodes of AF can lead to heart muscle damage over time. There is also an increased risk of stroke due to the formation of blood clots in blood pooling in the atria. AF patients tend to feel profoundly weak and tired during an AF episode. Patients may also experience confusion because less oxygen is getting to their brains.

Cardioversion, the synchronized delivery of a brief electrical shock to a fibrillating heart, usually restores a normal rhythm. For years, patients have had to visit a hospital to receive such shocks. Alternatively, they have learned to live with the transient condition and its long-term effects.

The Product

Guidant's VITALITY™ AVT® defibrillator, which comes with a handheld remote control called the PARTNER™ Rhythm Assistant, gives AF patients direct control over their heart rhythm (see Figure 31.1). When a patient feels the onset of AF, she holds the remote control close to their chest (see Figure 31.2) so that it can communicate via radio waves with the implanted defibrillator. Only if the patient is experiencing an atrial arrhythmia — a condition that the defibrillator is able to confirm — will the VITALITY™ AVT® transmit a

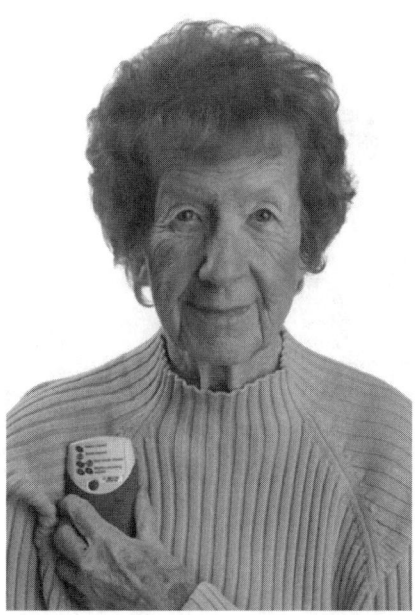

FIGURE 31.2
Woman holds the remote control where it can communicate electronically with the implanted defibrillator.

go-ahead for to the remote control to initiate a shock. In turn, the remote control employs spoken prompts to give the user the go-ahead. At that point, the patient can prepare himself or herself for the shock (e.g., sit down), hold down the deliver shock button for a few seconds, and then receive the shock within another few seconds (see Figure 31.3).

While the shock may be unpleasant, the benefits of quickly restoring a normal heart rhythm are profound. Rather than suffering the ill effects of AF for hours, days, or weeks, patients with the device can alleviate their symptoms in a relatively short period of time and continue with the day's activities.

User-Interface Development

User-Needs Research and Analysis

From the start of the project, Guidant recognized the need for comprehensive human factors engineering to ensure the development of a user-friendly and successful product. Initially, they engaged a human factors specialist to help

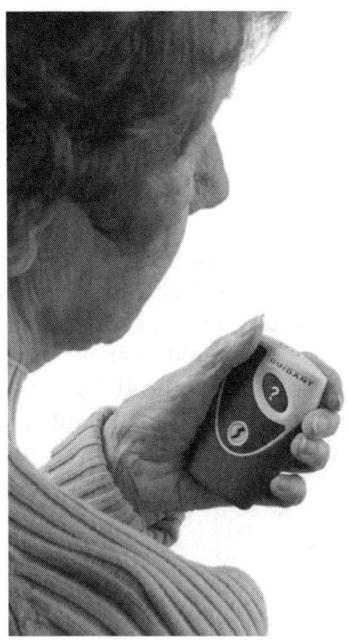

FIGURE 31.3
Woman listens to the remote control's spoken prompts while observing its controls.

define the basic requirements for their new product — specifically the handheld remote control — which was to be used primarily by older individuals. Together, the human factors consultant and Guidant staff established specifications for a device that individuals with a limited understanding of cardiac therapy and technology could operate effectively. Additionally, the consultant helped shape the development process to insure the effective application of human factors principles.

Guidant's next step was to engage a product development firm with a strong industrial design and human factors focus to conduct research into the users' needs and preferences regarding the remote control's shape, size, and interactive characteristics. The core research activity involved 15 heart patients at 3 separate treatment centers. During 30- to 120-minute interviews, each patient described their lifestyle, health management practices, and emotional, cognitive, and physical needs regarding the remote control.

Guidant's field research clarified that most of the prospective users favored spoken prompts over displayed prompts; that men preferred larger remote controls than women because they had larger hands; and that certain remote control shapes and button arrangements had a substantial influence on how the patients perceived the product's usability and dependability. The research also helped to determine the appropriate spacing between lighted icons (symbols) and an appropriate button arrangement to protect against accidental button actuation.

User-Interface Design

Drawing on the research findings, Guidant and its design consultants developed about a dozen design concepts, then narrowed the options to three alternative remote control forms, expressed as realistic-looking, nonfunctional models complemented by computer-based prototypes (created using Macromedia Director software) that simulated certain tasks. Guidant asked the 15 patients who participated in the initial research to evaluate the prototypes and suggest additional enhancements. After further design refinement, Guidant engaged a market research firm to collect even more design feedback on the prototypes from 150 prospective users living in the Minneapolis, San Diego, and Boston metropolitan areas.

Based on the stated preferences from the 165 prospective users, and considering many other engineering factors, Guidant finally converged on a preferred concept that was also practical to manufacture and would deliver reliable service over the product's expected lifetime. A period of intensive engineering ensued.

Usability Testing

Once Guidant produced its first prototype units intended for design evaluation purposes only, it took the proactive step of consulting with the FDA's Center for Devices and Radiological Health on a plan to verify the device's usability and related safety characteristics. Drawing support from a human factors firm specializing in the usability testing of medical devices, Guidant and the FDA settled on a usability test involving 55 older individuals (50 to 90 years of age).

Usability testing proceeded smoothly. Most of the test participants were able to perform a series of essential tasks, such as checking their heart rhythm and initiating a simulated shock, without significant problems (see Figure 31.4). The test showed that deliberately short voice prompts, such as "Check rhythm" and "Prepare for shock" were effective and reassuring. That said, the test revealed some residual opportunities for design enhancement, such as eliminating the need for patients to replace the remote control's batteries — a demonstrably difficult task.

As a final step to maximize the device's usability, Guidant prepared a quick reference card to augment the on-product instructions (see Figure 31.5).

Conclusion

During clinical trials of the PARTNER™ Rhythm Assistant, 72 patients received a total of 279 atrial shocks. All of the delivered shocks were considered medically appropriate and none of the shocks induced ventricular

Case Study: Remotely Controlled Defibrillator

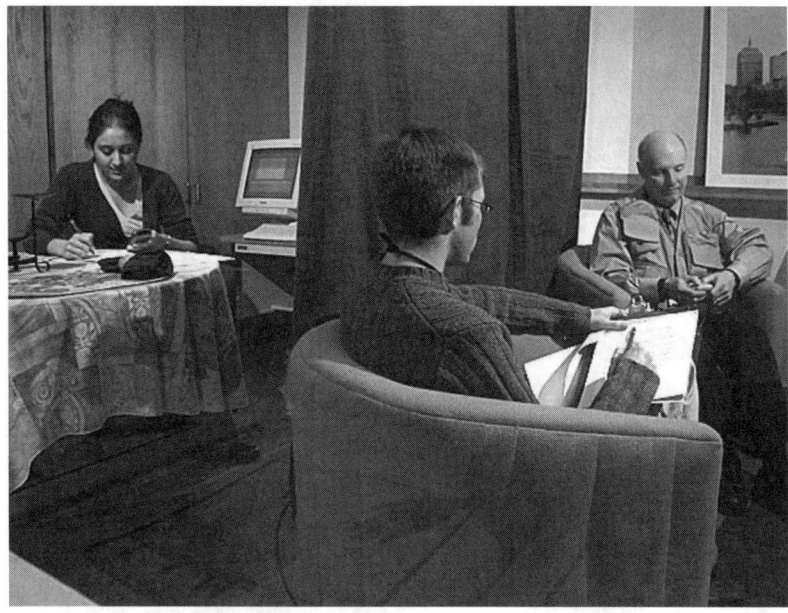

FIGURE 31.4
Researchers make note of a usability test participant's ability to administer a simulated cardioverting shock.

arrhythmia. As such, the clinical trial successfully demonstrated the product's safety and efficacy.

In 2003, Guidant introduced the PARTNER™ Rhythm Assistant as a companion to the VITALITY™ AVT® defibrillator. At the time this case study was written (April 2004), 16 patients were using the newly introduced product.

Usability is one of the product's defining features that pleases new users and fortifies the company's marketing efforts. After all, the primary customers — the clinicians — do not want their patients working too hard to use a medical device, particularly patients that may be feeling ill and easily confused.

Guidant's significant investment in user-centered design garnered the company a 2004 Medical Design Excellence Award.

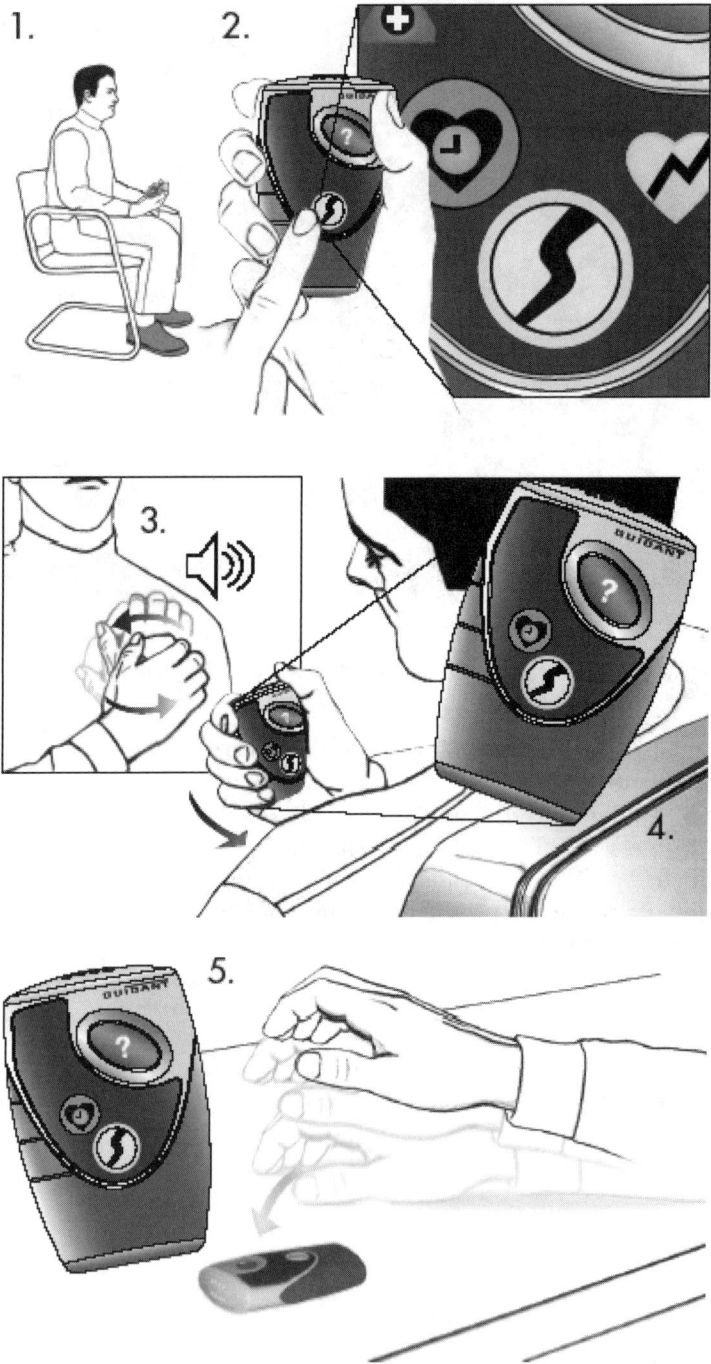

FIGURE 31.5
The product's quick reference card illustrates the sequence of steps leading to the delivery of a cardioverting shock.

Resources

Resources

General Human Factors

Burke, M., *Applied Ergonomics Handbook*, CCR Press, New York, 1991.

Department of defense design criteria standard: Human engineering, MIL-STD-1472F, Department of Defense, Philadelphia, PA, 1998.

Dreyfuss, H., *The Measure of Man and Woman Revised Edition*, John Wiley & Sons, New York, 2002.

Eastman Kodak Co., *Kodak's Ergonomic Design for People at Work*, John Wiley & Sons, New York, 2003.

Grandjean, E., *Fitting the Task to the Man*, Taylor & Francis, New York, 1991.

Salvendy, G., Ed., *Handbook of Human Factors and Ergonomics*, John Wiley & Sons, New York, 1997.

Sanders, M. and McCormick, E., *Human Factors in Engineering and Design*, McGraw-Hill, New York, 1993.

Woodson, W., Tillman, B., and Tillman, P., *Human Factors Design Handbook*, McGraw-Hill, New York, 1992.

Anthropometry and Biomechanics

Aghazadeh, F. and Mital, A., Injuries due to hand tools, *Applied Ergonomics*, 18, 4, 273–278, 1987.

Anthropometry of U.S. military personnel, DOD-HDBK-743A, Department of Defense, Philadelphia, PA, 1991.

Chaffin, D. and Anderson, G., *Occupational Biomechanics*, John Wiley & Sons, New York, 1991.

Garrett, J., The adult human hand: Some anthropometric and biomechanical considerations, *Human Factors*, 13, 7, 117–131, 1971.

Hall, S., *Basic Biomechanics*, McGraw-Hill, New York, 1999.

Hoag, L., Anthropometric and strength data in tool design, in Easterby, R., Kromer, K., and Chaffin, D., Eds., *Anthropometry and Biomechanics—Theory and Application*, Plenum Press, New York, 253–257, 1982.

Human body dimensions data for ergonomic design, vol. 2, no. 1, National Institute of Bioscience and Human Technology, Japan, 1994.

Lin, J., Radwin, R., and Richard, T., Dynamic biomechanical model of the hand and arm in pistol grip power hand tool usage, *Ergonomics*, 44, 3, 295–312, 2001.

Pheasant, S., *Bodyspace — Anthropometry, Ergonomics and Design*, Taylor & Francis, London, U.K., 1986.

Smith, S., Norris, B., and Peebles, L., ADULTDATA: The Handbook of Adult Anthropometric and Strength Measurements, Department of Trade and Industry, U.K., 1998.

Medical-Specific Human Factors

Berguer, R., Surgery and ergonomics, *Archives of Surgery*, 134, 9, 1011–1016, 1999.

Berguer, R., Forkey, D., and Smith, W., Ergonomic problems associated with laparoscopic surgery, *Surgical Endoscopy*, 13, 466–468, 1999.

Do it by design: An introduction to human factors in medical devices, Dept. of Health and Human Services, U.S. Food and Drug Administration, Office of Health and Industry Programs, Center for Devices and Radiological Health, Rockville, MD, 1996.

Garmer, K., Liljeren, E., Osvalder, A., and Dahlman, S., Usability evaluation of a new user interface for an infusion pump developed with human factors approach, Proceedings of the IEA, 128–131, 2000.

Goossens, R. and Van Veelen, M., Assessment of ergonomics in laparoscopic surgery, *Minimally Invasive Therapy and Allied Technologies*, 10, 3, 175–179, 2001.

Human factors design process for medical devices, ANSI AAMI-HE74-2001, Association for the Advancement of Medical Instruments, Arlington, VA, 1993.

Human factors engineering guidelines and preferred practices for the design of medical devices, ANSI AAMI-HE48-93, Association for the Advancement of Medical Instruments, Arlington, VA, 2001.

Medical electrical equipment — part 1-8: General requirements for safety — Collateral standard: General requirements, tests and guidance for alarm systems in medical electrical equipment and medical electrical systems, IEC 60601-1-8, International Organization for Standardization, Geneva, Switzerland, 2003.

Marcus, A., et al., User interface design for medical informatics: A case study of Kaiser Permanente, Proceedings of the 33rd Hawaii International Conference on System Sciences, 1–11, 2000.

Patkin, M. and Isabel, M., Ergonomics and laparoscopic general surgery, Annual Scientific Meeting of Royal Australian College of Surgeons, 1–8, 1991.

Wiklund, M., *Medical Device and Equipment Design: Usability Engineering and Ergonomics,* CRC Press, Boca Raton, FL, 1995.

Graphical User Interfaces and Usability

Baumann, K. and Thomas, B., *User Interface Design for Electronic Appliances,* Taylor & Francis, London, U.K., 2001.
Dunkley, L. and Smith, A., Cultural factors and user interface design, Proceedings of the IEA 6, 536–540, 2000.
Galitz, W., *The Essential Guide to User Interface Design,* John Wiley & Sons, New York, 1996.
Information technology — User system interfaces and symbols — Icon symbols and function, ISO/IEC 11581-6, International Organization for Standardization, Switzerland, 1999.
Jansen, J., The graphical user interface, *SGCHI Bulletin,* 30, 22–26, 1980.
Nielsen, J., *Usability Engineering,* Academic Press, New York, 1993.
Sawyer, D. and Talley, W., Display legibility guidelines: A design aid, *Information Display,* 13–16, 1987.
Ratner, J., Ed., *Human Factors and Web Development,* Lawrence Erlbaum Associates Publishers, London, U.K., 2003.
Wiklund, M., Ed., *Usability in Practice: How Companies Develop User-Friendly Products,* AP Professional, New York, 1994.
Zhao, C., Zhang, T., and Zhang, K., User interface design for the small screen display, Proceedings of the Human Factors and Ergonomics Society 45th Annual Meeting, 1548–1550, 2001.

Home Healthcare and Inclusive Design

The anthropometrics of disability: An international workshop, Rehabilitation Engineering Research Center on Universal Design, State University of New York, Buffalo, NY, 2002.
Bangor, A., Electronic text readability issues for the visually impaired, Proceedings of the Human Factors and Ergonomics Society 43rd Annual Meeting, 1372–1375, 1999.
Boussenna, M., Horton, D., and Davies, B., Ergonomics approach applied to the problems of two disabled people, *Applied Ergonomics,* 14, 4, 285–290, 1983.
Clarkson, J., Coleman, R., Keates, S., and Lebbon, C., Eds., *Inclusive Design — Design for the Whole Population,* Springer, New York, 2003.

Elkind, J., The incidence of disabilities in the United States, *Human Factors,* 32, 4, 397–405, 1990.

Fisk, A. and Rogers, W., *Handbook of Human Factors and the Older Adult,* Academic Press, New York, 1997.

Kanis, H., Operation of controls on consumer products by physically impaired users, *Human Factors,* 35, 2, 305–328, 1993.

Keates, S. and Clarkson, J., *Countering Design Exclusion — An Introduction to Inclusive Design,* Springer, New York, 2003.

Pirkl, J., *Transgenerational Design: Products for an Aging Population,* Van Nostrand Reinhold, New York, 1994.

Pirkl, J., Transgenerational design: Prolonging the American dream, *Generations,* 32–36, 1995.

Rowles, G. and Ohta, R., Ed., *Aging and Milieu: Environmental Perspectives on Growing Old,* Academic Press, New York, 1983.

Rubin, G., et al., A comprehensive assessment of visual impairment in a population of older Americans, *Investigative Ophthalmology & Visual Science,* 38, 3, 557–568, 1997.

Vanderheiden, G., Thirty-something (million): Should they be exceptions?, *Human Factors,* 32, 4, 383–396, 1990.

Index

Index

A

A-2000 Bispectral Index (BIS) Consciousness Monitor, 95
Abbott Laboratories
  Architect Laboratory Diagnostic Systems, 259–262
  company background, 257
  human factors goals, 258
  lessons learned, 267
  methods, 259
  potential pitfalls in development, 266
  product design process, 258
  Q2+ Cardiac Output Monitor, 262–266
Accidental actuation, 171–172
ACCU-CHEK VOICEMATE System, 216–217, 218
Accuracy, factors limiting recall, 52
Acute-care situations, in simulation exercises, 119
Adobe Illustrator, 107
AdvaMed, 253
Advanced features, simplifying use of, 161
Adverse events, xxvi, 3
  mitigating consequences of, xxxiii
Aircraft cockpits, shape coding of devices in, 170
Aksys, Ltd., company background, 283–284
Alarms, xxxi
  adjusting heart rate, 296
  advantages of color coding, 195–196
  avoiding annoying sounds in, 235
  preventing disablement of critical, 176, 179, 206–207, 213
  purpose of, 235
Allen, Amy, xix
Allocation of functions, 14–15
Alternative prompts, 223–224
Ambient sounds, 243
  recreating in signal design, 239
American Institutes for Research, xv, 188
American Institutes for Research and Design Science, xix

American National Standards Institute (ANSI), 191
  symbol acceptance criteria, 185
Amplification systems, 239
Anesthesia incidents, 33, 119
  malignant hyperthermia, 113
Anesthesia workstations
  color coding information on, 210
  controls preventing accidental actuation, 172
  design enhancements to, 170–171
  spaghetti cabling in, 175
Anesthesiology
  A-2000 Bispectral Index Consciousness Monitor, 95
  anesthesia workstation simulation, 121
  as separate OR culture, 67
Anesthesiology equipment, xxi, xxx
Anthropometric software, 79–81
Anthropometry, 15, 77–82
  documents containing, 77–78
Anthropometry databases, 82
Anthropometry of Infants, Children, and Youths to Age 18 for Product Safety Design, 78
Apple Computer, patent strategies, 132
Appliance Manufacturer, xi, xix
Architect Laboratory Diagnostic Systems, 259–262
Arsenault, Joy, xix
Arterial blood pressure
  advantages of color in displays of, 201
  visual representation of, 156
Artifact analysis, 86
Artificial arm, with voice activation technology, 220
Assistive devices, 228
  recruiting test users through retailers of, 232
Association for the Advancement of Medical Instrumentation, xi, xxi, 7, 22, 171
  Human Factors Engineering Committee, xix, xvi, 31
Atrial fibrillation, xxxiii, 308–314

323

Attention, devices requiring excessive user, xxix–xxx
Attention deficit disorder, 231
Attorney fees, in patenting process, 138
Auditory disabilities, 234
   design guidelines for persons with, 231
Auditory environment, 237
Auditory signals
   choosing sound frequencies, 239–241
   choosing sound patterns for, 241–242
   conspicuity of, 242
   criteria for success, 242
   designing usable, 235
   determining indicators for, 236
   distinctiveness of, 242
   freedom from annoyance, 242
   information gathering phase for, 237
   purpose of, 235
   recreating ambient sounds, 239
   sound reproduction equipment for, 241
   spectrum analysis for, 237–238
   testing candidate signals with users, 242–243, 243
   use of semi-musical sounds for, 239, 241, 243
   using sound-generation software for, 239–241
Automated external defibrillators (AEDs), 215–216
Automated receptionists, 215
Automated telephone prompts, 220
Automatic checks, 211
   designing into devices, 178, 179
Automatic teller machines (ATMs), softkey controls in, 182–183
Automation of functions, 209, 214
Automobile navigation systems, 215
Automotive industry
   early role of QFD in, 96
   human modeling software in, 81

B

Backward compatibility, 55
Bar-code medication management systems, xxi–xxii
Bar graphs, advantages of color in, 201
Berube, Karen, xix
Best-loved products, features of, 9
Beth Israel Deaconess Medical Center, 115
Bias, introduction of, 18
Biomechanical measurements, 18
Blaring music, 235

Blood chemistry analyzers, making user-friendly interfaces for, 151
Blood gas analyzers, use of color displays in, 193
Blood glucose monitors, 9
   with voice recognition technology, 216–218
Blood pressure monitors, 230
   display of trends, 296
Blood-warming devices, 121
Body dimensions, average *vs.* extreme, 78
Body scanning, 78–79
Boundary models, 81
Brainstorming, 146
Brand identity, 152
Breathing circuit diagrams, advantages of color in, 201
Breathing masks, 5
Bridging skills, 26
Brigham and Women's Hospital, 115
Building blocks, 87, 90
Button spacing, 105
   in patient-controlled defibrillator remote control, 311
   for persons with disabilities, 229
Buttons, 105

C

CAESAR Survey. *See* Civilian American and European Surface Anthropometry Resource (CAESAR Survey)
Canon Communications, xix
Cardiac catheterization labs, 70
Cardiac output measurement, 296
Cardiocap integrated patient monitors, 291–292
Cardiologists, 67
   unfamiliarity with programmers for defibrillators, 89
Cardioversion, patient controlled, 309–314
Care environment, xxiv–xxv
Caregivers
   designers adopting perspective of, 57
   feedback from professional, 286, 290
   responsibility of, 38
Carnegie Delicatessen Restaurant, xi–xii
Carnegie Mellon University, xvii
Carstensen, Peter B., 31
Case studies
   Architect Laboratory Diagnostic Systems (Abbott Laboratories), 259–262
   contrast medium injector system, 299–305
   patient monitor, 291–297

Index

personal hemodialysis system, 283–290
remotely controlled defibrillator, 307–314
Categorization tasks, 87
Cathode ray tubes, 194
Cell Robotics, 229
Cellular phones, software interface for, 149
Center for Medical Simulation, Inc. (CMS), 115–116, 117, 119, 123
   costs for using simulation facility, 120
Children's Hospital, 115
Chronic atrial fibrillation, 308–309
Civilian American and European Surface Anthropometry Resource (CAESAR Survey), 79
Civilian anthropomorphic data, 78
Class II/Class III medical devices, 22, 29
Clinical chemistry analyzers, 259
Clip appliers, 269
Co-training, 127, 129
Coaching, 17
Coded information, avoiding, 167
Cognitive disabilities, 227, 228, 234
   design guidelines for persons with, 230–231
Cognitive psychology, 15, 35, xvi
Color-coding information, 173, 174, 209, 211
   in Abbott Laboratories products, 262
   as advantage of color displays, 195–196
   warning messages, 194
Color displays, 193–194
   in Abbott Laboratories products, 265
   advantages of, 194–201
   in integrated patient monitors, 291, 293
Color palette, limiting in interface design, 155
Color vision, impaired, 198
Commodity syndrome, 94
Communication, enhanced by color displays, 194, 201
Communications skills, importance to industrial designers, 129
Company image, and use of color displays, 197
Competitive edge, 38
   afforded by color displays, 196, 202
   excellence in user manuals as, 248, 254
   provided by visual elegance, 12
Competitors' products, 63
Complexity
   controlling in interface design, 161–168
   degrees of product, 164–165
   discouraging to innovation, 99, 101
   reducing by eliminating extra features, 212
   strategies for controlling, 168
Computer-based learning, 245–246
   potential of, 252, 254

Computer-based prototype software files, 23
Computer-based user manuals, 245–246
Computers, as cause of product quality decline, 36
Conceptual design, 17
Conceptual inquiries, 48
Configuration stability, 206, 213
Congressional oversight hearings, 33
Congruous hues, 155
Connections, simplifying and ensuring, 173–175, 179
Connectors, keying, 174
Consensus standards, xxiii
Consistency of design, xxx, 158–159, 208–209, 213
   in labeling of important features, 166–167
   for talking medical devices, 222
Consistent syntax, 156
Constructive interaction, 17
Consumer research, role of verbal behavior in, 51
Content
   separating with empty space, 152
   simplified updating with computerized manuals, 251
Context, 72
   impact on responses to questions, 65
   importance of considering, 71
Continuous taping, *vs.* time-lapse samples, 73–76
Contrast medium injector system, 299
   design process for, 302–303
   ethnographic research for, 302–303
   manufacturer background, 299–300
   product description, 301–302
   product development, 303–305
Controlled environments, patient simulators in, 122
Controls
   excessively dense, 151–152
   labeling with symbols, 46
   logical arrangement of, 167–168
   lower-force for disabled persons, 228
   minimizing need for sustained pressure on, 230
   for screen navigation, 152–153
   value of large, 208
   value of standardized, 208
Copyright protection, of software user interfaces, 133
Corporate human factors programs
   Abbot Laboratories, 257–267
   Ethicon Endo-Surgery, Inc., 269–279
Corporate lore, 12
   stifling innovation by, 98

Corporate structure, implications of user-centered design for, 276
Corporate subculture, 57
Cost savings, of computerizing documentation, 248, 251, 254
Crash carts, 7
Creativity, 97
Crisis situations, xxix
Critical actions, requiring confirmation of, 172, 179
Critical care monitors, 294
Critical controls, guarding, 170, 171–172, 179
Critical information, legibility/readability of, 172–173, 179
Critical symbols, reinforcing with language-specific text labels, 186
Criticare Systems, 212
CRT screens, simulating hardware devices on, 109
CT scanning, contrast medium injector system development for, 299–305
Cultural anthropology, 57, 58, 59, 62
Custom label kits, 188
Customer choice, preference for color displays, 198
Customer expectations, meeting with color displays, 197
Customer learning styles, 250–251

D

Data input, ease of, 107
Datex Medical Instrumentation, 188
Datex-Ohmeda, 188, 190, 196, 250
  patient monitor case study, 291–297
DaVinci Surgical System, 220
Default values, preventing automatic return to, 177
Defibrillators, xxxiii, 8, 56, 57, 67
  case study, 307–314
  programmers for communicating with, 89
  remotely controlled by patients, 307–314
Deleterious outcomes, 52
Demonstration mode, xxviii, 177
Density
  See also Screen density
  and advantages of color displays, 196
Department of Health and Human Services, 78
Design, consistency of, xxx, 160
Design brief, 12
Design by consensus, 99
Design control process, 25, 47–48
  at Abbott Laboratories, 258

Design drawings, 23
Design excellence, 5. *See also* Medical product design excellence
  at Ethicon Endo-Surgery, Inc., 270
Design guidelines
  confirming critical actions, 172
  guarding critical controls, 171–172
  including automatic checks, 178
  indicating operational modes, 177
  limiting number of modes, 177
  making critical information readable, 172–173
  for persons with auditory deficits, 231
  for persons with cognitive disabilities, 230–231
  for persons with mobility/dexterity disabilities, 229–230
  for persons with visual deficits, 232
  presenting information in usable format, 176–177
  preventing automatic resetting, 177
  preventing disabling of critical alarms, 176
  preventing negative transfer, 177–178
  simplifying connections, 173–175
  for talking medical devices, 221–224
  using tactile coding, 176
Design history file, 48–49, 274–275
Design inadequacies, potential consequences of, 3–4
Design inconsistencies, 158–159
Design patents, 132–134, 140
  exclusion from provisional applications, 134
Design problems
  manufacturer recalls due to, 33
  screen density, 151–152
Design process, 13
  at Abbott Laboratories, 260
  design freezing, 303
  including experts in, 232
  including people with disabilities in, 232
  systematic, 21
Design Science, xvi
Design templates, 157
Design tips
  avoiding information coding, 167
  display size, 167
  extraneous feature handling, 163
  important *vs.* unimportant features, 163
  incorporating protective mechanisms, 166
  labeling features, 166–167
  limiting number of modes, 166
  logical arrangement of controls, 167–168
  minimalistic design, 162–163
  operational status indicators, 163–164

Index

Designer-as-stylist model, 97
Development budgets, limited, 103
Development engineers, no substitutes for product users, 266
Development steps, FDA-mandated, 4
Development time
    shortened with prototyping software, 106
    for VisualBasic *vs.* C++, 108
Device abandonment, reasons for, 228
Device categories, problematic, 37
Device configurability, problematic nature of, 213
Device integration, and choice of color *vs.* monochrome displays, 200
Device labeling, creative approaches for global marketing, 182–188
Device limitations, disabled patients' inability to overcome, 228
Device maintenance, 57
Device manuals, xxxi. *See also* Documentation; User manuals
Device misuse, xxvi
Device recalls, 28
Device resets, preventing automatic, 177
Device testing, in intended use environment, xxv
Devices, overly complex, xxxi
Dexterity problems, 227, 229–230, 234
Diagnostic scanners, 5
Diagnostic tasks, xxii
Dialysis machines, xv, xxv, 3, 24, 56
    making user-friendly interfaces for, 151
Diary and workbook studies, 88
Digitized speech technology, 217–220, 220, 224
Disabilities
    simulating in design process, 233, 234
    types of, 229–232
    understanding users' needs, 232–233
Disabled users
    designing home healthcare products for, 227–228
    reasons for device abandonment, 228
    strategies for meeting needs of, 234
Display design, 35, 104–105, 111
    value of large displays, 203, 207
Display size, 167
Disposable cameras, 87
Distractions and interruptions, xxv, xxx
Division of labor, 71
Documentation, xxxi–xxxiii. *See also* User manuals
    in Ethicon Endo-Surgery product development, 271–273
    FDA-mandated, 4
    relative importance over patient safety, 70

Dose calculators, 212
Double labeling schemes, 186
Drawings
    in patent application process, 134, 135
    in vision statement formulation, 147–148
Due diligence, 47
Duracell EasyTab hearing-aid batteries, 231
504DX Portable Pulse Oximeter, 212

E

Eagle Patient Simulator, 116
Early twentieth-century music, as source of auditory signals, 239, 241, 243
Ease of manufacture, 275
Ease of use
    for cardiologists, 67
    in Ethicon Endo-Surgery products, 270
    for feature-laden products, 168
    inverse relationship to product complexity, 161, 162
Economic risk, *vs.* innovation, 100
Economy of scale, and choice of color *vs.* monochrome displays, 200–201
Efficacy issues, 38
Efficiency issues, 38
Egocentrism, in user-centered medical product development, 55
Electrical engineers, 67
Electroluminescent panels (ELPs), 194
Electromedical equipment, safety of, 44
Empirical testing, in body measurements, 82
Empty space, 152
End stage renal disease (ESRD), 283–284
End-user involvement, 35
End-users, interviewing, 62
Enforcement measures, 22
Engineering algorithms, misplaced importance on, 56
English-only labels, 187–188
Entropy measurement, 292
Environments of use, 62, 63–64, 72
    in development of integrated patient monitors, 294
    recording and analyzing sound from, 237–238
    testing auditory signals in, 242–243
Ergonomics, 34, 35
    textbook guidelines for designers, 171
Error recovery, xxxiii
Ethicon Endo-Surgery, Inc.
    background, 269
    design history files, 274–275
    design process, 270–271

goals, 270
lessons learned, 275–279
methods, 271–274
observational and interview research, 273–274
technical documents, 271–273
usability testing, 274
Ethnographic field research, 62–66, 72
in development of contrast medium injector system, 302–303
Ethnography, 57
in new product development, 61–72
Evolutionary product development, 48
Expectations, discovering users/, 67
Experience, adverse effect on seeing user's point of view, 55, 59
Extraneous features
avoiding in talking medical devices, 222–223
eliminating, 163, 212, 213–214
reducing in user interface, 287

F

Facial expressions, 64
Failure, punishing, 98, 101
Fatigue, 179
as factor in use error, 169
FDA. *See* U.S. Food & Drug Administration
Feature creep, 163
Feature wars, 196
Features war, 99
Feeding equipment, 257
Field inspections, 23–25
Field observation, 86
Field research, 12–14, 20
ethnographic, 62–66
methodology of, 66–71
Fine motor control disabilities, 229
Firsthand knowledge, 64
Foamcore models, 109
Focus groups, 35, 48, 72
role in vision statement formulation, 146, 148
vs. usability testing, 266
Force limits, 273
Frame-by-frame viewing, 75
French, Brian, 248
Full-body scanning systems, 79
Functional associations, 176
Functional requirements, 3, 7
Functional testing, xxviii
Functionality, unused due to elaborate nature of, 57

G

Gaba, David, 116, 121
Gas analyzers, in patient simulators, 116
GE Medical Systems Information Technologies, 249
acquisition of Datex-Ohmeda by, 291
Gender, in talking medical devices, 223
Gene chip arrays, xxii
Gestures, 64
Gitlin, Laura, 228
Global hardware designs, 191
tradeoff with device usability, 181–182
Global user interfaces, designing, 181–191
Goals
discovering users', 67
for manufacturers and clinicians, 39
Good manufacturing practices, xxiii
Goodrich, Christopher, 188, 190, 196
Goodrich, Kristina, xix
Government requirements, xiii
Governmental restraints, xxv
Graphic design software, 107
Graphic designers, in medical product development, 127
Graphic elements
in Abbott Laboratories products, 261
patents for, 131
in PHD Personal Hemodialysis System, 287
reducing size of, 152
refining icons, 158
simplifying in interface design, 152
Graphic simplicity, of color *vs.* monochrome displays, 195, 202
Graphics file formats, 107
Graphics handling, ease of, 107
Grip architectures, 273
Group ideology, 69
Group purchasing contracts, 38
Guidance documents, 39
for auditory signals, 237, 243
Guidant, 307–314

H

Halasey, Steve, xix
Hamilton, Ward, 217–218
Hand movements, 64
multicultural meanings of, 183
Hands-on training. *See also* In-service training
for IV infusion pumps, 247
user preference over manual reading, 245, 246

Index 329

Handwritten labels, 187
Hardware elements, eliminating for international use, 182
Hardware engineering
 building common versions for multinational users, 181
 vs. software engineering, 12
Harmonic Scalpel UltraCision ultrasonic devices, 269
Hasler, Rodney A., 31
Headers
 in interface design, 152
 use of simple language in, 156–157
Heart rate, visual representation of, 156
HeartStart FR2 SEMI-Automatic External Defibrillator, 206
HeartStart Home Defibrillator, 8
Heilman, Dr. Stephen, 299
Hemodialysis machines. *See also* Dialysis machines
 personal automated, 283–290
Heuristic design criteria, 233
Hewlett-Packard Component Monitoring System, 293
Hidden cameras, 86
Hidden modes of operation, xxviii, xxxi
Hierarchical labels, 155–156, 157, 160, 266
High priority messages, advantages of color in, 201
Home healthcare products, 233
 applying inclusive design principles to, 227–228
 ethnographic research for, 66
 personal hemodialysis system, 283–290
 remotely controlled defibrillator, 307–314
Hospital auditory environment, 235
Hospital beds, prominent labels on, 207
Human-computer interface
 guidance in written standards, 42
 problematic nature of, 36
Human error, study of, 33
Human factors
 at Abbott Laboratories, 260
 in alarm/auditory signal design, 237
 co-training in, 127, 129
 definition, 31
 in development of remotely controlled defibrillator, 307–314
 international efforts promoting, 44
 need to sell concept of, 277
 and patient simulators, 123
 reinforced by marketplace, 52
Human factors analysis, 15
Human Factors and Ergonomics Society, 49

Human factors consultants, 49, 294
 at Abbott Laboratories, 258
Human Factors Design Process for Medical Devices, 7
Human factors design standards, xi
Human factors engineering, xii, 161, 162, 171
 in design of personal hemodialysis system, 285–286
 integration with industrial design team, 270, 279
 and medical devices, xxii–xxiii
 process training at Abbott Laboratories, 258
 for remotely controlled patient-activated defibrillator, 310–312
Human Factors in Alarm Design, 237
Human Factors in Auditory Warnings, 237
Human factors practices, 170–171
 reducing use error by integrating, 169
Human factors program, 21
Human factors program plan, 23
Human factors research, xxi
Human factors roundtable
 regulatory issues, 31–41
 standards development and implementation, 41–53
Human factors studies, xiii
Human factors teleconferences, 39
Human modeling software, 79–81
Human Patient Simulator, 117, 123
Human simulators, 119. *See also* Patient simulators
Hydromorphone, xxiii
Hypoxic brain injury, reduction in occurrence of, xxxi
Hypoxic gas mixtures, xxx

I

Icons, 191
 in diagnostic device example, 184
 in hospital beds, 185
 labeling of, 166, 167
 maximizing comprehension of, 158
 patents for, 131
 refining and harmonizing, 158, 160
 sparing use of, 183–186
 value of standardizing, 208–209
Ideological responses, vs. authentic reactions, 69
iLook Personal Imaging Tool, 96
Image quality, enhanced with color displays, 194, 202
Imaging, patent protection for, 132

Immunoassay analyzers, 259
Impaired color vision, 198
Implementation issues, 41–53
Important features, making prominent, 212
In-service training
    altering to prevent risks, xxiv
    limitations of, 204, 213
    user preference for, 245, 246
In vitro diagnostic devices (IVDs), 257
Inclusive design, 233
    for home healthcare devices, 227–228
Indigo Laser System, 269
Industrial design, 20, 127
    importance of communication skills to, 129
    importance to medical product development, 127
    integration with human factors engineering, 12–18, 270, 279
    role of renaissance persons in, 125
Industrial designers, treating as stylists, 97
Industrial Designers Society of America (IDSA), xix, xvi
Industry conventions, identifying, 178
Ineffective implementation, xxviii
Information flow, in talking medical devices, 221
Information gathering, for auditory signal design, 237
Infusion pumps, 37, xv, xxv
    hands-on training for, 247
    intravenous, 36
    making user-friendly interfaces for, 151
    proneness to use errors, xxiii
    protective mechanisms for, 166
    testing by patient simulators, 114
    use of color displays in, 193
Inhaled medications, 116
Innovation
    barriers to, 93
    crucial role in development, 93, 100
    discouraging, 93
    misapplication of QFD discouraging, 95–97
    morale-building nature of, 94
    role in product success, 93–95
    vs. design by consensus, 99
Innovation, xi, xvi
Input devices, 105–106, 111
Institute of Medicine, 41
Integrated patient monitors, 291–297
Integrated software/hardware design, 12, 109
Integrated teamwork, in patient simulation, 118
Intellectual property issues, 128
IntelliVue MP40 patient monitor, 173

Intended use environment, designing for, xxiv–xxvi
Intended viewing distance, 35
Intensive care unit
    device integration in, 200
    simulated, 119
    spaghetti cabling in, 174
Interaction times, longer in ethnographic methodology, 69
Interactive CD-ROM manuals, 245, 250–251
Interactive devices
    problematic nature of, 37
    talking medical devices, 215–216
Interdisciplinary training, 270
    importance for medical product designers, 126–127
Interface design, xxviii. *See also* Design tips; User interface design
    grid structure for, 153–154
    hierarchical labels in, 155–156
    limiting color palette in, 155
    refining and harmonizing icons in, 158
    simplifying typography in, 155
    style guide maintenance for, 159
    use of simple language, 156–157
    visual balance in, 154–155
International Council of Societies of Industrial Design, xvi
International efforts, 44–45
International Electrotechnical Commission, 28, 185
    IEC 60601-1, 44
    standard symbols for medical devices, 181
International perspectives, 28
    use of icons instead of text, 167
Interviews, 72
    advantages of, 65
    of end-users, 62
    in vision statement formulation, 146
Intravenous drug administration, testing with patient simulators, 117
Intuitive design, 203–204
    caregiver's perspective, 204–205
Intuitive Surgical, 220
Inventions, patent applications for, 134–137
Israelski, Edmond W., xix, 257

J

Jack human modeling software, 80
Jancsurak, Joe, xix
Jargon, 55, 71
    in talking medical devices, 223–224
Joysticks, 105

Index

K

Keyboards, 105
Keypads, 105
King, Karen, xix
Kingsley, Patricia A., 252
Knopp, Stephanie, xix
Knowledge, adverse effect on seeing user's point of view, 55, 59
Knowledge retention, greater with computerized manuals, 251

L

Labeling strategies, 182
    developing multilingual labels, 186
    eliminating hardware elements, 182
    providing custom label kits, 188
    using English-only labels, 187–188
    using softkeys, 182–183
    using symbols sparingly, 183–186
Labels
    creative approaches for global marketing, 182
    handwritten language-specific, 187
    large text for disabled users, 228
    multilingual, 186
    redundancy of, 157
    text for icons, 158
    use of hierarchical, 155–156
    using prominent, 205–206, 213
Laboratory-based testing, *vs.* patient simulators, 123
Language issues, 46
    language-dependent text labels, 182
    simplifying in interface design, 156–157, 160
    use of icons to overcome, 167
Language menus, 188
Laparoscopic surgical instruments, 271–273, 276
Laparoscopic surgical suite, 12–14
Lasdun, Sir Denys, 277
Laser scanning, of body dimensions, 78
Laser stripe method, 79
Learnability, 15
Learning time, reduced with computerized manuals, 251
Leclerc, Kristin, xix
Legal action, xxiv
    exposure to, 47
Legal restraints, xxv
Legibility
    enhancing for critical information, 172–173

optimizing for personal hemodialysis system, 288
Liability claims, 21, 28
    avoiding future, 50
    reducing exposure with patient simulators, 114
Licensing fees, deriving from patent protection, 140
Life-critical alarms, preventing disablement of, 176, 179
Limb control, loss of, 229
Linear thinking, 97
Liquid crystal displays (LCDs), 193, 194, 265
Listening skills, 72
    in ethnographic field research, 70–71
Literacy issues, 46
Localization issues, 189–190
    in talking medical devices, 223
Logos, reducing size in interface, 152
Lonsinger, Nancy, 218
Look and feel, patents for, 131
Lower-skilled personnel, xxii

M

Macintosh operating system, 104
Macromedia Authorware, 107, 108, 111
Macromedia Director, 107–108, 111
Macromedia Freehand, 107
Magnetic resonance, contrast medium injection systems for, 299–305
Malcolm Baldridge National Quality Award, 299
Malignant hyperthermia, simulating, 113
Mammotome breast biopsy devices, 269, 278
Management support, required for user-centered design, 275
Mannequin programs, 80
Manufacturer awareness, 39
Manufacturing cost
    as competing product goal, 275
    target, 55
Market advantages, patents, 131
Market research, 49
Marketing/engineering design brief, 12
Marketing research, *vs.* usability testing, 266
Marketing surveys, xxviii
Massachusetts General Hospital, 115
Mathematical functions, 107
Measurements, in usability testing, 18
Mechanical breakdown, 71
Mechanical engineering, 127
    co-training in, 129
Mechanical ventilators, xxv

Medical assistants, lack of training, xxii
Medical conventions, color palette appropriateness for, 155
Medical Design Excellence Awards, xi, xix, 52, 313
   logo of, 8
Medical Device & Diagnostic Industry, xi, xix, xvi, 31
Medical Device Amendment of 1976, 32
Medical Device and Ergonomic Design: Usability Engineering and Ergonomics, xv
Medical device designers
   responsibility of, 170
   solemn responsibility of, 7
Medical device user interfaces, xxii
Medical devices
   Class II/Class III, 22
   designing error-resistant, 169–179
   grid structure for, 153–154
   and human factors engineering, xxii–xxiii
   migration from medical facilities to homes, 227
   user-friendly interfaces for, 151–160
Medical Education Technologies, Inc., 117
Medical error, 41
   equipment contributions to, xxii
Medical information management systems, xv
Medical product design excellence, 3–9
Medical product development
   crucial role of innovation in, 93
   ethnographic field research in, 72
   problem of egocentrism in, 55–59
   role of patient simulators in, 122
   role of renaissance persons in, 125
Medical technology design, xi
Medical training, via patient simulators, 113–124
Medical use environment, xxiv
Medrad, Inc., 299–305
Methodology, in ethnographic research, 66–71
Mice, as input devices, 105
Microcontrollers, 104
   support for serial displays, 104
Microprocessor-controlled medical devices, xxviii
   as cause of quality decline, 36
   design of, xxxi
   standards offering guidance on, 42
Microprocessors, embedding into models, 111
Microsoft Corp.
   patent strategies, 132
   User Interface Design Guidelines for Windows 95, 159
Microsoft Visual Basic, 107

Military standards, as model for medical device design, 171
Minimally invasive surgical instruments, 269
Minimum drug concentration, xxiii
Minor changes, 214
   avoiding, 210
Mobility problems, 227, 229–230, 234
Model-building tasks, 88
Modification, ease of, 106–107
Modifications, to existing equipment, 48
Monochrome displays
   availability problems for, 200, 202
   disadvantages of, 194–201
   replacement of, 265
Monopoly, importance to success, 93–94
Morale, role of innovation in building, 94
Morphine administration, xxiii
Motorola, patent strategies, 132
MRI systems, patients' reactions to old *vs.* new style, 57–58
Multi-generational product planning, 270
Multidisciplinary approach, importance in medical product development, 125
Multilingual labels, 186
Multiple-camera recording systems, 74
Muto, William H., xix, 257

N

National Patient Safety Foundation, 33
Navigation cues, 152–153, 160
Negative transfer, reducing potential for, 177–178, 179
Nonadverse events, difficulty of counting, 52
Nondirectional microphones, 237
Nondomain experts, limited usefulness as test subjects, 121
Nonobviousness, as criteria for patent protection, 132, 133
Nonprovisional patent applications, 135
Nonverbal expression, 86, 87–88
Novelty, as criteria for patent protection, 132–133
Novice users, 100
Nuclear power plants, critical controls design in, 170
Nurses
   attitudes toward user manuals, 245–248, 252
   observation in initial design phase, 265
   as primary users of medical devices, 252
   responsibility for defibrillator programming, 89

Index

O

Observational research, 86
   in Abbott Laboratories product design process, 265
   careful, 72
   as discovery tool, 86
   in Ethicon Endo-Surgery product development, 273–274
Obstacles, benefits of removing, 203–204, 213
Off-the-shelf products, for simulation purposes, 109
Offhand verbal statements, 64
Office of Device Evaluation (ODE), 253
Office of Surveillance and Biometrics, 29
Omron HEM 712C blood pressure monitor, 230
On-site interviews, 48, 88
   advantages of, 65
Online help, 208
   in Abbott Laboratories products, 262
Open Ergonomics, 81
Operating room environments, 62–63
   blaring music in, 235
   device integration in, 200
   integrated patient monitors designed for, 291
   sound environment in, 236
Operating room equipment, xxi
Operating room simulation, 124
Operational modes
   indicating and limiting number of, 177
   limiting number of, 166, 179
Operational status, indicators for, 163, 166
Opiate drug administration, xxiii
Optimized configuration, 206
Organizational culture, xxv
   catheterization labs, 71
Outcomes
   counting deleterious, 52
   as goal for manufacturers and clinicians, 39

P

Pacemakers, 67
   programmers for communicating with, 89
Page numbering, in interface design, 152
Palm-based computer, 104
Paper-based user manuals, 253
   vs. electronic versions, 248–250
Parallel ports, 104
Partial melodies, usability of, 241
PARTNER Rhythm Assistant, 309–314
Password access, 172
Past experiences, inability to recall accurately, 62, 86
Patent Assistance Center, 139
Patent claims, number permitted, 132–133
Patent pending status, 134
Patent protection
   assistance for, 139–140
   claim writing for, 138, 141
   common mistakes in, 138
   costs related to, 137–138
   critical nature of timing, 138
   design vs. utility patents, 132–134
   duration of, 132–133
   example device, 135–136
   licensing fees deriving from, 140
   maintenance fees for, 138
   medical companies' use of, 132
   nonprovisional applications, 135
   patent application process, 134–137, 141
   philosophical and strategic issues, 139–140
   provisional application, 134
   scope of, 133
   small investor status, 138
   for software user interfaces, 131–132
Patent searches, 133
   costs of, 138
Path specification, 15
Patient-bed designers, 57
Patient-controlled analgesia (PCA), use errors in, xxiii
Patient identification bracelets, xxi–xxii
Patient injury, due to device use errors, xxiv
Patient mannequins, 116, 124
Patient monitors, xv, 5, 6
   with color vs. monochrome screens, 199
   Datex-Ohmeda case study, 291–297
   entropy measurement via, 292
   IntelliVue MP40, 173
   making user-friendly interfaces for, 151
   modular, 293
   use of hierarchical labels in, 155
   user's guide for, 249
Patient-programmable devices, 172
   personal hemodialysis system, 286–287
   remotely controlled defibrillator, 307–314
Patient safety
   as goal for manufacturers and clinicians, 39
   relative importance of, 70
   vs. global hardware design, 181
Patient simulators, 113–114
   clinician's viewpoint on, 121–122
   costs associated with, 119–120, 122, 123
   environment for, 118–119

participant experiences with, 120–121
realistic testing with, 114–115
role in medical device development, 122
running, 118
technology behind, 115–118
use for medical training purposes, 113
Web sites pertaining to, 122–123
Patients, designers adopting perspective of, 57
Patterned behavior, safety risks of, 177–178
Patterned light projection, 79
Payoff, for usability investment, 50
PC platform, 104
PDAs, 104, 111
Pennsylvania State University, xvii
PeopleSize software, 81
Percentile person, 78, 80, 82
Perceptual disabilities, 228
Personal hemodialysis system, case study, 283–290
Personal Lasette, 229
PHD Personal HemoDialysis System, 283–290
Philips Medical Systems, 173
  Component Monitoring System, 293
Physical anthropology, 77
Physical constraints, xxx
Physical disabilities, 228
Physiological measurements, 18
Physiological monitors, xxix, xxviii
Plain wording, in voice prompts, 222
Platform, 111
  selecting appropriate, 103–104
Police sketch method, 87
Pop-up controls, 152
Portable usability testing equipment, 261
Ports, keying, 174
Post-market surveillance, 23, 26–28, 41
Preference testing, xxviii
  as stifling to innovation, 99–100, 101
  vs. usability testing, 266
Preliminary product definition, 14
Preliminary software/hardware prototyping, 17
Premarket review process, 21, 25–26, 39, 40
Price point, 55
  differences between monitor and color displays, 194
Prior art, 133
Procedural maps, 274
Procedural violations, underreporting of, 41
Product development costs
  minimizing with color *vs.* monochrome displays, 201
  reducing for color/monochrome displays, 198
Product failures, 98

Product geometry, 77
Product goals, competing, 275
Product reviews, FDA-conducted, 23
Product simulations, testable, 103–111
Product success, role of innovation in, 93–95
Professional culture, xxv
Programmed infusion rate, 211
Progressive image, afforded by color displays, 197, 202
Prominent labels, 205–206
Prompts. *See also* Voice prompts
  benefits of short, 222
  suitable pacing of, 221
  suitable volumes for, 221–222
  synchronizing with user actions, 221
  tailoring to specific customer needs, 224
  value of extensive, 205
  voice, 218–220
Proprietary technology, 140
  advantages and disadvantages, 131
Protective mechanisms, incorporating in design, 166
Prototypes, 15
  at Abbott Laboratories, 261, 265
  in ethnographic field research, 63
  low-fidelity hardware and software, 110
  of personal hemodialysis system, 288–289
  preliminary, 17
  testable, 103–111
Prototyping software. *See also* Software prototyping tools
  VisualBasic for contrast medium injection system, 303
Psychologists, xii, xvi
Psychology of language, xvi
Pulmonary arterial pressure, visual representation of, 156
Pulse generators, in time-lapse video recording systems, 74
Pulse oximeters, 24
  auditory signals of, 235

Q

Q2+ Cardiac Output Monitor, 262–266
QFD design system, 276
Quality control, *vs.* innovation, 96
Quality function deployment (QFD), 95–97, 101
Quantitative analyses, time-lapse video advantages in, 74
Quick reference cards, 250
  for remotely controlled defibrillator, 314

Index

R

Raemer, Dan, 115
RAMSIS human modeling software, 81
Rapid prototyping tools, 17, 20
Rapport, developing with users, 68–69
Readability, 35
    of critical information, 172–173
    and left text justification, 153
    of screen content, 160
Realistic testing, 114–115, 124
Recordkeeping, importance of real-time, 71
Reese, Will, 72
Regulations, xxv
    marketplace driven nature of, 34
Remote control size, gender preferences for, 311
Renaissance person, role in medical product development, 125
Respiratory depression, xxiii
Respiratory rate, visual interface for, 156
Respiratory therapy devices, 3
Response time, of actual device *vs.* prototype, 104
Retrospective testing, 18
Reversibility, of undesirable actions, xxx
Rickard, Peg, 250
Roche Diagnostics, 216, 218
Rolla, Joseph, 132
Rotary controls, 105

S

Safety issues, xii, 179
    electromedical equipment, 44
    inconsistent design compromising, 158–159, 159
Safework human modeling software, 80–81
Sales opportunities, 38
Sample sizes, small in usability testing, 267
Satisfaction issues, 38
Sawyer, Dick, 31
Screen density, 160
    reducing, 151–152
Secondary information, presenting via pop-ups, 152
Self-referential designs, avoiding, 266
Semi-musical sounds, use in auditory signals, 239, 241, 243
Serial ports, 104
Shape coding, 170, 174, 209
    color coding outperforming, 195

Shelf life, of color *vs.* monochrome displays, 198
SimMan Universal Patient Simulator, 123
Simulation alternatives, 109–110, 111
    patient simulators, 113–124
Simulation exercises, 119
Simulation mode, 210
Simulator Center at Stanford University, 123
Situational awareness, loss of, 163
Six-Sigma design system, 276
Size coding, 195
Slang, 71
Slow-motion video, 75
Social-political attitudes, xxv
Socrates Telecollaborative System, 220
Softkeys, 191
    using, 182–183
Software-driven products, 12–18, 20
Software engineering
    role in medical product development, 127
    vs. hardware engineering, 12
Software operating system, 55
Software options, 107–108
Software prototyping tools, 17, 106–107
Software user interfaces
    developing vision statements for, 148–149
    patenting, 131–132
    shifting controls from hardware to, 182
    tailoring to local/international markets, 188–190
Sound degradation, 239
Sound-generation software, 239–241
Sound patterns, 241–242
Sound playback, 239
Sound reproduction equipment, 241
Spaghetti cabling, managing/reducing, 173–175
Speaker systems, 239, 242
Speaking aloud, 18
Special use environments, 59
Specialization, overemphasis on, 125
Spectrum analysis, 237–238
Speech
    as input mode for visually disabled users, 232
    lack of correlation with behavior, 86
Speech technologies, 217–220
Spinal implants, 257
Split-screen recording systems, 74
Spreckelmeier, Larry, 269
Stakeholder groups, 25
Stamps, embedding in prototypes, 109, 111
Standardization, in equipment manufacture and controls, xxx

Standards, xxiii, 32
  AAMI HE74: 2001 Human Factors Design Process for Medical Devices, 22, 29, 40, 42
  AAMI HE74, Human Factors Design Process for Medical Devices, xvii
  ANSI/AAMI HE75, 237
  ANSI/AAMI HE49-1993, 237
  Association for the Advancement of Medical Instrumentation, xi
  for auditory signals, 235, 237, 243
  development of, 22, 41–53
  HE48 1993, 42
  IEC 60601-1-8, 237
  international, 44–45
Start and stop buttons, advantages of color in, 201
Start-ups, role of innovation in, 100
State transition diagram, user-centered, 15–16
Stellant CT Injection System, 303–304
Stereo photogrammetry, 79
Stress levels, increased by auditory signals, 235
Supply problems, avoiding with color displays, 200
Surgical linear cutters/staplers, 269
Surgical procedures, observation of, 273–274
Surgical stapler, 279
Surveys, 72
  differentiation from ethnography, 69
Swift method, 88–89, 90
Symbol acceptance criteria, 185, 191
Symbol labels
  for proper connections, 175
  using sparingly, 183–186
Symbol-laden products, decreased usability of, 181
Synthesized speech technology, 217–220, 220, 224
System factors, xxv
System states, for auditory signals, 236

T

Tactile coding, 176
  for persons with auditory deficits, 231
  for persons with visual deficits, 232
Tactile cues, xxx
Tactile feedback, 105
Tactile landmarks, for visually impaired users, 232
Talking glucose meters, 216–218
Talking medical devices, 215
  design guidelines for, 221–224
  sample applications, 215–217
  technology behind, 217–220
  two-way communication in, 220
Talking RX Prescription Reader, 219–220
Task analysis reports, 23
Task flow, for talking medical devices, 221
Task practice, value of, 210
Task speed, 204
  increased by extensive prompting, 205
Teaching hospitals, 115
  use of patient simulators in, 114
Technical writers, 245, 249
Technological constraints, xxxi
Technology creep, xxv–xxvi
Temporal sound patterns, 240–241
Testable product simulations, 103–111
Text
  centered justification, 153
  labeling proper connections with, 175
  left justification and readability, 153
  patent protection for, 133
  reducing amount in interface design, 152
  refining icons with, 158
  riverbank effect, 153
Text handling, ease of, 107
The Measure of Man and Woman, 77, 82
The Military Handbook: Anthropometry of U.S. Military Personnel, 78
Therapeutic tasks, xxii
Third-party applications, and choice of color *vs.* monochrome displays, 200
Three-dimensional body scanning, 78–79
Throw-away coding, 303
Tight schedules, 103
Time-lapse video, 73–76
Time pressures, 179
  as factor in use error, 169
Time to market
  crucial role in prototyping, 110
  overemphasis on, 97–98, 101
  as product goal competing with user-centered design, 275
  shortened with good design, 50
Timing
  impact on responses to questions, 63
  in patent application process, 138
Timing functions, 107
Titles, meaningful in interface design, 152
Tone, suitability in talking medical devices, 223
Total quality management (TQM) movement, 145–146
Touch pads, 105

Index

Touch screens, 105
   in Abbott Laboratories products, 261, 263–264
   in PHD Personal Hemodialysis System, 286
   in Stellant CT Injection System, 304
Train-the-trainer approach, 204
Training, xxxi–xxxiii
   limitations of in-service, 204, 213
Translations, in talking medical devices, 223
Travel distance, 105
Trial-and-error learning, 114, 124
Triggering force, 105
Trocars, 269, 271
Troubleshooting guides, 250
Trust, 68
Tufts University, xv
Tulane University, xvii
TÜV, 28
Two-way communication, 220, 225
Typography, simplifying in interface design, 155

U

Ultracision harmonic scalpel, 278
Ultrasound imaging, 96
   contrast medium injection systems for, 299–305
Unanticipated use environments, xxvi
Unauthorized actuation, 171–172
Unimportant features, 163
Universal design, for home healthcare devices, 228
University of California, San Diego, xxi
University of the Arts, xvii
U.S. Defense Logistics Agency Apparel Research Network program, 79
U.S. Food & Drug Administration, xix, xxii
   21 CRF 820.30, 270
   Center for Devices and Radiological Health, 312
   field inspections, 23–25
   guidance documents by, 39
   human factors regulations, 286
   human factors teleconferences, 39
   legal requirement for paper-based user manuals, 246, 253
   mandated development steps and documentation, 4
   measures to maximize awareness, 39
   Office of Device Evaluation, 51
   post-market surveillance, 23, 26–28
   premarket reviews, 25–26
   product reviews, 23
   recall study by, 33
   regulation and enforcement of human factors design, 171
   requirements, 6–7
   scrutiny of human factors programs, 21
   stance on enforcement, 40
   Web site, 27
U.S. Patent and Trademark Office (PTO), 132
   Web site, 139
Usability
   best-in-class, 258
   enhanced by color displays, 194
   tradeoff with common hardware version, 181
Usability claims, credible, 114
Usability in Practice, xv
Usability test plans, 48, 258
   for complexity, 168
Usability test reports, 23
Usability testing, xv, 15, 17–18, 18–19
   for AS/3 integrated patient monitors, 296
   for auditory signals, 242–243
   early-stage, 275
   for Ethicon Endo-Surgery products, 274
   FDA-mandated, 171
   measurements in, 18
   for patient-controlled defibrillator, 312
   portable equipment for, 261
   small sample sizes acceptable in, 267
Use environment, 100
Use error, xxiii–xxiv
   anticipating, xxx
   factors leading to, 170
   incidence in medicine, 169, 179
   limiting consequences of, xxx–xxxi
   minimizing likelihood of, xxxiii, 22
   preventing/mitigating through device design, 170, 205
   recovery from, 295
   reducing through device design, 169–179, 213
Use scenarios, 274
User-centered design, xii, xxvi
   at Abbott Laboratories, 257
   at Ethicon Endo-Surgery, Inc., 269–279
   ethnographic methods in, 61
   management support required for, 275
   process and principles of, xxviii–xxx, 13
   role of testable prototypes in, 103–111
   for talking medical devices, 221
User-device interactions, 203
   talking medical devices, 215–225

User error
   and design consistency, 199
   vs. use error, xxiii–xxiv
User-friendly interfaces, 151–160
   reducing use error through, 169–179
User input
   importance of early, 275
   soliciting, xxvii
User interface design. *See also* Design tips;
      Interface design
   AS/3 integrated patient monitor, 294–296
   developing user friendliness, 151–160
   navigation cues for, 152–153
   for patient-controlled defibrillator, 310–312
   personal hemodialysis system, 285–290
   PHD Personal Hemodialysis System,
      287–290
   style guides for, 159
   TQM and, 146
User-interface research, xv
   at Abbott Laboratories, 261
User interfaces, 47
   contribution to medical error, xxii
   improved by color displays, 196
   for pacemaker programming, 67
   patenting, 131–141
   style guide, 23
User issues, not in conscious awareness, 62
User manuals, xxxii. *See also* Device manuals;
      Documentation
   benefits of computerization, 251–252
   current industry practice, 246
   European preference for reading, 247
   as extension of device labeling, 254
   hybrid strategy, 250–251
   negative reinforcement loop, 247–248
   paper-based *vs.* electronic, 248–250
   quick reference cards, 250
   regulatory perspective on, 252–253
   shift toward computer-based, 245–246
   troubleshooting guides, 250
   valuation of excellence in, 247–248, 254
   waste of development effort, 247
User needs/preferences
   for AS/3 integrated patient monitor
      development, 294–296
   for patient-controlled defibrillator, 310–311
   researching, 44, 286–287
   role in vision statement formulation, 146
User requirements specifications, 23
User research reports and videotapes, 23
User testing
   of auditory signals, 242–243
   in body measurements, 81–82
   of icons, 158

   structured approach to, xxvii
   to validate voice prompts, 224
Users
   fallibility of, xxiv
   hypothetical, 274
   involving in design process, xii
   understanding, xxvi–xxviii
Utility patents, 132–134, 140

V

Vacuum fluorescent displays, 194
Validation testing, xxx
Values and norms
   discovering users', 67
   dominant, 70
Vascular devices, 257
Ventilators, 37
   making user-friendly interfaces for, 151
   use of color displays in, 193
Verbal behavior
   fallibility of, 85, 86
   limitations of, 61
Verbal techniques, improved, 88–89
Video documentation, 64, 72
   advantages of, 73–74
   alteration of speed of, 86
   in Ethicon Endo-Surgery product
      development process, 273–274
   searchable, 274
   slow-motion, 75
   time-lapse, 73–76
Video output, 104
Viewing distance, intended, 35
Virtual control panels, 182
Virtual fitting studies, 81
Vision statements
   benefits of, 150
   origins in TQM movement, 145
   process example, 148–149
   for product design, 145
   sketching product for, 147–148
   steps in formulating, 146–147
   unified vision of, 149
   from user and developer perspectives, 147,
      149
Visual appeal
   of color displays, 194–195, 202
   with intuitive design, 203–204
Visual balance, 154–155, 160
Visual codes, 195
Visual cues, xxx
   for persons with auditory deficits, 231

Index

Visual deficits, 234
    design strategies for persons with, 232
    optimizing screen legibility for, 288
Visual design elements, design patents for, 132
Visual elegance, 12
Visual perception research, xvi
Visual programming tools, 108
VisualBasic, 108, 111
    software interface prototyping with, 303
VITALITY AVT defibrillator, 309–314
Voice activation technology, 220
    for persons with mobility/dexterity disabilities, 229
Voice-enabled medical devices, 224. *See also* Talking medical devices
Voice output, 205
Voice prompts
    consistent terminology and syntax for, 222
    design guidelines for, 221–225
    importance of clear direction, 222–223
    multilingual considerations, 223
    preferred by older individuals, 311
    providing alternative, 223–224
    for remotely controlled defibrillator, 312
    terse, 218
    use of plain wording in, 222
Voice recognition technology, 217
Voice recording and playback technology, 219–220
Voice talent, hiring, 218
Volume adjustability, 231

W

Wagner, Debra, 249
Warning letters, 25
Warning messages, color-coding of, 194
Web-based learning, 245, 251
Web sites, on patient simulators, 122–123
Weinger, Matthew, xix, xxi, 31, 121–122
Wharton School of the University of Pennsylvania, xvii
White noise, 235
Wiklund, Michael E., xv, 3, 21, 31, 113, 131, 145, 151, 161, 169, 181, 193, 203, 215, 245
Wilcox, Stephen B., xvi, 55, 61, 85, 227, 235
Windows operating system, 104
Worldview, understanding others', 66–71
Write It Right: Recommendations for Developing User Instruction Manuals for Medical Devices Used in Home Health Care, 252

Y

Yue, Li, 110

Z

ZEUS Robotic Surgical System, 94
ZOLL AED Plus, 216
ZOLL Medical Corporation, 216, 217